IMPORTANT ✍ W9-AGE-695

HERE IS YOUR REGISTRATION CODE TO ACCESS
YOUR PREMIUM McGRAW-HILL ONLINE RESOURCES.

For key premium online resources you need THIS CODE to gain access. Once the code is entered, you will be able to use the Web resources for the length of your course.

If your course is using **WebCT** or **Blackboard**, you'll be able to use this code to access the McGraw-Hill content within your instructor's online course.

Access is provided if you have purchased a new book. If the registration code is missing from this book, the registration screen on our Website, and within your WebCT or Blackboard course, will tell you how to obtain your new code.

Registering for McGraw-Hill Online Resources

To gain access to your McGraw-Hill web resources simply follow the steps below:

1. USE YOUR WEB BROWSER TO GO TO: **register.dushkin.com**
2. CLICK ON **FIRST TIME USER**.
3. ENTER THE REGISTRATION CODE* PRINTED ON THE TEAR-OFF BOOKMARK ON THE RIGHT.
4. AFTER YOU HAVE ENTERED YOUR REGISTRATION CODE, CLICK **REGISTER**.
5. FOLLOW THE INSTRUCTIONS TO SET-UP YOUR PERSONAL UserID AND PASSWORD.
6. WRITE YOUR UserID AND PASSWORD DOWN FOR FUTURE REFERENCE. KEEP IT IN A SAFE PLACE.

TO GAIN ACCESS to the McGraw-Hill content in your instructor's **WebCT** or **Blackboard** course simply log in to the course with the UserID and Password provided by your instructor. Enter the registration code exactly as it appears in the box to the right when prompted by the system. You will only need to use the code the first time you click on McGraw-Hill content.

Thank you, and welcome to your McGraw-Hill online Resources!

REGISTRATION CODE

ux6hj-95ky-m987-pt24

0-07-292167-6 T/A **FIELDS: DRUGS IN PERSPECTIVE, 5/E**

Fifth Edition

Drugs in Perspective

A Personalized Look at Substance Use and Abuse

Richard Fields, Ph.D.

Director/Owner, Faces Conferences

Private Counseling Practice

Bellevue, WA

Tucson, AZ

Boston   Burr Ridge, IL   Dubuque, IA   Madison, WI   New York   San Francisco   St. Louis
Bangkok   Bogotá   Caracas   Kuala Lumpur   Lisbon   London   Madrid   Mexico City
Milan   Montreal   New Delhi   Santiago   Seoul   Singapore   Sydney   Taipei   Toronto

Higher Education

DRUGS IN PERSPECTIVE: A PERSONALIZED LOOK AT SUBSTANCE USE
AND ABUSE, FIFTH EDITION

Published by McGraw-Hill, a business unit of The McGraw-Hill Companies, Inc., 1221 Avenue of
the Americas, New York, NY 10020. Copyright © 2004 by The McGraw-Hill Companies, Inc. All
rights reserved. Previous edition(s) 2001, 1998, 1995, 1992 No part of this publication may be
reproduced or distributed in any form or by any means, or stored in a database or retrieval system,
without the prior written consent of The McGraw-Hill Companies, Inc., including, but not limited
to, in any network or other electronic storage or transmission, or broadcast for distance learning.

Some ancillaries, including electronic and print components, may not be available to customers
outside the United States.

This book is printed on acid-free paper.

Domestic   2 3 4 5 6 7 8 9 0 DOC/DOC 0 9 8 7 6 5 4

ISBN 0–07–255690–0

Vice-President/Editor-in-Chief: *Thalia Dorwick*
Executive editor: *Vicki Malinee*
Freelance Developmental editor: *Gary O'Brien*
Senior marketing manager: *Pamela S. Cooper*
Project manager: *Mary Lee Harms*
Production supervisor: *Enboge Chong*
Designer: *George Kokkonas*
Photo research coordinator: *Alexandra Ambrose*
Photo researcher: *Toni Michaels*
Senior supplement producer: *David A. Welsh*
Media technology producer: *Lance Gerhart*
Compositor: *ElectraGraphics, Inc.*
Typeface: *Times*
Printer: *R. R. Donnelley & Sons Company/Crawfordsville, IN*

Credits: Page 3: © Jack Spratt/The Image Works; Page 22: © Universal Studios. Photo Courtesy
of the Academy of Motion Pictures Arts and Sciences; page 36: © Richard Hutching/Photo
Researchers; page 65: © Michael Siluk; page 78: DEA/Department of Justice; page 79 (top): The
Bettmann Archive/Corbis; page 79 (bottom): Courtesy of Wiener Press Bilbbienst; page 84 (all),
87, 96: DEA/Department of Justice; page 99: The Bettmann Archive/Corbis; page 112, 113:
AP/Worldwide Photos; page 197: © Michael Siluk; page 223; PhotoDisc.

Library of Congress Cataloging-in-Publication Data

Fields, Richard.
　Drugs in perspective: a personalized look at substance use and abuse / Richard Fields.—5th ed.
　　p. cm.
　Includes index.
　ISBN 0-07-255390-0 (alk. paper)
　1. Drug abuse. 2. Alcoholism. 3. Drug abuse—Prevention. 4. Alcoholism—Prevention. 5. Drug
abuse—Treatment. 6. Alcoholism—Treatment. I. Title.
HV5801.F48   2004
362.29'17—dc21

2003048742

www.mhhe.com

Contents

Preface

The major emphasis in the fifth edition of *Drugs in Perspective* is on a multidimensional approach that emphasizes confounding variables—biological, psychological, social, and family systems. Within the past decade and at the beginning of the new millennium we have seen an emerging awareness of the impact of alcohol/drugs on the individual, the family, and the community.

The 11 chapters are designed to give readers as full an understanding of the dynamics of chemical dependency as possible. Each chapter is developed to integrate concepts that build on each other.

The goal of the book is to help readers develop an effective perspective on the multifaceted aspects and problems associated with alcohol/drug use, abuse, and addiction.

�ख Acknowledgments

Thanks to you, the readers, who have on occasion come up to me at conferences to let me know how much you appreciate the book and how you use it in your learning and clinical setting. Thanks to the numerous teachers and counselors who have adopted the book for students and clients.

A special thanks to all my private clients who have taught me about having compassion, humility, strength, courage, spirituality, connectedness, and vision. Thanks for enjoying my sense of humor.

Thanks to the staff at McGraw-Hill—Gary O'Brien, Vicki Malinee, and Mary Lee Harms.

Thanks to Nancy at the Alcohol and Substance Abuse Institute (ASAI) library at the University of Washington.

Introduction

✖ The Myth of the Simple, Magical Solution

Drug use, abuse, and dependence are not easily understood. Too often, people search for that simple solution to an epidemic problem or for a simple explanation. Philosopher H. L. Mencken remarked that "any solution to a big problem that is simple, is usually wrong."

Having spent more than 25 years working with individuals and their families, I still struggle case by case to try to find some common patterns and new insights into what works in treatment. I am constantly questioning what may have caused alcohol/drug problems and how best to engage, motivate, and approach clients with drug abuse and dependence. For some, the solution is abstinence and strong involvement in self-help groups; for others, it is a different path. For many, it is the acceptance of the "disease," while others label their alcohol/drug use as an "allergy" or a problem with tolerance. Some individuals can stay sober for a month or two and then experience a "binge relapse," while others can abstain for several years. Many, through the help of Alcoholics Anonymous, Narcotics Anonymous, a sponsor, and a recovery support group, can maintain sobriety as a life choice.

This book attempts to give a relatively unbiased view or reporting of the literature on alcohol/drug prevention, intervention and treatment. It is biased in that it is influenced by my clinical work with substance abusers, addicts/alcoholics, and their families over the past 25 years. The fifth edition of the book is different from previous editions. The material has been updated, the design and order changed, and new material added and older material deleted, but it also reflects changes in my own understanding and thinking about substance abuse and addiction.

This book can help you better understand the confounding variables of substance abuse and dependence and develop prevention, intervention, and treatment techniques and skills. I hope it will help you explore your own personal perspective about drugs, and it won't give you a "simple solution."

✖ Approaches to Alcohol/Drug Abuse

Historically, we have failed dramatically in our responses to the alcohol/drug problem in the United States. From the 1930s to the 1960s, public and private responses to alcohol/drug abuse caused tremendous damage, which we are still trying to overcome. These approaches were riddled with emotional and political biases, which denied the real dimensions of the problem. Scare tactics—a politically biased approach that alienated young people—began in 1937 and continued for the next 30 years in a variety of forms. For example, the following marijuana scare story appeared in the July 1937 issue of *American* magazine:

> An entire family was murdered by a youthful marijuana addict in Florida. When officers arrived at the home, they found the youth staggering about in a human slaughterhouse. He had ax murdered his father, mother, two brothers, and a sister. He seemed to be in a daze. He had no recollections of having committed the multiple murders. The officers knew him ordinarily as a sane, rather quiet young man; now he was pitifully crazed. They sought the reason. The boy said he had been in the habit of smoking something with youthful friends called "muggles," a childish name for marijuana.

The co-author of this article was Henry J. Anslinger, then commissioner of the Federal Bureau of Narcotics and Dangerous Drugs. After reviewing this single case and a study of the paranoid schizophrenic reactions of heavy hashish smokers in India, Anslinger expounded on the evils of marijuana. He described marijuana as a drug that would consistently result in violent, aggressive, paranoid behavior, as evidenced in the Florida case.

Another scare tactic example is the 1936 movie *Reefer Madness.* This movie's serious intent to discourage marijuana use backfired because the situations were so absurd that audiences viewed it as a humorous farce.

Those using scare tactics assumed that, if young people were frightened by adverse reactions to drug use, they would be too frightened to use the drug. For the young people who perceived drug use as incongruent with their values, goals, and lifestyle, scare tactics were effective. For most young people, however, scare tactics proved to be an ineffective approach because much of the information was exaggerated, overgeneralized, or sensationalized. As a result, young people did not perceive the source of such information as credible. What young people heard did not bear any resemblance to what most users experienced. All in all, scare tactics alienated young people, heightened their curiosity, and increased rather than decreased their experimentation with drugs.

In the late 1960s and early 1970s, President Richard Nixon declared his famous war on drugs. Even though an all-out warlike effort was needed and money was readily available to fight drug addiction, no one knew how to tactically fight this war on drugs. Drug use had spread to epidemic proportions. Also, President Nixon was not the ideal general for this war, having already alienated young people during another war, in Vietnam.

During this same time period, the government was also duped by treatment programs, which mismanaged funds for treatment. At that time, there were few experts and little, if any, clear direction to the battle. The failure of Nixon's war on drugs left a bitter taste in the mouths of government funding sources. Money for treatment programs was cut each year thereafter, and the focus shifted to prevention. Realizing that the war was being lost, the government developed a new, more positive approach: if we can reach the kids before they become dependent on drugs, we will prevent a future generation of drug casualties.

These early prevention efforts emphasized drug-specific information. The assumption was that, if young people were to receive credible drug-specific information, they would then wisely decide not to use drugs. Unfortunately, the reverse held true. Drug-specific approaches heightened curiosity and alleviated the fears associated with drug use, resulting in increases of drug use by young people.

Throughout the ensuing years, U.S. administrations continued to fail to develop a comprehensive and cohesive drug policy. Most of the administrations put a major emphasis on the supply side of the drug problem and significantly neglected the demand side. Emotional and political biases of these administrations caused them to be blind to the many causes of drug dependence and resulted in an adherence to "a simple, magical solution" that was politically advantageous. Administration after administration adhered to a strong supply-side approach, without addressing the reasons for the demand that perpetuated the problem. The Clinton administration repeated this cycle, and the Bush administration has been distracted by international issues, all these administrations focused on the politically expediate supply-side approach of trying to stop drug trafficking, with little effort toward the "demand side" of the problem.

✬ What Is the Trend in Drug Use by Secondary School Students?

The Monitoring the Future National Survey reported that drug use by high school students had stabilized in 1999 and that this might predict a future downturn in adolescent drug use. The reality is, this downturn in adolescent drug use in the new millennium never occurred. Instead there was a shift in the use of various drugs.

In 2001, use of some drugs increased, while use of others decreased or stabilized. Although drug use by high school students peaked in the mid 1990s, there has been no significant decreasing trend in overall drug use. This on-line generation might have more information about drugs, but they are still choosing to use drugs.

The 27th Monitoring the Future national survey (2001) of high school seniors and the 10th national survey of 8th- and 10th-graders had a sample size of 44,000 students in 424 public and private secondary schools throughout the United States.

The survey reported student drug use, availability of drugs, and the students' ratings of risk involved in using particular drugs for students in grades 8, 10, and 12. Perceived risk is thought to be a predictor of drug use. The more the perceived risk of drug use outweighs the perceived benefit of use, the less likely the student is to use the drug. Also, the more easily and readily available the drug is to students, the more drug use will increase. Table 1 provides an overview of trends in drug use by students in grades 8, 10, and 12.

Ecstasy (MDMA)

Increased Use of Ecstacy for All Grade Levels—1998–2001 (see Table 2)

The most alarming finding of the Monitoring the Future study is the sharp increase of the use of Ecstasy (MDMA) since 1998. Table 2 shows the recent trend in Ecstasy use by students in grades 8, 10, and 12. The use of Ecstasy increased for all grade levels, peaking in 2001, and then decreasing in 2002. A similar increase was found in a follow-up survey when the former students were 19 to 26 years old.

Increase in Availability (see Table 3)

The survey reported that the availability and easy access to Ecstasy for 12th graders had increased quite dramatically from 1999–2001. Table 3 shows availability of

TABLE 1

Trends in Drug Use by High School Students

	Use	Availability	Perceived Risk
MDMA	Up	Up	Up
LSD	Down	Slightly down	Down
Alcohol	Stable since 1990s— all grade levels		
Marijuana	Stable all grade levels		
Cocaine	Down (10th) Stable (8th and 12th)	Down	Down
Cigarettes	Down	N/A	Up
Amphetamines	Down (8th, 10th) Stable (12th)	Stable	Up
Meth and Crystal	Stable	N/A	N/A
Inhalants	Down	Universally available	Up
Barbiturates	Stable (8th, 10th) Up (12th)	Slight decrease	Stable
Anabolic Steroids	Stable (8th, 10th) Up (12th)	N/A	N/A

TABLE 2

MDMA (Ecstasy—Percentage of Students Who Used in the Last Year

	1996	2000	2001	2002
8th-graders	N/A	3.1	3.5	2.9
10th-graders	4.6	5.4	6.2	4.9
12th-graders	4.6	8.2	9.2	7.4

TABLE 3

MDMA Availability—Percentage Saying "Fairly Easy" or "Very Easy" to Get

	1999	2000	2001	2002
8th-graders			23.8	22.8
10th-graders			41.4	41.0
12th-graders	40.1	51.4	61.5	59.1

Ecstasy to students in grades 8, 10, and 12. The good news is the rate of increased use of Ecstasy is beginning to slow in 2002.

Increased Students Perceived Risk in Using MDMA Once or Twice (see Table 4)

Ecstasy, even used once or twice, is perceived by students as a "great risk" and has increased from 1990 to 2002. (See Table 4.) "While we are seeing a continuing increase again this year, we are also seeing evidence of deceleration of this rise, as a growing proportion of students are coming to see this drug as dangerous" (Lloyd Johnston, press release, December 19, 2001).

The two major dangers that students see associated with use of Ecstasy are neurological/brain damage and contaminants (i.e., substances that may be mixed in with Ecstasy, or unknown substances passed off as being Ecstasy).

In December 1999, the National Institute on Drug Abuse (NIDA) launched a campaign on the dangers of Ecstasy. Materials disseminated in this $54 million initiative included postcards showing a brain scan of a normal brain next to a brain scan of a brain damaged by Ecstasy. The postcards were based on neurotoxicity research that compared brain scans of 14 Ecstasy users with those of nonusers. Marsha Rosenbaum, in her article "Ecstasy: America's New 'Reefer Madness'" (2002), notes that "Although the research was preliminary, and provoked more questions than answers, it effectively set in motion the current 'this is your brain' campaign." As Rosenbaum describes, a national panic arose over Ecstasy use, and the media sounded alarm. The dominant tone was similar to the scare-tactics approach to marijuana use that had been so ineffective in earlier decades. Following are some typically alarmist print headlines:

- "Raves about 'Club Drugs' Cause Worry" (*USA Today,* December 7, 1999)
- "The Dangers of Being Young, Hip and High" (*U.S. News and World Report,* December 13, 1999)
- "Party-Drug Scene: 'E' Trade Spreads Largely Unchecked" (*Christian Science Monitor,* May 1, 2000)
- "Too High a Price" (reporter.com, May 23, 2000)
- "The Poisoning of Suburbia" (Salon.com/Health, July 6, 2000)
- "Alarm of Spreading Ecstasy" (*Washington Post,* August 1, 2000)
- "In New Drug Battle, Use of Ecstasy Among Young Soars" (*New York Times,* August 2, 2000)

TABLE 4

MDMA Perceived Risk—Percentage Seeing "Great Risk" in Using Once or Twice

	1999	2000	2001	2002
8th-graders			35.8	38.9
10th-graders			39.4	43.5
12th-graders	35.0	37.9	45.7	52.2

- "Agony of Ecstasy: Providers Brace for Treatment Challenge" (*Alcoholism and Drug Abuse Weekly,* August 14, 2000)
- "Ecstatic About Ecstasy—But at What Cost?" (*Journal of Addictions and Mental Health,* September–October 2000)

Rosenbaum makes the point that although the government continued these "scare tactics" and increased penalties for possession and distribution of Ecstasy, cooler heads were prevailing. Examples were the *New York Times* article "Distilling the Truth in the Ecstasy Buzz" (Feurer 2000), and a *Time* magazine story that provided a more comprehensive look (Cloud 2000). In the fall of 2001, the Food and Drug Administration (FDA) approved the first study of MDMA's efficacy in the treatment of post-traumatic stress disorder. This may result in opening up research into the therapeutic uses of Ecstasy.

Fishbein et al. (2002) described a "boomerang" effect from the scare-tactic public service announcements regarding Ecstasy: "Beginning with the 'fried egg' commercials ("This is your brain on drugs"), American youth have been bombarded with antidrug public service announcements since they were small children. The effectiveness of such messages is problematic at best, and may well be counterproductive." When the "truth," or whole story, about Ecstasy is discovered by young people, it is quite possible that we will see a further rise in Ecstasy use in the future.

The problem of the drug being contaminated with other substances, or other substances being passed off as Ecstasy, has been a problem with many illicit drugs. Originally this was a problem with cocaine, yet as time has gone on the purity of cocaine has increased. If this new market of young Ecstasy users develops, the sellers will develop more reliable forms of Ecstasy. So the story of Ecstasy may enter a new phase of increased use in the ensuing years, requiring education, prevention, harm reduction, and treatment, not just scare tactics.

Another interesting finding of the survey regarding Ecstasy use by students is that 12th-grade African American students tried Ecstasy significantly less (2 percent use) than 12th-grade white and Hispanic students (10 percent use). We know that, historically, when Caucasian children have been involved with drugs, the alarm has sounded, monies have become available for prevention, and legislation has increased the legal penalties. Unfortunately, if Ecstasy were used largely by African American youth and less by white youth, the likelihood is that the alarm would not be sounded.

LSD

At the same time as Ecstasy use by high school students is increasing, LSD use is decreasing. (See Table 5.) The authors of the Monitoring the Future Study suggest that this decrease reflects the fact that many former LSD users have switched to Ecstasy.

LSD use peaked in 1996 and has gradually been declining since then. The annual prevalence of LSD use by high school students has remained below 10 percent for the last 26 years. In 2001, use had decreased for both 8th- and 10th-graders, and had approximately held steady for 12th-graders.

Availability of LSD peaked in 1995 and 1996 and has gradually decreased since then. Table 6 shows availability of LSD for students in grades 8, 10, and 12.

Students' perceptions of the risk of using LSD have been declining. (See Table 7.) This further supports the theory that LSD users are switching to Ecstasy.

TABLE 5

LSD Use—Percentage Who Used in the Last Year

	1996	1999	2001	2002
8th-graders	3.5	2.4	2.2	1.5
10th-graders	6.9	5.9	4.1	2.6
12th-graders	8.8	7.6	6.6	3.5

TABLE 6

LSD Availability—Percentage Saying "Fairly Easy" or "Very Easy" to Get

	1995	1996	2001	2002
8th-graders	23.5	23.6	17.6	15.2
10th-graders	39.8	41.0	31.2	26.8
12th-graders	53.8	51.3	44.7	39.6

TABLE 7

LSD Perceived Risk—Percentage Seeing "Great Risk" in Using Once or Twice

	1995	1996	2001	2002
8th-graders	36.7	36.5	31.6	29.6
10th-graders	44.7	45.1	41.3	40.1
12th-graders	36.4	36.2	33.2	36.7

Alcohol

Alcohol is the most widely used licit drug and it continues to be used and abused by high school students. Four out of every five students (80 percent) have consumed alcohol (more than just a few sips) by the end of high school; and about half (51 percent) have done so by 8th grade. In fact, nearly two-thirds (64 percent) of the 12th-graders and nearly a quarter (23 percent) of the 8th-graders in 2001 reported having been drunk at least once in their life. To a considerable degree, alcohol trends have tended to parallel the trends in illicit drug use—including a modest increase in binge drinking (defined as having five or more drinks in a row at least once in the past 2 weeks) in the early part of the 1990s, but a proportionally smaller increase than was seen for most of the illicit drugs. Fortunately, binge drinking rates leveled off 3 or 4 years ago, just about when the illicit drugs began to turn around.

Marijuana

Marijuana has been the most widely used illicit drug for the 26 years of the Monitoring the Future Study. Annual rates for marijuana use peaked in 1996 for 8th-graders, and peaked in 1997 for 10th- and 12th-graders (see Table 8).

Since the study began in 1975, from 83 to 90 percent of every senior class have said they could get marijuana fairly easily or very easily (Table 9).

Perceived risk of regular marijuana use peaked in 1990 and has tended to decline since then (Table 10). Perceived risk for occasional marijuana use might be much lower.

Cocaine

Cocaine use by high school students peaked in 1998 and 1999 (Table 11). However, recently cocaine use has dropped in all grades.

Availability has also decreased over the past few years. Availability peaked in 1989, with a resurgence of availability in 1992 and 1998 (Table 12).

High school students' perceptions of the risk of cocaine use have been declining over the last few years. Cocaine-related deaths and cocaine addiction in entertainers and athletes certainly have had an impact on young people's perception of cocaine. Cocaine is no longer seen as the "in" drug, as it was in the 1980s. Table 13 shows perceived risk of cocaine use for students in grades 8, 10, and 12.

TABLE 8

Marijuana Use—Percentage Who Used in the Last Year

	1996	1997	2000	2002
8th-graders	18.3	17.7	15.6	14.6
10th-graders	33.6	34.8	32.2	30.3
12th-graders	35.8	38.5	36.5	36.2

TABLE 9

Marijuana Availability—Percentage Saying "Fairly Easy" or "Very Easy" to Get

	1975	1990	2000	2002
8th-graders	N/A	N/A	47.0	46.6
10th-graders	N/A	N/A	77.7	75.9
12th-graders	87.8	84.4	88.5	87.2

TABLE 10

Marijuana Perceived Risk—Percentage Seeing "Great Risk" in Using Regularly

	1975	1990	2000	2002
8th-graders	N/A	N/A	74.8	71.7
10th-graders	N/A	N/A	64.7	60.8
12th-graders	43.3	77.8	58.3	53.0

TABLE 11

Cocaine Use—Percentage Who Used in the Last Year

	1998	1999	2001	2002
8th-graders	3.1	2.7	2.5	2.3
10th-graders	4.7	4.9	3.6	4.0
12th-graders	5.7	6.2	4.8	5.0

TABLE 12

Cocaine Availability—Percentage Saying "Fairly Easy" or "Very Easy" to Get

	1989	1992	1998	2002
8th-graders	N/A	25.7	25.7	22.5
10th-graders	N/A	35.0	36.8	31.8
12th-graders	58.7	52.7	51.3	44.6

TABLE 13

Cocaine Perceived Risk—Percentage Seeing "Great Risk" in Using Regularly

	1990	2000	2001	2002
8th-graders	N/A	43.3	43.9	43.2
10th-graders	N/A	48.8	50.6	51.3
12th-graders	59.4	51.1	50.7	51.2

❈ Adolescent Cigarette Smoking

Similar to the patterns of adolescent drug use, in the Monitoring the Future study, cigarette smoking peaked in 1996 among eighth- and tenth-graders nationwide and in 1997 among twelfth-graders.

Cigarette use peaked in 1996 at grades 8 and 10, capping a rapid climb of some 50 percent from the 1991 levels (when data first were gathered on these grades). Since 1996, current smoking in these grades has fallen off considerably (by 42 percent and 30 percent, respectively), including the further decline in 2001. Overall increases in perceived risk and disapproval of smoking appear to be contributing to this downturn.

Consistent with the Monitoring the Future Study, the Centers for Disease Control report that tobacco use is the leading cause of preventable death in the United States, and more than 3,000 teens in the United States became established daily smokers each day. Gilpen, Choi, Berr, and Pierce (1999) suggest that "smoking uptake by adolescents is at levels that warrant aggressive public health efforts to circumvent a continued epidemic of smoking-related diseases."

❈ Organization and Content of the Fifth Edition

The fifth edition has been expanded with the goal of helping students and counselors understand the multidimensional aspects of substance abuse. The text's strong family-systems approach makes it unique. The text is organized so that each chapter builds upon earlier chapters.

The reader can now learn even more about causes of substance abuse, assessment, prevention, intervention, treatment, and relapse prevention. This fifth edition has been expanded and updated to make it a contemporary text with drug-specific information and interactions. More clinical case examples have been included to help the reader understand teaching points and counseling skills with substance abusers. Discussion questions help focus the reader's thinking about the cases.

The fifth edition has many tables that can easily be adapted for educational presentations to the general population and for counseling substance abusers.

This fifth edition would not have been possible without the feedback from our reviewers. This fifth edition's editing, redesign, and updates in content and orientation are based closely on the significant input of our reviewers. Many thanks to our reviewers, who have helped make this text to be what we consider to be the best in the field:

John R. Bourdette
Western New Mexico University

Roland LaMarine
California State University—Chico

Steven E. Meier
University of Idaho

I would also like to thank the staff at McGraw-Hill for their faith in this project, their input, editing, and production support, and most importantly their energy in getting the book out to you, the student and the counselor in the field.

Reference

Fishbein, M., et al. 2002. Avoiding the boomerang: Testing the relative effectiveness of antidrug public service announcements before a national campaign. *American Journal of Public Health* 92(2): 238–45.

I dedicate this book to my wife Deborah and son Matthew

Understanding Substance Abuse

Etiology
A Better Understanding of Models of Drug Dependence and Addiction

❖ Chapter in Review

Drugs will always be used for a variety of purposes, including altering consciousness; regulating mood (affective states); relieving stress, negative feelings, and boredom; stimulating thought or action; and disconnecting or connecting.

In 1957 the American Medical Association declared alcoholism a disease, based on three criteria: (1) There is a known etiology (cause), (2) the symptoms get worse over time, and (3) alcoholism has known outcomes.

Devor (1994) describes alcoholism in terms of a developmental-genetic model. He proposes that "alcoholism no longer be thought of as a single disease, but as a group of illnesses in which the influences of genes and environment ebb and flow over the course of the at-risk lifetime."

Adoption studies and twin studies support the view that there is a genetic predisposition to alcoholism.

Various personality traits are more pronounced in addicts/alcoholics. The two primary personality disorders that are related to substance abuse are antisocial personality disorder and borderline personality disorder. Risk-taking behavior and impulsivity are also personality traits of substance abusers.

According to the self-medication model of drug use, drug use is purposeful and drug users choose specific drugs for their desired effects.

Drugs are used to regulate mood and affect (feeling). Feelings of depression, isolation, and emotional pain are often temporarily sedated by drugs. Ironically, patterns of substance dependence and addiction lead to a spiraling pattern of depression, interpersonal problems, feelings of isolation, and developmental problems.

Tension-reduction models are the most highly researched models and are the foundation for a number of treatment approaches. According to this model, drugs are used to counter tension, stress, anxiety, conflict—any aversive emotional state.

The family model is strongly emphasized in this textbook. According to this model, dependence on alcohol or other drugs is a "family disease" and family plays a major role in how family members deal with drugs.

The models described in this chapter present an overview of prevailing theories, research, and clinical observations in the field of alcohol and drug use and abuse. The models are intended to help individuals who are entering or already working in the field gain a better understanding of substance abuse.

I encourage you to study and explore all of these models. Don't discount any of them due to your current biases—try applying each model in

---

The case studies in this chapter are based on a composite of many clients. Names and circumstances have been changed to maintain anonymity.

your work in the field. In the classroom, discuss the application and validity of these models, taking into account each student's individual experiences.

Unfortunately, no one model explains all substance abuse or fits all users' reasons for using. In the spirit of the old adage "If you are a hammer, everything else is a nail," many people want to find a single variable, approach, or model that will predict all cases of substance abuse—when the reality is that there are many confounding variables. Clients/patients are all different, with different coping skills, family histories, physical traits, affective temperaments, personality traits, and developmental histories. Studying the models will make you aware that factors that play a major role in one individual's substance abuse might play no role at all in another person's drug problems—one size does not fit all.

All people consciously or subconsciously alter their states of consciousness. Some common ways children achieve this are through daydreaming, rolling downhill, tumbling, and spinning.

Maybe someday we will have medical tests that accurately predict substance abuse—a simple blood test, or a test for patterns of neurotransmitter activity that correlate with risk, for instance. Or maybe one of the models you're going to study in this book will be proven to be more correct than the others. For now, our best resource is to study the available models and understand how each can be used to prevent, intervene in, and treat substance abuse.

It's peer pressure. . . . No, it's poor self-concept. . . . It's just because it's fun and pleasurable. . . . It's the hopelessness of our society. . . . It's due to the dishonesty and hypocrisy of our institutions. . . . No, it's our inability to connect with each other and establish effective relationships. . . . It's the parents. . . . It's the media that promote instant pleasure, short-term goals, and alcohol use. . . . It's the ineffectiveness of the school system and other institutions. . . . It's the avoidance of pain and hedonism of modern society. . . . It's the lack of caring for our fellow humans. . . . It's stress, pressure, and the breakdown of the family. . . . It's socioeconomic inequities. . . . It's just available. . . . Why not?

✖ Why Do People Abuse Alcohol/ Drugs?

Our Innate Drive to Alter Consciousness

It has been said that there are four primary drives: hunger, thirst, sex, and our desire to alter our consciousness. Drugs have been used throughout history to alter consciousness and will continue to be used in this way in the future.

Some feel drugs open avenues to unconscious issues, conflicts, and possibly an awareness or perception new to the user's life. On the downside, drugs can easily become traps that keep us from using our minds in positive ways. Drug use becomes unrealistic and neurotic when it becomes an addiction. People who are addicted to drugs tend to be passively dependent and destructive. Their nervous system becomes less functional, and the addicted person is less able to function in active, constructive, and interesting ways. Our society is becoming more aware of positive ways to alter consciousness while avoiding addictions to alcohol/drugs, food, gambling, television, work, and many other activities.

Drug Use as a Passive Activity

Many people are passive procrastinators and conflict avoiders. In my private counseling practice, I often see clients who deny the painful issues that initially brought them to counseling. Once they get some immediate relief, they avoid the real issues. Nonetheless, growth involves working through painful conflicts. Our search for the magic pill or cure for the pain of the human condition has created a modern marketplace for alcohol and drug elixirs.

Using alcohol or other drugs is a passive activity; individuals take pills, powders, or liquids and wait for the desired effect—an alteration of their consciousness. In some cases, such as freebasing cocaine or injecting drugs (e.g., heroin), the desired effect is almost instantaneous. Instead of facing and working through their feelings of boredom, sadness, stress, and loneliness, the individual passively changes what he or she feels by using alcohol/drugs. Changing your mood by more active approaches involves more effort and motivation. This is frequently a learning process, especially if the individual has a lifelong pattern of either avoiding feelings or self-medicating feelings with alcohol/drugs. We will explore such proactive approaches in Chapter 11.

✖ Models of Alcohol/Drug Dependence and Addiction

We cannot isolate one specific cause of alcoholism and other drug addictions. There are often multiple, confounding reasons for addiction, just as there are numerous causes for cancer and other medical diseases. Many theories and models of causality exist. Early models of alcoholism labeled alcoholics as inherently weak or unable to control or tolerate their consumption of alcohol. One test of manliness was the ability to "really hold his liquor." Other early models focused on individual psychopathology, arguing that alcoholics used alcohol in a pathological manner to block out memories of unpleasant, traumatic personal experiences that brought with them unmanageable feelings. As time went on, a physiological model of alcoholism developed as scientists searched for a biochemical link to, or genetic marker of, alcoholism.

Today, those of us in the alcohol/drug field generally accept the fact that alcoholism and drug addiction have multiple causes, or etiologies. Clearly, a matrix of both genetic and environmental factors can cause an individual to develop problems with alcohol and drugs. "Evidence has accumulated to indicate that alcoholism is a heterogenous entity arising from multiple etiologies" (Tabakoff and Hoffman 1988). We will discuss some of the causality models later in this chapter.

Disease Model of Alcoholism

In 1957, the American Medical Association declared alcoholism a disease on the basis of three criteria: (1) Alcoholism has a known etiology (cause), (2) the symptoms get worse over time, and (3) alcoholism has known outcomes. The outcomes of alcoholism are dependence, physical symptoms, and eventual death. For more than 30 years, research has indicated an increasingly strong case for a genetic component of alcoholism; this validates the disease model.

The disease model is the foundation of Alcoholics Anonymous and many other self-help programs. The increased acceptance of this disease model is due to continuing research linking alcoholism to genetic markers, the model's effectiveness as a recovery tool, and its reduction of the shame-based stigma associated with problems of alcohol/drug dependence and addiction. (See Chapter 11 for more information on the advantages and drawbacks of Alcoholics Anonymous.)

Genetic Model of Alcoholism

In January 1990, researchers at the University of California, Los Angeles, and the University of Texas, San Antonio, identified a link between the receptor gene for the neurotransmitter dopamine and alcoholism (Blum et al. 1990). Although these findings need to be replicated with a larger sample, they establish more clearly the significance of a genetic factor predisposing people to alcoholism. Ernest Noble of UCLA said that this research "more firmly establishes alcoholism as a disease, and adds to evidence that genetic factors are as important as environmental factors in predisposing people to the disease." The general opinion is that alcoholism is related to several genes, however, and that no one gene can be a genetic marker to identify individuals at risk for alcoholism.

Devor (1994) describes a developmental-genetic model of alcoholism. He proposes that "alcoholism must no longer be thought of as a single disease with a cause that is either genetic or environmental but as a group of illnesses in which the influences of genes and the environment ebb and flow over the course of the at-risk lifetime." The logical conclusion is that treatment for alcoholism would be individually designed and fine-tuned to consider both pharmacological and behavioral therapies.

Adoption Studies

Donald W. Goodwin (1971) conducted a series of adoption studies in Denmark, indicating that sons of alcoholics are four times more likely to become alcoholics than are sons of nonalcoholics. In the study, the results held true whether the sons were raised by nonalcoholic foster parents or their own biological parents, thus supporting the genetic component of alcoholism. Cloninger, Bohman, and Sigvardsson (1981) conducted detailed and extensive adoption studies that confirmed the earlier work of Goodwin in demonstrating the following:

1.   Adopted sons of alcoholic biological parents are four times more likely to become alcoholics than adoptees whose biological parents are not alcoholics.

2. Sons of alcoholic biological parents are more likely to be classified as alcoholics at an earlier age than their peers.
3. Daughters of alcoholic fathers, although not demonstrating a greater incidence of alcoholism, exhibit a high incidence of somatic anxiety and frequent physical complaints.

Twin Studies

Studies of identical (monozygotic, or MZ) and fraternal (dizygotic, or DZ) twins have supported a genetic factor. Because identical twins are genetically identical but fraternal twins have no more genes in common than nontwin siblings, research should show a higher rate of alcoholism in MZ twins than in DZ twins. Kaij (1960) examined 174 sets of twins and demonstrated that, indeed, the MZ twins had a 71 percent concordance rate, and the DZ twins had only a 32 percent concordance rate. In 1981, Hrubec and Omenn again demonstrated a higher concordance rate in MZ twins (26 percent) than in DZ twins (12 percent). A 1984 study by Gurling and associates, however, did not support the previous studies' results.

Currently, no significant genetic research is exploring drug abuse due to the many research design problems with illicit drugs. The assumption is that the genetic factors for drug addiction are comparable with the genetic research findings on alcoholism.

Personality and Substance Abuse

It's my personality. . . . I'm compulsive. . . . I drink/drug to quiet my temper. . . . It quiets my moodiness. . . . I use because I'm bored.

Addictive Personality

For quite some time, the media have emphasized the concept of an **addictive personality.** This simplistic approach makes the mistake of labeling all alcoholics and other addicts as possessing a particular personality that leads to addictive and compulsive behavior. It is more accurate to recognize that many personality traits can make an individual vulnerable to the diseases of alcoholism and drug addiction, but to conclude that there is a particular addictive personality is beyond the scope of modern medicine. It is more accurate to say that such individuals have **psychological vulnerability:** a prior psychological factor that makes a pattern of substance dependence more likely to develop (Jellinek 1960).

It is difficult to identify the relationship of alcoholism and drug addiction to particular dimensions of personality, because many personality traits overlap. Cloninger's (1987) three-dimensional model of personality has been applied to the research literature on alcohol use disorders. Cloninger identifies three temperament constructs that correlate with alcohol-use disorders:

1. Harm avoidant—cautious, apprehensive, fatigable, inhibited
2. Reward dependent—ambitious, sympathetic, warm, industrious, sentimental, persistent, moody
3. Novelty seeking—impulsive, excitable, exploratory, quick-tempered, fickle, extravagant

TABLE 1.1

Drugs and Their Effects

Drugs	Effects
Narcotic analgesics	Kill pain, numb, shut out, slow down
CNS depressants (e.g., alcohol)	Decrease activity, relaxation
CNS stimulants	Increase activity, excitation
Hallucinogens	Change the user's view of the world
Marijuana	Relaxation, stimulation of senses, stimulation of thought

Self-Medication Motive for Drug Use

People use drugs to get a variety of desired effects, such as pleasure, relaxation, excitation, relief from negative emotional states, and enhancement of positive emotional states (Table 1.1). For example, opiates (narcotic analgesics—e.g., heroin, morphine) are used to kill pain, numb, shut down, or shut out the world. In contrast, stimulants (e.g., cocaine, amphetamines) are used to increase stimulation, activity, and action. Unfortunately, continued drug use creates a negative cycle of abuse, dependence, and addiction.

Edward Khantzian (1985) makes the case that drug use is not a random phenomenon. Instead, he says, it is a purposeful attempt by the user to assuage painful affective states and manage psychological problems and disorders:

> Rather than simply seeking escape, euphoria, or self-destruction, addicts are attempting to medicate themselves for a range of psychiatric problems and painful emotional states. Although most such efforts at self-treatment are eventually doomed, given the hazards and complications of long-term, unstable drug use patterns.

Khantzian observed more than 200 narcotics addicts with lifelong problems of rage and violent behavior, and concluded that these addicts used opiates primarily for the drugs' anti-aggression and anti-rage action. In his work with cocaine addicts, he found that these addicts tended to take cocaine to medicate themselves against chronic depression, hyperactivity, restless syndrome, attention deficit hyperactivity disorder (ADHD), and two mood (affective) disorders—cyclothymic disorder and bipolar disorder (see definitions of these disorders in Chapter 10).

Clearly the importance in exploring the self-medication motive is to help users identify why they are taking drugs and then learn how to better cope with the affective states and psychological problems they find so unbearable. The ability to identify and label emotional states, and then to "work through" these feelings, is a foundation of drug prevention with young people and of treatment for those who are experiencing drug abuse, dependence, and addiction.

Personality Traits

Many researchers and clinicians have described various personality traits of alcoholics/addicts. These personality traits include the following:

- High emotionality
- Anxiety and overreactivity
- Immaturity in interpersonal relationships
- Low frustration tolerance
- Inability to express anger adequately
- Anger over dependence and ambivalence to authority
- Low self-esteem with grandiose behavior
- Perfectionism
- Compulsiveness
- Feelings of isolation
- Sex role confusion
- Depression
- Dependence in interpersonal relationships
- Hostility
- Sexual immaturity
- Rigidity and inability to adapt to changing circumstances
- Simplistic, black-and-white thinking

Personality Disorders

> I'm angry and drugs quiet me. . . . It's hard for me to get close to others without drugs. . . . I feel anxious and fearful, so the drugs relax me.

Of all the personality disorders, the one with the strongest relationship to substance abuse is antisocial personality disorder (ASPD). The personality disorder with the second highest correlation to substance abuse is borderline personality disorder. (For more information on these disorders, see Chapter 10.)

Risk-Taking Behavior—Impulsivity/Disinhibition

> It seemed like a good idea at the time.

Impulsivity/disinhibition includes personality traits such as sensation seeking and aggressiveness. I refer to some substance abusers as "edgewalkers"—people who are living on the edge of danger or risk. Impulsive/disinhibited individuals are at increased risk for alcohol-related problems (Caspi et al. 1997; Schukit 1998), and the traits of impulsivity/disinhibition are elevated in the children of alcoholics (Alterman et al. 1998; Scher 1991).

Alcohol/drug use involves taking the risks involved in using. There have always been individuals who, when told no, are curious and perhaps contrary and translate that no into yes. This is especially true of adolescents. Alcohol/drug use affects each individual's physical and emotional balance; for some, that balance is very delicate, even before they start to use alcohol/drugs. Individuals who have a need to be in control usually have a negative reaction when they use alcohol/drugs. People who enjoy losing control and are looking for an altered state of consciousness that approaches their outer limits of effective functioning become more involved in alcohol/drug use. Some thrill seekers may go further, to substance dependence and addiction.

The alcoholic/drug addict lifestyle, subculture, and environment are the most alluring features of addiction for some. Scoring drugs, hanging out in bars, associating with users, stealing, and engaging in other antisocial behaviors all reinforce the actual use of alcohol/drugs. The risk-taking behavior itself creates feelings of rebellion, aggression, rage, self-destructiveness, and "aliveness" (i.e., the adrenaline rush accompanying danger and fear).

The problems that result from these risk-taking behaviors lead to a vicious cycle of taking more alcohol/drugs to alleviate the feelings of pain, anxiety, and depression. This debilitating cycle continues until users recognize their own powerlessness and destructive behavior, or until they are in jail or dead.

Mood and Affect (Feeling) Disorders

Drugs quiet the pain of my depression. . . . Drugs are catalysts to my mania.

Disturbances in affect, mood, and depression are common causes of substance abuse and addiction to medical and nonmedical psychoactive substances, especially in women (Whitlock et al. 1967).

Individuals who are experiencing problems in regulating their affect and mood may self-medicate with alcohol/drugs. Alcohol/drugs may be used to alleviate and self-medicate feelings of anxiety or panic, as well as other negative emotional states, including melancholia, depression, and even mania. Major depression, dysthymic disorder, cyclothymic disorder, atypical depression, and bipolar disorder (manic-depressive illness) are the primary affective, or feeling, disorders associated with self-medicating with alcohol/drugs (for more information on these disorders, see Chapter 10).

Major depression and dysthymia occur one and a half to two times more commonly in alcoholics (Helzer and Pryzbeck 1988). Female alcoholics have a tenfold increased incidence of mania, and male alcoholics have a threefold increased incidence of mania (Hesselbrock, Meyer, and Keener 1985).

Patients with major depression who experience intermittent or chronic dysphoria may come to value the powerful, though brief, euphorigenic effects of opioids or cocaine. Patients with bipolar or cyclothymic disorder who use cocaine may discover that the drug not only can bring them out of their depressive episodes but also can enhance their endogenously produced highs (Marin and Weiss 1986). Seasonal affective disorder (SAD) is another form of depression that leads to increased alcohol/drug use, especially during the "sunless" winter months in certain environments.

The person who starts taking alcohol or other drugs to assuage the negative effects of a mood or affect disorder can be led by those drugs into a spiraling pattern of isolation and interpersonal distancing. This isolation exacerbates the affective disorder. The pattern can lead to social phobia and paranoid ideations (see Case Study 1.1).

Some Feelings That Contribute to Drug Abuse
Feelings of Hopelessness

It is hard to identify a single factor that leads to feeling hopeless, so hopeless that the person gives up (even if only temporarily) and stops trying to grow, achieve, and develop. Many clients feel as if they are getting nowhere, despite their continued efforts. It could be the hopelessness of poverty or financial disaster or of other socioeconomic loss. It could be the shattering of idealism in one's work or relationships.

Case Study 1.1

Jerry: Drugs, Depression, and Developmental Gaps in Relationships

As an adolescent, Jerry was a social outcast. He was a poor athlete, the last one chosen for any team. He wanted to be anonymous and not stand out, but he was very tall, overweight, and poorly coordinated. He was also extremely intelligent and well read. He tried to hide his intelligence, but the teachers would always call on him because he was one of the only students who read the assignments and understood them. At home, his alcoholic parents were unavailable and distracted by their drinking parties and drinking friends. They ignored Jerry's bouts of depression and periodic outbursts of rage, labeling them "an adolescent thing," and figuring he would grow out of it as he got older.

Drugs seemed to be the perfect answer for Jerry to self-medicate his feelings and deal with being an outcast at home and at school. He knew some college kids down the block, and with their help he began using and then dealing marijuana. He was transformed overnight from Jerry the "fat nerd" to Jerry the dope dealer. He began to dress differently and was invited to parties because he always had the best dope. Jerry functioned at the parties by getting so wasted he just sat and observed everyone. He developed a reputation as a stoner and a guy who could get you any drugs you wanted. For the first time in his life, Jerry felt empowered and felt as if he had a place in the group.

Discussion and Epilogue

During his adolescence, Jerry didn't fit into his peer group. He was physically, emotionally, and intellectually different, and he was shamed by his peers for these differences. These negative experiences were compounded by his parents' alcoholism and his own feelings of sadness and isolation.

Drugs not only made Jerry feel better physically and emotionally, but also gave him an identity within his peer group that he felt was acceptable. He was no longer the shy, overweight, introverted "nerd"; now he was the "stoner." He sat in the corner at parties in a blue haze of smoke, or blazed on hallucinogens, or in an alcoholic stupor.

Discussion Questions

What role does "peer group" have in alcohol/drug use?

Do you think kids could intervene when a peer develops an alcohol/drug problem?

Do you think "connection" by a positive peer group could help overcome alcohol/drug abuse?

Describe the possible influence of a mentor (teacher, coach, pastor, etc.) in dissuading a young person from using/abusing alcohol/drugs.

Describe the developmental lags that occur with adolescent substance abuse.

It could be the frustration of blocked goals and aspirations in employment, career, or interpersonal relationships. It could be the devastation of physical health, disease, physical injury or the loss of a loved one. It could be the hopelessness of not knowing how to read or other blocks in learning or achievement. It could be the continual shame and loss of pride from emotional, physical, or sexual violation. It could be a single or continued exposure to a traumatic event or great loss that leads to feelings of hopelessness. One or all of these can lead to hopelessness, which can lead to increased drug use, alcohol/drug problems, and addiction.

Pessimism

Many of my clients recovering from alcohol/drugs described their fathers as "pessimists." Their fathers (and sometimes their mothers) were extremely negative, sarcastic, shaming, critical of others, judgmental of their spouses and other family members, and pessimistic about the world in general. This pessimistic attitude was not limited to the fathers. Some family members were fearful and worried, expressing the philosophy that others would take advantage of people and "rip you off," either financially or emotionally. They viewed the world as hostile. As a result, they approached the world defensively, expecting to get hurt, looking for the negative. Some of these parents were alcoholics/addicts; some led lives that were limited, isolated in social and emotional connection, not trusting or getting close to others.

Unfortunately, this pessimistic attitude contributes to alcoholism/addiction and is detrimental to recovery. Pessimistic individuals can maintain abstinence from alcohol/drugs, but they have difficulty trusting others or being vulnerable and real enough to get close to others, and they struggle with giving to others or attaining a spiritual sense of self. Developing and maintaining a support system for alcoholism/drug addiction is an integral element of recovery. However, developing the skills to overcome pessimism, and the mistrust of others and the world in general, is an ongoing developmental process.

Pessimism and Learned Optimism   Martin Seligman, in his book *Learned Optimism* (1991), describes pessimists as having a very negative view of the world and interpreting events as being **permanent, pervasive, and personalized.** These three *P*s of pessimism color the individuals' thoughts, beliefs, and attitudes about themselves and the world. Pessimists have these distorted thoughts about the world and over time continually approach situations with this distorted thinking process. They interpret a loss as permanent, verbalizing the all-or-none perception that "it will never get better, it will always be this way," making shaming self-statements, and seeing the world as hard, cruel, and uncaring. The pessimist takes one negative incident or a few negative situations or encounters and generalizes that they are pervasive (e.g., one or a few rejections lead to "No one loves me, there is nothing lovable about me, all of me is ugly"). Of course, the pessimist personalizes everything ("It was my fault," "If only I were . . ."). Most cognitive-behavioral therapists encourage their clients to take up these distorted thoughts by *disputing* the distorted reality and by *distracting* themselves from the incessant cycle or focus of these thoughts. This process of disputing and distracting from the distorted thoughts is a common strategy for cognitive-behavioral change. Seligman describes some disputes to some universally distorted thoughts:

> Distorted thought—"I can never be loved or find love."
> Dispute—"Love is precious but rare."
> Distorted thought—"No matter how hard I try, I can't ever be successful."
> Dispute—"Success is doing my best."

TABLE 1.2

Optimism and Pessimism

Dr. Seligman describes pessimists as thinking that a "negative event or interaction" is **permanent, pervasive** (in all parts of one's life), **and personalized** (caused by your own inadequacy).

Whereas, an **optimists'** reaction to a negative event or interaction as being very **temporary, specific** (related to this one event), and **external** (does not reflect their internal self).

Pessimism and Optimism	
Pessimism	**Optimism**
Permanent	Very temporary
Pervasive	Specific
Personalized	External

Source: Learned Optimism by Martin Seligman, Pocket Press, 1991

TABLE 1.3

Optimism

. . . is the hopeful positive attitude of accurate perception and passionate action

. . . is an attitude, that properly harnessed and directed can lead to tremendous awareness, growth and fulfillment

Pessimists think about bad events or situations as being
    Permanent
    Pervasive
    Personalized

Three major characteristics of optimism:
    The situation is very temporary
    It is specific
    It is external

Source: Learned Optimism by Martin Seligman, Pocket Press, 1991

Seligman defines success as "talent/skill + drive + optimism." In his book, he has a test on optimism. I was very proud of how well I did on the test, soon to find out as I read the next page that even a little bit of pessimism can sabotage all the optimism you have.

Seligman says that an optimistic individual views setbacks, mistakes, and failure as *very temporary,* often confined to a *specific* situation, and *external,* or outside of oneself (i.e., not an internal personalized flaw). Another term that many prevention specialists use to describe the optimistic personality is *resiliency.* Despite negative situations, resilient individuals challenge themselves to improve and don't think

Case Study 1.2

Allan: Heroin, a Refuge That Killed

Music was Allan's refuge while he was growing up. He spent many nights alone in his room, playing his guitar, writing music, listening to his favorite artists—and drowning out his father's constant yelling at his mother. At times his father's yelling escalated beyond verbal abuse to physical violence. His father was an alcoholic who often got fired from his jobs. He would blame the company, his boss, or his wife for his own failures, and Alan got tired of the routine.

As a result, Allan tried to avoid conflict with others. He was liked by his friends, his teachers, and people in general. His affable style and musical talent led him to be the lead singer in an up-and-coming band. As time went on, the band was becoming popular and Allan and the band were "going places." They were about to sign a record contract and they were planning a road tour. However, Allan was using heroin. The other band members were concerned that his heroin use was getting out of control and feared that he would blow the record contract and the tour. So they and their agent sent Allan in for a drug evaluation. At the evaluation Allan was up-front about his heroin use, admitted he was out of control, and agreed to enter an inpatient drug treatment program.

Allan did great in treatment and followed up with his aftercare. He was drug-free and feeling great, having 100 days of sobriety. The band was about to sign their record contract and were preparing for the tour. Despite the fact that he was doing well, with excellent support, Allan tried shooting heroin, just one more time, and it was his last. A fan gave him some heroin. The heroin was of high purity and Allan's tolerance was low, having been drug-free for 100 days. He overdosed and never regained consciousness.

Discussion Questions

Describe some positive alternative activities that helped you cope with family problems and conflicts.

What could have been done to avoid a "drug overdose"?

What personality traits contributed to Allan's problems?

What role does music play in alcohol/drug use (i.e., Drugs, Sex and Rock n' Roll)?

What role do you think the family plays in addiction?

---

of themselves as victims. Optimists develop a plan to overcome the negative obstacles in their lives. They persevere through adversity (see Tables 1.2 and 1.3).

You can certainly see how pessimism is a major characteristic of and contributing factor to alcoholism/addiction. The alcoholic/addict's sarcasm and sarcastic sense of humor underly a negative worldview. Procrastination about organizing, cleaning up, or dealing with one's life is an ongoing aspect of this pessimistic view (see Case Study 1.2).

Poor Future Orientation

Michael Yapko, in his book *Breaking Down the Patterns of Depression* (1997), describes depression as having its roots in a "poor future orientation." Individuals who see their future as negative might abuse drugs, having a short-range view. Many addicts/alcoholics report that they don't expect to live very long. Thinking that their life span is limited, they are not concerned about having good physical health. As one client put it, "I might as well party hearty, since I will die young, anyway."

Many adolescents have a poor future orientation because of a continued pattern of academic failure or a difficult family situation. Academic failure, especially in the late elementary grades, highly correlates with early antisocial behavior and alcohol/drug abuse (Johnston et al. 1978; Kandel, Kessler, and Margulies 1978; Robins 1978). Many of these children fail to develop the skills necessary to learn, integrate concepts, and succeed in school. Many exhibit learning disabilities, emotional problems, and attention deficit disorder. These children's parents are frequently in denial of these emotional and learning disabilities, and the school system may not adequately address these problems, resulting in educational failure for the children. Some of these children do well during adolescence, some barely escape alcohol/drug problems, some develop addictions, and some die in alcohol/drug–related accidents and overdoses.

Some young adults might be frustrated that their careers are not developing. Middle-aged persons may be realizing that they face limitations and may not accomplish what they had intended. Older adults may have the existential despair about aging, future health problems, or death itself.

All of these issues may cause a person to have a poor future orientation. The adolescent, the young adult, the middle-aged person and the elder may choose to abuse alcohol/drugs to cope with these discouraging issues. The obvious goal, whether the difficulty is poor future orientation, pessimism, or hopelessness, is to address these issues and to find new ways to enjoy life and relationships.

Tension-Reduction Models

> It's stress. . . . I just drink to calm down. . . . I need to relax. . . . I'm so tense. . . .
> It lets me worry less. . . . I can avoid the conflicts. . . . It makes decisions easier. . . .
> I can do the tedious work easier. . . . I can summon energy. . . . It reduces the
> tension. . . . It allows me not to think so much. . . . It makes me feel better. . . . It
> is pleasurable.

These are common rationalizations people give for using drugs—whether with a martini at the end of a busy workday, or marijuana, cocaine, or another drug.

The tension-reduction theory (TRT) is one of the most widely researched theories of drug use. Early research focused on tension reduction and relief from stress as a primary reason for alcohol and drug use. Today, the tension-reduction theory is considered one aspect of drug use. Individuals consume drugs for a variety of reasons, including the sheer pleasurable feelings that accompany drug use.

> Not only has tension reduction theory (TRT) been successful in the amount and
> range of research that it has engendered, but also it is clearly the theoretical
> progenitor of many of the theories that have developed over the past 50 years. The
> progress and extensions of TRT encompass most of the psychological approaches
> to alcohol. As a field, we seem to have accepted the notion that alcohol is
> reinforcing because it reduces tension, and we have been undaunted in our pursuit
> of evidence of this basic precept.

The tension-reduction model involves the concept of homeostasis, or balance. The individual will use alcohol/drugs to counteract (or balance out) stress, anxiety,

*Average tension level (ATL) varies with each individual.
**Average amount of stimulation(s) required to produce convulsion.

FIGURE 1.1   *Average Tension Level*

SOURCE: From *Facts About Drug Abuse,* 1975, National Institute on Drug Abuse, U.S. Department of Health and Human Services.

emotional tension, and conflict—any aversive emotional state. Alcohol/drugs are therefore used as tension reducers.

Tension has been defined as any state that is an aversive source of motivation, causing feelings of fear, anxiety (vague fear), conflict, and frustration due to blocked goals (see Figure 1.1). Stress is just a modern version of tension. Here is one definition of stress, from *Merriam Webster's Collegiate Dictionary*: "a physical, chemical, or emotional factor that causes bodily or mental tension and may be a factor in disease causation." The tension-reduction theory of alcohol use has two major assumptions: alcohol reduces tension, and individuals drink alcohol for its tension-reducing properties (Blane and Leonard 1988). Genetically predisposed individuals may find that alcohol or other drugs have effects that buffer, or reduce, stress for them.

A noted authority on alcohol and drugs, Stanley Gitlow, emphasizes an etiological model that focuses on discomfort and tolerance to stress as a major factor in the decision to use alcohol/drugs. Gitlow believes that we have biological variations in our levels of tolerance to stress and stimulation. "The initiating stimulus could well be perceived by one individual as minimally inconvenient, while another individual would perceive that same stimulus as agonizingly urgent. The overriding determinant and major variable of appetite regulation is most likely the intensity of the individual's perception of need for relief" (Gitlow 1985). Petrie (1960) identified three basic classifications in dealing with stimuli: (1) *stimulus reducers* perceive and react to a stimulus as if that stimulus were less than it is; (2) *stimulus moderators* perceive and react to the stimulus as it is; (3) and *stimulus augmenters* perceive and react as if that stimulus were more than it is. "A perceptual characteristic, such as stimulus augmenting, leading to an overly sensitive need for relief from any discomfort, appeared to be a possible and intriguing genetically determined CNS factor" (Gitlow 1985). In 1984, Lynne Hennecke reported a significantly higher incidence of stimulus augmenters in the sons of alcoholic fathers than in the sons of nonalcoholic fathers. Hennecke suggests that, in stimulus augmenters, alcohol is used to shut down the stimulation overload from the environment.

Gitlow (1972) describes alcoholism as a biochemical defect. The individual possessing this defect is easily agitated by stimuli, becomes uncomfortable, and uses alcohol for its sedating effect. Unfortunately, withdrawal from alcohol creates an agitating effect, and the individual must drink again to relieve this discomfort.

Figure 1.2 shows various reactions to alcohol and their relationships to stress. Anyone ingesting alcohol or other sedative hypnotics goes from the normal level of functioning to a level of reduced inhibitions. As that person continues to consume alcohol, the effect becomes more pronounced, as indicated by loss of motor control and loss of coordination. Excessive levels of alcohol ingestion can cause alcoholics to pass out, become comatose, and die. As an alcoholic stops using alcohol, the withdrawal symptoms follow the same progression. At low ingestion levels, the withdrawal may be minor anxiety or aggressive behavior. Figure 1.3 shows the changes after approximately an hour of alcohol consumption. There is a reduced inhibition (change S^1), followed by anxious/aggressive behavior from withdrawal (change S^2). After one hour of alcohol consumption, the human body takes from 6 to 8 hours to get back to its normal average tension level.

When more alcohol is consumed, the withdrawal symptoms are stronger—hangovers, delirium tremens, convulsions, and death. Figure 1.4 shows that after 5 to 7 hours of alcohol consumption, the human body takes 16 to 20 hours to get back

FIGURE 1.2   *Reaction to Sedative Hypnotics (Particularly Alcohol)*

SOURCE: From *Facts About Drug Abuse,* 1975, National Institute on Drug Abuse, U.S. Department of Health and Human Services.

S^1 Reduced tension level due to sedative/hypnotic consumption.
S^2 Increased tension due to psychomotor stimulation.

FIGURE 1.3   *Tension Changes Due to Alcohol Consumption*

SOURCE: From *Facts About Drug Abuse,* 1975, National Institute on Drug Abuse, U.S. Department of Health and Human Services.

FIGURE 1.4   *Effects of Higher Dosages of Alcohol*

SOURCE: From *Facts About Drug Abuse,* 1975, National Institute on Drug Abuse, U.S. Department of Health and Human Services.

FIGURE 1.5   *Tension Levels Produced by 48 Hours of High-Level Alcohol Consumption*

SOURCE: From *Facts About Drug Abuse,* 1975, National Institute on Drug Abuse, U.S. Department of Health and Human Services.

to its average tension level. Figure 1.5 describes a 48-hour binge pattern of alcohol consumption, which requires a recovery time of approximately 600 hours, or 25 days.

Withdrawal from alcohol is far more dangerous than withdrawal from other drugs (see Chapter 3). As Figure 1.6 illustrates, each time the drinker is about to go to the normal range and suffer withdrawal, he or she consumes more alcohol to avoid experiencing withdrawal. To ward off withdrawal, alcoholics often resort to the "hair of the dog." Figure 1.7 shows how, after an entire evening of alcohol consumption, drinking the traditional Bloody Mary the next morning temporarily takes the edge off a hangover. We could develop similar figures for stimulants, hallucinogens, marijuana, and a variety of other drugs to illustrate the effects on an individual's stress levels and normal functioning.

Conditioning and Substance Abuse

> I use drugs because it feels good. . . . Drugs make for a goodtime. . . . I expect to feel good under the influence. . . . There is no "guesswork" here—take the drug for the desired effect. . . . It's modern chemistry. . . .

A strong reinforcing factor in alcohol/drug use is the memorable feeling attached to the first use. A first-time experience with a drug or alcohol-induced altered state of consciousness is a new and unforgettable awareness. This first or early experience with alcohol/drugs is so reinforcing that time after time the individual attempts to

FIGURE 1.6 *The Built-Up Effects of Additional Alcohol Consumption*

SOURCE: From *Facts About Drug Abuse,* 1975, National Institute on Drug Abuse, U.S. Department of Health and Human Services.

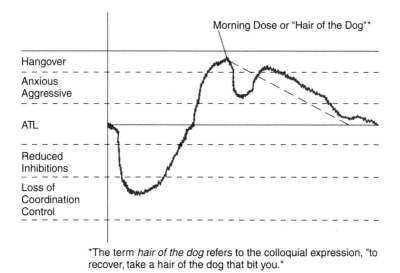

*The term *hair of the dog* refers to the colloquial expression, "to recover, take a hair of the dog that bit you."

FIGURE 1.7 *Hair-of-the-Dog Effect*

SOURCE: From *Facts About Drug Abuse,* 1975, National Institute on Drug Abuse, U.S. Department of Health and Human Services.

reproduce or recapture that original memorable experience. Heroin smokers call it "chasing the dragon." This can be similar to one's first romantic involvement or to the extremely pleasurable yet painful romantic associations of unrequited love. Alcohol/drugs can become that first love, like no other experience ever felt before. Unfortunately, it is impossible to duplicate that feeling. The cycle of addiction has begun: the individual tries to repeat an experience that cannot be recaptured because by definition it was the first. This is the reason addicts continue using alcohol/drugs even though the feeling and behavioral experiences clearly have become negative and unpleasant. They hope that somehow the next time will be different.

Frequently, alcoholics and addicts have **euphoric recall** of the pleasant experiences they had during earlier, excessive uses of alcohol/drugs. They forget the negative consequences and dangerous situations that they barely escaped. The human mind defends against the overwhelming fear and shock of these negative experiences and instead recalls the good times. Thus, alcoholics and addicts forget how destructive and dangerous their experiences with alcohol/drugs can be.

If illicit drugs were legal, imagine the unlimited advertising campaigns that could be developed for their sale, based on these characteristics:

> Feeling down and depressed? Lack the energy to do even the most basic things? Suffer from lowered sex drive, sleep disturbances, or have difficulty with interpersonal relationships? Not making the kind of money you would like to, need a vacation, a general lift? Wondering what life is all about or if it is even worth it? Try Zippy, the new nonnarcotic wonder medication brought to you by the What's Happening Now, Don't Worry, Be Happy Institute of Living Life.

Expectancy and cognitive models assert that alcohol/drug use is an anticipatory response to a pleasure state, conditioned by previous use. This may describe the obsessive-compulsive aspect of chemical dependency.

Biobehavioral models focus on the conditioning, reinforcement, stimulus situations (triggers), and pleasure and withdrawal states associated with alcohol/drugs.

Attention Deficit Hyperactivity Disorder (ADHD)

The media have recently given some attention to ADHD in adults, especially adults who might be substance abusers. The three key features of ADHD are inattention, impulsivity, and hyperactivity. The syndrome more commonly affects males (the male-to-female ratio is estimated at between 3-to-1 to 10-to-1). It is very possible that individuals with ADHD will use alcohol/drugs to self-medicate and manage their symptoms.

The symptoms of inattention include not completing tasks, being easily distracted, being unusually disorganized, forgetting daily activities, and losing things. Signs of impulsivity can include saying and doing things without considering others' feelings, interrupting others, and generally acting without considering the consequences. The symptoms also describe hyperactivity.

There have been thousands of studies of ADHD in children and adolescents, but relatively few involving adults. In establishing a diagnosis of ADHD in adults, it is imperative to determine if the symptoms were present during childhood. "To qualify for a diagnosis of ADHD, the key features should be persistently present, pervasive and causing a substantial impairment to the individual's life. This is different from the occasional inattentiveness, restlessness, or impulsivity that everyone experiences" (Varley 1995).

More research is clearly needed to demonstrate the linkage between adult ADHD and alcoholism/drug addiction.

Psychoanalytic Models

The traditional psychoanalytic view of alcohol/drug dependence focused on a fixation at the oral stage of development, resulting in an oral and narcissistic premorbid personality. Otto Fenichel (1945) theorized that individuals use psychoactive drugs "to satisfy the archaic oral longing which is a sexual longing, a need for security, and need for the maintenance of self-esteem simultaneously." Menninger (1963) believed that alcohol may function as a coping device to alleviate stress and that the primary psychoanalytic root is a mother's denial of milk (security) in infancy. Other psychoanalytic theories suggest drinking as a strategy for allaying anxiety over masculine inadequacy (Machover et al. 1959). Analytical theories also suggest that abusers use alcohol/drugs to suppress latent homosexuality and ego-dystonic feelings of homosexuality (i.e., the person's ego is not compatible with the possibility of being homosexual).

The dominant psychoanalytic explanation of alcohol/drug use today is that it is caused by "a structural deficit in object relations." This means that individuals have a hard time establishing effective interpersonal relationships due to their difficulty in managing their affect (feeling) and impulse controls. They often establish their defense mechanism of denial by defensive grandiosity. In 1986, James Donovan outlined psychoanalytic descriptions used by various researchers in identifying this difficulty in object relations:

H. Krystal and H. A. Raskin (1970)—indicated a defective stimulus barrier and an inability to desomatize emotions

Chein et al. (1964)—described drug use to cope with painful feelings and overwhelming responsibilities in the outside world

L. Wursmer (1974)—emphasized the maladaptive narcissism of the addict, a defensive stance against the potentially overwhelming feelings of rage and loneliness

E. J. Khantzian (1978)—pointed to the impoverished self-esteem, the lack of capacity for self-care, and the poor emotional regulation of the alcoholic

Khantzian (1982) and Khantzian, Halliday, and McAuliffe (1990)—described an inability to handle emotions and behavior characterized by swings from overcontrol to undercontrol. Feelings are often vague, ill defined, and confusing when expressed

Wursmer (1987)—suggested drugs may be used to deny or "overthrow" a particularly burdensome and chafing inner authority figure

Psychoanalytic Meaning

Sometimes the choice of a particular drug is related to the meaning that drug has, both consciously and subconsciously, for that person.

Alcohol/Drugs as Power

Alcohol/drugs frequently denote power or feeling powerful to users. The expression *getting high* symbolizes feeling above others or above one's usual sense of self. Ironically, despite the original reason for using drugs to feel powerful, the ultimate state

Although cocaine may give users feelings of power, cocaine use can actually have many negative effects on personality and can quickly lead to addiction for some people.

in the cycle of addiction makes the individual powerless. Cocaine is a drug that has a symbolic meaning of power. As a power drug, cocaine is attractive because of its status as well as its physical and psychological effects. An energizing stimulant, cocaine produces a sublime feeling of well-being; users describe being on top of the world, in control, able to accomplish a great deal, able to have tremendous capabilities and insights, and able to stimulate sexual arousal and performance. However, the reality today is that cocaine is one of the most addicting drugs, and one of the fastest addicting drugs, and it ultimately renders users powerless (see Case Study 1.3).

Alcohol and other drugs symbolize power in the forms of sensuality and sexuality; potency; the feeling of being supernatural, pleasure, sensitivity, insensitivity, or not feeling pain; productivity; rebelliousness; high energy; and so forth. Our review of the research on why adolescents initially used marijuana indicated the following reasons: for pleasure; contentment; the joy of being high; relaxation and recreation; to facilitate social interactions; to achieve status in one's peer group; friendship leading to better understanding; to defy authority, seek thrills, and flirt with danger; for curiosity and excitement; escapism; enhancement of activity; to enhance aesthetic appreciation or sexual stimulation; to alleviate a sense of alienation; to make life better and more tolerable; to understand or find oneself; to expand one's mind for religious insights; to improve oneself.

Alcohol/Drugs as Self-Destruction

Alcohol/drugs can also have a powerful meaning as weapons of self-destruction and ultimately death. In *Family Therapy of Drug Abuse and Addiction,* M. Duncan Stanton and associates (1982) describe the addict as "part of a continuum of self-destruction." Stanton et al. report that, compared with the general public, addicts have a higher death rate, a shorter than average life expectancy, and a greater than normal incidence of sudden death. Compared to nonaddicts, addicts also have a more positive and potent view of death and are more likely to express a wish for death.

A number of clinicians have described alcoholism and drug addiction as an unconscious death wish. Self-destructiveness is the failure of ego functions involving self-care and self-protection. "We are all subject to our instincts, drives, and impulses, and if they are expressed indiscriminately, we are subject to hazard and danger" (Gottheil 1983).

Alcohol/Drugs in Seduction and Sexuality

Alcohol/drugs have important symbolic seduction and sexuality meanings. Practically all drugs and alcohol have been described at some time as aphrodisiacs.

Case Study 1.3

George: Recovering from Alcohol but Dying from Cigarettes

George had been in recovery from alcoholism for more than 2 years and recognized the benefits of sobriety. His financial situation was manageable and improving, he was losing weight gradually, he had a better relationship with his daughter, and even got along with his ex-wife.

When confronted in group therapy about his continued habit of smoking cigarettes, George maintained that he was going to smoke for one more year and then quit. His father had died of a heart attack at age 50, and George was now 49. He espoused a distorted belief that he had held for most of his life—that he was going to die by age 50. He rationalized that if he made it to 50, he would then stop smoking.

Discussion

Poor future orientation often involves limitations in one's view of future events and possibilities, whether financial, interpersonal, employment-related, or health-related. Poor future orientation is a major factor that exacerbates mood, often leading to depression.

This case illustrates George's pessimism about his own future health and his expectation and fear that he will (as his father did) die at age 50. George is living his life based on this belief, which is a distortion of reality. Although George is in recovery from alcohol and sees the benefits of his sobriety and working a recovery program, he is not committed to quitting smoking. Exploring his belief that it may not be worth working on smoking cessation is an integral element to his taking action.

Discussion Questions

Do you think the addiction to "cigarettes" should be addressed when the person is in alcohol/drug treatment?

Do you think self-help meetings (e.g. Alcoholics Anonymous, and Narcotics Anonymous) should be smoke-free?

How hard do you think nicotine addiction is to overcome, compared to other drugs?

Do you think people are still not in recovery, if they are smoking cigarettes compulsively? Explain.

Unfortunately, no drug is truly an aphrodisiac. Alcohol/drugs may reduce inhibitions and stimulate sexual arousal at low doses; however, alcohol and other drugs impair sexual performance, especially with prolonged use.

The symbolic seduction and sexuality meanings of alcohol/drugs are exploited in advertisements for tobacco and alcohol products. If such advertising were legal, it would probably be used to advertise illicit drugs, too.

Whether celebrating an important event with a traditional toast of wine, champagne, or alcohol; passing around a pipe filled with marijuana; or sharing cocaine, heroin, or other drugs, the symbolic meaning is a shared altered state of consciousness (see Case Study 1.4).

Case Study 1.4

Lyn: Marijuana and Seduction

Lyn is a female client in outpatient therapy who successfully stopped smoking marijuana 10 months ago. At a party, a male acquaintance flirts with Lyn from across the room. She is very interested so she returns the seductive eye contact. When they eventually make it to the same part of the room, they begin a conversation. He asks her out to the balcony where it is quieter. Even though Lyn has not smoked marijuana in 10 months and has a history of marijuana dependence, she accepts and smokes the marijuana he offers her, without much thought.

Discussion

Drugs are often linked to seduction and sexuality. For Lyn, the seductive nature and excitation of this new relationship was too powerful a draw for her to refuse the marijuana. She knew that marijuana had had significant negative consequences in her life, but the trigger of seduction overcame this awareness. Often people will say, "It seemed like a good idea at the time," rather than recognize the long-term consequences.

Discussion Questions

What role do alcohol/drugs play in seduction and sexuality?
Do you think alcohol/drugs can be cross-addicting with sexuality?
Explain the interaction dynamic of alcohol/drugs and sexuality (i.e. "Drugs, Sex, and Rock n' Roll").
What developmental problems can occur when alcohol/drugs are used to facilitate sexuality, and intimacy?

Family Model

I drink/drug because I come from a "dysfunctional family.". . . My mom drank a lot. . . . I felt neglected. . . . I was abandoned. . . . I was abused. . . . I was shamed, violated, and traumatized.

The family model is the model most emphasized throughout this book; it includes all aspects of family life. Some examples of factors contributing to alcohol/drug use in the family include the following:

- Imbalance in parenting
- Marital discord
- Alcoholic/addict behavior
- Imbalanced and dysfunctional family interaction
- Significant trauma and stress in the family
- Physical, emotional, sexual, and psychological violation
- Inappropriate boundaries
- Shame, abandonment, rejection

The family model of chemical dependency is developed in more detail throughout this book.

Family

According to the family model of alcohol/drug use, alcohol and drug addiction and dependence are **family diseases.** The genetic predisposition to alcoholism is well documented. The probability of developing the disease of alcoholism and drug addiction is 4 times higher for those individuals who have one alcoholic or drug-addicted parent. The probability increases to 8 times higher if both parents are alcoholics or addicts.

Children from alcoholic, dysfunctional, and shame-based family systems are at greater risk for developing problems with alcohol/drugs. The modeling of family members who use alcohol/drugs also greatly influences the development of alcohol/drug dependence. Exhibiting poor communication, the alcoholic/addict family has specific "no talk, no feel, no trust" rules (see Chapter 7). Such a family system breeds childhood traumas of fear, rejection, abandonment, and sometimes violation. (see Chapters 5 and 6.)

Parents with substance-abuse problems have extreme difficulty in being effective parents. "Parenting is a difficult, time-consuming, complicated task. Staying on top of the situation requires quick, sensitive, and intuitive judgment of that which works best" (Kempher 1987). Parents with alcohol/drug problems are ill-equipped to provide the kind of patient, dedicated care necessary for children to develop and grow. Their parenting styles tend to be rigid and insensitive to the needs of children. These parents tend not to be nurturing and available. They often use coercive or abusive parenting techniques they learned from their own parents.

Poor Self-Concept

The most frequently generalized risk factor for problems with alcohol/drugs is a poor self-concept. Parents and schools talk about children's general underachievement, shyness, and aggressive or antisocial behavior as being a result of this lack of self-concept. Report cards and progress reports include comments such as "does not work up to his/her potential," "has difficulty finishing assignments and staying on task," "fails to participate in class, daydreams," and "more concerned with peers than teacher." It should be no surprise that the same evaluations occur for adults who have difficulty with work relationships and general achievement.

There are so many definitions of self-concept that isolating this variable as a causative factor for alcohol/drug problems is impossible. While exploring all of these definitions of self-concept, I developed a more workable behavioral definition that better explains what we are talking about. Instead of using the label *self-concept,* which implies something one gets from outside of oneself and is, therefore, beyond one's internal ability to develop, I relabeled it as a **sense of self.** A sense of self is less static than self-concept, involves more choices by the individual, and is active rather than passive. A sense of self comes from within to the outside world, rather than the outside world's defining who the individual is. This important point has implications for individuals who develop codependent relationships with addicts and alcoholics. (See Chapter 7.) Under this definition, a person with a sense of self is

1. A unique, worthwhile individual with emerging talents and skills
2. An individual who can accomplish things (e.g., develop, prioritize, and achieve goals; solve problems; resolve conflicts; accept and carry out responsibilities; and have the maturity to develop and grow)

3. An individual who can trust and be trusted, one who sets appropriate boundaries for intimacy in relationships

In his article "Beyond Drug Education," Paul Robinson (1975) argued that the goal is "not to convince people not to do drugs" but to empower them to enhance their development of self. Robinson suggests that we need to emphasize educational programs that help students acquire this sense of self, by helping students develop the skills to

- Control their destructive impulses
- Understand their values, needs, and desires
- Make wise decisions
- Resist peer pressure when it endangers their welfare or inhibits their growth
- Find nonchemical means of fulfillment and satisfaction
- Think intelligently and rationally

By focusing on programs that teach children and adults to develop and enhance a sense of self, we make them less at risk for alcohol and drug problems.

The more time I spend working in the fields of alcohol/drug recovery and mental health, the more clearly I see that a poor sense of self is a strong predictor of problems with alcohol/drugs. Families that do not promote the child's sense of self cause those children to be emotionally disabled (i.e., they develop a poor sense of self). In later chapters we will discuss these specific family issues in more detail.

Encouraging potential alcoholics and addicts to develop a sense of self is just one aspect of the problem; other factors must also be addressed. Even children and adults who possess a wonderful and creative sense of self can be at risk. Improving the sense of self is a preventive inoculation but is neither a cure nor a guarantee against having alcohol/drug problems. (See Chapter 10.)

Adolescence

As children enter adolescence, they are at risk for alcohol/drug problems. In *Drugs and Drinking* (1985), Jay Strack classifies five major factors in adolescent abuse of drugs, using the mnemonic *PEACE:*

P—pressure (peer pressure)
E—escape
A—availability (of alcohol/drugs)
C—curiosity
E—emptiness

Psychosocial Models—Social Learning Theory

> It's fun to use and be with friends. . . . It's peer pressure. . . . It's cool to use and chill out. . . . I can use drugs and belong. . . . I can connect with others when we are together. . . . Sex is better. . . .

A variety of models can be considered psychosocial or social learning models. The key element of these models is the social learning aspect of alcohol/drug use. Social learning theory also incorporates other models, such as the tension-reduction model.

For example, the young child who sees Dad drink his martini at the end of the day and witnesses the relief of tension may come to see drinking alcohol as an extremely positive experience. Children often experience their parents as more approachable and positive after they have used drugs or alcohol. Nathan (1983), describes alcohol use as a socially acquired, learned behavior pattern, maintained by antecedent cues (classical conditioning and expectancies), consequent reinforcements (operant conditioning and tension reduction), cognitive factors, modeling influences, and the interaction of behavioral and genetic mechanisms.

Marlatt and Gordon (1985) emphasize certain social learning and cognitive-behavioral points about addiction:

- Addictive behaviors are a category of "bad habits" (or learned maladaptive behaviors). Biological factors may contribute to predisposing an individual to alcohol problems, but specific patterns of use are learned.
- Addictive behaviors occur on a continuum of use—that is, behavior such as alcohol abuse is not categorical (e.g., present or absent) but instead varies in quantity and frequency of occurrence.
- All points along the continuum of addictive behavior are influenced by the same principles of learning. Therefore, the same mechanism that may be applied to explaining alcohol use can be invoked to explain alcohol-use disorder.
- Addictive behaviors are learned habits that can be analyzed in the same way as any other habit.
- The determinants of addictive behaviors are situational and environmental factors, beliefs and expectations, and family history and prior learning experiences with the substance or activity. Emphasis also is placed on the consequences of addictive behavior to understand its reinforcement and punishing features.
- Besides the effects of alcohol (or another substance or activity in question), it also is important to discern the social interpersonal reactions that the individual experiences before, during, and after engaging in the addictive behavior. Social factors are important, both in the acquisition and later performance of the addictive behavior.
- Frequently, addictive behaviors are exhibited under conditions that are perceived as stressful. To that degree, they represent maladaptive coping behaviors.
- Addictive behaviors are strongly affected by the individual's expectations of achieving desired effects of engaging in the addictive behavior. Furthermore, self-efficacy expectancies (i.e., expectations of being able to use behavioral skills to cope with a situation without engaging in the addictive behavior) are important. If self-efficacy in a situation is low, and the individual believes (expects) that engaging in the addictive behavior would help him or her cope with it, then the likelihood of engaging in the behavior increases.
- The acquisition of new skills and cognitive strategies in a self-management program can result in changes in addictive behavior to new, more adaptive behaviors, which come under control of cognitive processes of awareness and decision making. Accordingly, the individual can assume and accept a greater degree of responsibility for changing the addictive behavior.

Sociocultural Models

In his review of cultural and cross-cultural studies, Bales (1946) identified factors in the influence of a culture or sociological organization on rates of alcoholism:

1. The degree to which a culture causes acute needs for adjustment of inner tension in its members
2. The attitudes toward drinking that the culture produces in its members
3. The degree to which the culture provides substitute means of satisfaction

Societies, cultures, communities, socioeconomic groups, and even neighborhoods offering few or limited alternatives to drinking and drugging as tension relievers are more susceptible to addiction. The more these groups produce acute inner tensions (shame), suppressed or acted-out aggression, extreme conflict, dilemmas, mixed messages, sexual tensions, and the condoning of attitudes about alcohol/drugs as the normal, accepted way of relieving these tensions, the more prone individuals are to develop alcohol/drug dependence. When there is no limit on supply and distribution, attitudes are liberal, and cost is relative, the incidence of alcohol and drug abuse is high.

The attitude of the culture and ethnic customs may also facilitate patterns of alcohol/drug use. "The Irish and the American Indian groups positively sanction men's drinking to intoxication away from home; in these cultures the rates of alcoholism are high. Drug/alcohol dependence and addiction are influenced by sociological factors such as age, occupation, social class and subculture, and religious affiliation. In the United States, for example, young, single, unemployed urban men have a high incidence of abuse" (Donovan 1986).

Individuals who feel alienated from a larger society and who have no sense of belonging may feel that the society's rules and values about alcohol and drugs don't apply to them. This feeling of alienation from a larger social body may result in more favorable attitudes about alcohol/drugs. The application of this social model of alcohol/drug use is evidenced by the crack cocaine epidemic.

The lack of opportunity or hope that one can achieve the American Dream can contribute to feelings of despair that lead to alcoholism and/or drug addiction. This despair is most prevalent in the ghettos in America's inner cities. However, this sense of despair can occur in any locale, in any socioeconomic setting. From the blue-collar bars, to the shooting galleries in abandoned buildings, to middle-class suburban high schools, to the plush boardrooms of major corporations, drugs and alcohol infest our society.

References

Alterman, A. I., et al. 1998. Personality pathology and drinking in young men at high and low familial risk for alcoholism. *Journal of Studies on Alcohol* 59:495–502.

Bales, R. 1946. Cultural differences in rates of alcoholism. *Quarterly Journal of Studies of Alcohol* 6:480–99.

Benward, J., and J. Densen-Gerber. 1975. Incest as a causative factor in antisocial behavior: An exploratory study. *Contemporary Drug Problems* 4:323–40.

Blane, Howard T., and Kenneth E. Leonard, eds. 1988. *Psychological theories of drinking and alcoholism.* New York: Guilford Press.

Blum, Kenneth, et al. 1990. Allelic association of human dopamine D2 receptor gene in alcoholism. *Journal of the American Medical Association* 263(15):2055–60.

Caspi, A., et al. 1997. Personality differences predict health-risk behaviors in adulthood: Evidence from a longitudinal study. *Journal of Personality and Social Psychology* 73:1052–63.

Chein, I., et al. 1964. *The road to H.* New York: Basic Books.

Cloninger, C. R. 1987. A systematic method for clinical description and classification of personality variants. *Archives of General Psychiatry* 44:573–88.

Cloninger, C. R., M. Bohman, and S. Sigvardsson. 1981. Inheritance of alcohol abuse. *Archives of General Psychiatry* 38:861–68.

Devor, Eric. 1994. A developmental-genetic model of alcoholism: Implications for genetic research. *Journal of Consulting and Clinical Psychology* 62(6): 1108–15.

Donovan, James M. 1986. Etiological model of alcoholism. *American Journal of Psychiatry* 143:1–11.

Fenichel, Otto. 1945. *The psychoanalytic theory of neurosis.* New York: W. W. Norton.

Gitlow, S. E. 1972. The pharmacological approach to alcoholism. *Journal of Drug Issues* 2(3): 32–41.

Gitlow, S. E., and Herbert S. Peyser. 1988. *Alcoholism: A practical treatment guide.* Philadelphia: Grune & Stratton.

Goodwin, D. W. 1971. Is alcoholism hereditary? A review and critique. *Archives of General Psychiatry* 25:545–49.

Gottheil, Edward, ed. 1983. *Etiological aspects of alcohol/drug abuse.* Springfield, Ill.: Charles C. Thomas.

Gurling, H. M., et al. 1984. Genetic epidemiology in medicine: Recent twin research. *British Medical Journal* 288:3–5.

Hammond, D. C., G. Q. Jorgenson, and D. M. Ridgeway. 1979. *Sexual adjustment of female alcoholics.* Salt Lake City: University of Utah.

Helzer, J. E., and T. R. Pryzbeck. 1988. The co-occurrence of alcoholism with other psychiatric disorders in the general population and its impact in treatment. *Journal of Studies on Alcohol* 49:219–24.

Hennecke, Lynne. 1984. Stimulus augmenting and field dependence in children of alocholic fathers. *Journal of Studies on Alcoholism* 45:486–92.

Hesselbrock, M. N., R. E. Meyer, and J. J. Keener. 1985. Psychopathology in hospitalized alcoholics. *Archives of General Psychiatry* 42:219–24.

Hrubec, Z., and G. S. Omenn. 1981. Evidence of genetic predisposition to alcoholic cirrhosis and psychosis: Twin concordance for alcoholism and its end points by zygosity among male veterans. *Alcoholism* 5:207–15.

Jellinek, E. M. 1960. *The disease concept of alcoholism.* New Haven, Conn.: Hillhouse Press.

Johnston, L. O., et al. 1978. Drugs and delinquency: A search for causal connections. In *Longitudinal research on drug use,* edited by D. B. Kandel. Washington, D.C.: Hemisphere.

Kaij, L. 1960. *Alcoholism in twins: Studies in the etiology and sequelae of abuse of alcohol.* Stockholm: Alonquist & Winkell.

Kandel, D. B., R. Kessler, and R. Margulies. 1978. Antecedents of adolescent initiation into stages of drug use: A developmental analysis. In *Longitudinal research on drug use,* edited by D. B. Kandel. Washington, D.C.: Hemisphere.

Kempher, Carol. 1987. Special populations: Etiology and prevention of vulnerability to chemical dependence in children of substance abusers. In *Youth at high risk for substance abuse.* Washington, D.C.: U.S. Department of Human Services.

Khantzian, E. J. 1982. Psychopathology, psychodynamics, and alocholism. In *Encyclopedia handbook of psychiatry,* edited by E. M. Pattison and E. Kaufman. New York: Gardner Press.

Khantzian, E. J. 1985. The self-medication hypothesis of addictive disorders: Focus on heroin and cocaine dependence. *Journal of Psychiatry* 142(11): 1–39.

Khantzian, E. J., K. S. Halliday, and W. E. McAuliffe. 1990. *Addiction and the vulnerable self.* New York: Guilford Press.

Krystal, H., and H. A. Raskin. 1970. *Drug dependence: Aspects of ego functions.* Detroit: Wayne State University Press.

Machover, S., et al. 1959. Clinical and objective studies of personality variables in alocholism: An objective study of homosexuality in alcoholics. *Quarterly Journal of Studies in Alcohol* 20:528–42.

Marin, Steven, and Roger D. Weiss. 1986. Psychiatric comorbidity in drug and alcohol addiction. *Journal of Drug Education.*

Marlatt, A., and J. Gordon. 1985. *Relapse prevention: Maintenance strategies in the treatment of addictive behaviors.* New York: Guilford Press.

Menninger, K. 1963. *The vital balance.* New York: Viking Press.

Miczek, K., Elise M. Weerts, and Joseph F. Debold. 1992. Alcohol, aggression, and violence: Biobehavioral determinants. In *Alcohol and interpersonal violence: Fostering multidisciplinary perspectives,* edited by Susan E. Martin. NIAA Research Monograph 24. Washington, D.C.: U.S. Dept. Health and Human Services.

Petrie, A. 1960. Some psychological aspects of pain and the relief of suffering. *Annals of the New York Academy of Sciences* 86:13–27.

Robins, L. W. 1978. Sturdy childhood predictors of adult antisocial behavior: Replication from longitudinal studies. *Psychology Medicine* 8:617–22.

Robinson, Paul E. 1975. Beyond drug education. *Journal of Drug Education* 5(1): 183–91.

Scher, K. J. 1991. *Children of alcoholics: A critical appraisal of theory and research.* Chicago: University of Chicago Press.

Scher, K. J., and T. H. Trull. 1994. Personality and disinhibitory psychopathology: Alcoholism and anti-social personality disorder. *Journal of Abnormal Psychology* 103:92–102.

Schukit, M. A. 1998. Biological, psychological, and environmental predictors of alcoholism risk: A longitudinal study. *Journal of Studies in Alcohol* 59:485–94.

Seligman, Martin E. P. 1991. *Learned optimism: How to change your mind and your life.* New York: Pocket Books.

Stanton, M. Duncan, et al. 1982. *The family therapy of drug abuse and addiction.* New York: Guilford Press.

Strack, Jay. 1985. *Drugs and drinking: What every teen and parent should know.* Nashville: Nelson.

Tabakoff, Boris, and Paula L. Hoffman. 1988. Genetics and biological markers of risk for alcoholism. *Public Health Report* 103(6): 690–98.

Turner, S., and F. Colao. 1985. Alcoholism and sexual assault: A treatment approach for women exploring both issues. *Alcoholism Treatment Quarterly* 2(1): 91–101.

Varley, Christopher. 1995. Hyperactive adults. *Professional Counselor.* December.

Whitlock, F. A., et al. 1967. Drug dependence in psychiatric patients. *Medical Journal of Australia* 1:11–57.

Wursmer, L. 1974. Psychoanalytic considerations of the etiology of compulsive drug use. *Journal of the American Psychoanalytic Association* 22:820–43.

Wursmer, L. 1987. Flight from conscience: Experience with the psychoanalytic treatment of the compulsive drug abuser. *Journal of Substance Abuse Treatment* 4:169–79.

Yapko, Michael D. 1997. *Breaking the patterns of depression.* New York: Doubleday.

Alcohol/Drugs in Our American Society
Major Problems and Perspectives

❖ **Chapter in Review**

Alcohol abuse and alcoholism are major problems that are often minimized or overlooked as not being a part of "the war on drugs."

Binge drinking is a significant problem on college campuses. Research indicates that 40 to 45 percent of college students binge drink; the significant negative consequences include academic problems, property damage, sexual assault, personal injury, and death. At least half of the sexual assaults on college campuses involve alcohol consumption by the perpetrator, the victim, or both.

Alcohol is estimated to be involved in 25 to 50 percent of intimate partner violence. Drinking by men seems to be a stronger predictor of such violence than drinking by women is.

Drinking and driving is still a major problem but has decreased over the past decade, especially among young drivers.

Tobacco is responsible for more than 400,000 deaths annually from lung cancer and cardiovascular disease. It is estimated that 40 million adults and 3 million adolescents are active smokers. Eight out of every 10 alcoholics is a smoker.

Denial of family problems (such as parental alcoholism and addiction), academic failure, and trauma, violence, and violation are some of the risk factors for problems with alcohol/drugs.

The following systemic problems make it hard to address prevention of substance abuse:

- An emphasis on the supply side and neglect of the demand side in the "war on drugs"
- Academic failure, and schools' failure to address the learning and motivational needs of their students
- A long history of neglecting the treatment needs of people of color
- A breakdown in family, neighborhood, and community support
- Socioeconomic inequities

There are many perspectives on alcohol/drug use. These include: the moral/legal perspective, which is primarily the viewpoint of law enforcement and the criminal justice system; the medical-health perspective of the medical and health fields; the psychosocial perspective of alcohol/drug and mental health treatment agencies; and the social-cultural perspective, which is held by most social agencies and social institutions (e.g., regarding housing and employment).

❈ Major Problems

Alcohol Abuse and Alcoholism

Alcohol is the most devastating drug we know of to-day in terms of the sheer numbers of people it af-fects. Estimates indicate that there are more than 12 million alcoholics in the United States and that a significant number of other people meet the criteria for alcohol abuse and alcohol dependence. (See Chapter 4 for diagnostic criteria for substance abuse and substance dependence.)

Alcohol is integrated into the fabric of the mainstream American lifestyle, causing many people to minimize its impact and cost to our society. It has been estimated that business and industry lose more than $136 billion each year due to time lost at work due to absenteeism, illness and/or personal problems, reduced productivity, and health care costs related to alcohol.

However, the production, distribution, and sale of alcohol are also very big business in the United States. This side of the economics of America's developed taste for alcohol often deters our legislators from supporting new and creative ways to address the problems related to alcohol abuse and addiction. The tendency has been to emphasize the "war on drugs" and to exclude alcohol as a target of that war. Many established institutions in the United States agree that we must do something about the "drug" problem, yet they deny, ignore, or neglect addressing the larger problems related to the abuse of alcohol. This section identifies major problems related to alcohol abuse and addiction.

Binge Drinking on College Campuses

> Binge drinking is at once the most important public health problem on our
> campuses and a critical challenge to institutional mission. (Keeling 2002)

In the 1990s, binge drinking by college students gained national publicity because of significant problems it was causing on campuses. Unfortunately this trend still continues into the new millennium: Binge-drinking college students continue to cause property damage, personal injury, and deaths.

Alcohol use on college campuses was first reported to be a problem on college campuses half a century ago (Straus and Bacon 1953). Today, studies clarify the extent of the problems of binge alcohol use on college campuses. The Harvard School of Public Health's College Alcohol Study (CAS) (O'Malley and Johnston 2001) found that 40 to 45 percent of college students binge drink. They also found an alarming increase in the prevalence of frequent binge drinking among women—from 5.3 percent in 1993 to 11.9 percent in 2001 for women enrolled in all-women colleges, with a smaller increase in coed colleges (see Table 2.1). More underage students on college campuses reported having been drunk on three or more occasions in the past 30 days. (See Figure 2.1.)

Binge Drinking on campus has many negative consequences for students, including these:

TABLE 2.1

Percentage of Prevalence of Binge Drinking on College Campuses

	1993	1997	1999	2001
Total (%)	43.9	43.2	44.5	44.4
Female (%)	39.0	38.4	30.4	40.9
Male (%)	49.2	48.5	50.02	48.6

Source: O'Malley and Johnston 2001.

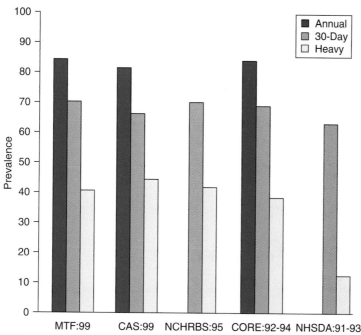

FIGURE 2.1   *Prevalence of Annual 30-Day and Heavy Alcohol Use Among College Students (MTF, CAS, NCHRBS, CORE, NHSDA)*

SOURCE: O'Malley and Johnston 2002.

- Academic difficulties
- Antisocial behaviors
- Psychosocial problems
- High-risk sexual behaviors
- Other risk behaviors (e.g., drinking and driving)

Accidental injury is the leading cause of death among older adolescents and young adults, and binge drinking is involved in many of these accidents (Table 2.2).

Schools with patterns of heavy or binge drinking have more incidents of verbal, physical, and sexual assaults and property damage.

Sexual assault is defined as any act that includes forced touching or kissing, verbally coerced intercourse, or physically forced vaginal, oral, or anal penetration. Rape is any behavior that involves some type of vaginal, oral, or anal penetration due to force or threat of force, a lack of consent, or an inability to give consent due to age, intoxication, or mental status (Abbey 2002).

At least half of the sexual assaults on college campuses involve alcohol consumption by the perpetrator, the victim, or both (Abbey 2002).

There is general agreement that programs aimed at preventing binge drinking need to address both the students and the kind of institutions they are attending. The prevention program should address the college environment, student campus culture, and individual factors to reduce high-risk alcohol use (Presley, Meilman, and Leichliter 2002). The key elements for successful prevention programs on campus involve

---

TABLE 2.2

Potential Negative Consequences of College Student Drinking

Damage to Self

    Academic impairment

    Blackouts

    Personal injuries and death

    Short- and longer-term physical illnesses

    Unintended and unprotected sexual activity

    Suicide

    Sexual coercion/rape victimization

    Impaired driving

    Legal repercussions

    Impaired athletic performance

Damage to Other People

    Property damage and vandalism

    Fights and interpersonal violence

    Sexual violence

    Hate-related incidents

    Noise disturbances

    Institutional Costs

Property damage

    Student attrition

    Loss of perceived academic rigor

    Poor "town-gown" relations

    Added time demands and emotional strain on staff

    Legal costs

Source: Perkins 2002.

"changing the campus social environment by encouraging student participation and involvement, using educational and informational processes, and engaging in campus regulatory and physical change efforts" (Ziemelis, Bucknam, and Elfessi 2002).

Alcohol and Violence

Many problems associated with alcohol use involve violence (see Figure 2.2).

Intimate Partner Violence

It is estimated that alcohol is involved in 25 to 50 percent of cases of intimate partner violence (IPV) (Leonard 2000). The psychophysiological effects of alcohol use can lead directly or indirectly to IPV. Alcohol consumption can result in impaired judgment, cognitive impairment, loosened inhibitions, and numerous physical effects that can lead to violence. Alcohol abuse can also lead to exacerbation of already dysfunctional marital or partner relationships (Leonard 2000) and have negative ef-

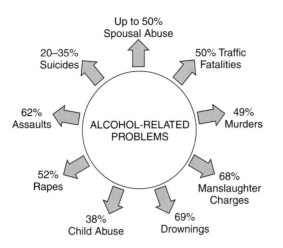

FIGURE 2.2   *Americans Have a Big Problem with Alcohol, the Number One Drug of Abuse*

SOURCE: Office for Substance Abuse Prevention, modified. Data derived from the National Institute on Alcohol Abuse and Alcoholism. In Carroll, Charles R., Drugs in Modern Society, Brown & Benchmark, 1993.

fects on family life, which increases the probability of violence (Steinglass et al. 1987).

Drinking by men seems to be a stronger predictor of IPV than drinking by women. This suggests that prevention and treatment programs aimed at problem drinking among young men would reduce IPV (White et al. 2002).

Women entering substance-abuse treatment were found to have a history of physical violence with a family member or significant other (Easton, Swan, and Sinha 2000; Bennett and Lawson 1994). Alcohol use by offenders and/or victims is found in approximately one-third to two-thirds of rape incidents (Abbey 1991).

Alcohol—Drinking and Driving

Drinking alcohol and driving continues to be a major problem as evidenced by the many traffic fatalities while people are under the influence of alcohol. The relative risk of a fatal single-vehicle crash with blood alcohol (BAC) levels of 0.08 to 0.10 percent, varies from 11 percent (for drivers age 35 and older) and 52 percent (for male drivers ages 16–20). The highest driver fatality rates where alcohol is involved is found among the youngest drivers. Among male drivers younger than 21, a BAC increase of just 0.02 percent more than doubles the relative risk for a single-vehicle fatal crash. (National Institute for Alcohol Abuse and Alcoholism, Alcohol Alert, April, 2001)

A number of factors contribute to young drivers' greater crash risk. These include:

- A lack of driving experience
- Overconfidence
- The presence of other teenagers in the car (encouraging risky driving)

As a result, many states are instituting stricter guidelines for younger drivers— such as no other young people in the car for the first year of driving, and provisional licenses that are suspended with any traffic violation.

Although drinking and driving is still a major problem, research shows that drinking and driving in the United States has decreased over the past decade, especially among young drivers. The proportion of all traffic fatalities that are alcohol-related has also decreased (NIAAA, 2001). This decrease is due to a number of strategies:

- The National Highway Traffic Safety Administration estimates that raising the minimum legal drinking age to 21 years of age has reduced traffic fatalities by 13 percent (for 18- to 20-year-olds).
- Twenty-seven states have now approved legislation to lower BAC limits to 0.08 percent.
- The state of Maine has lowered BAC levels to 0.05 for anyone who has been convicted of driving under the influence (DUI).
- Media campaigns and high school and college prevention programs have increased.
- There is more enforcement and surveillance for driving under the influence, especially during weekends and holidays.

See Figure 2.3 for a comparison of alcohol consumption and blood alcohol level.

Tobacco: The Most Deadly Drug

Tobacco is responsible for more than 400,000 deaths annually, mostly related to lung cancer and cardiovascular disease. Cigarettes kill more Americans than AIDS, accidents, fires, illegal drugs, and suicide combined. Smoking tobacco is the single most preventable cause of death.

> Almost 35% of young people aged 12 to 17 reported smoking at least once during their lifetime. (NIDA 2002)

A study of children's beliefs about smoking (Rogers et al. 2001) found that fourth-graders held very negative beliefs about smoking and were strongly antismoking. Yet many children change their beliefs as they become adolescents. Young children have strong all-or-nothing, black-and-white, concrete beliefs about things. It appears that this is true of fourth-graders. However, adolescents tend to the gray on issues, and their beliefs are less concrete and rigid. Although adolescents see smoking as being somewhat risky, they admire some aspects of smoking. Two primary aspects of cigarette smoking that adolescents viewed as favorable were solidarity with friends and providing relief from boredom (Loughlin et al. 2001).

According to the 2000 National Household Survey on Drug Abuse, 67 percent

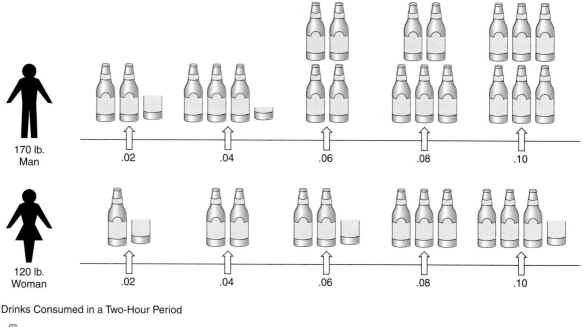

170 lb.
Man

.02   .04   .06   .08   .10

120 lb.
Woman

.02   .04   .06   .08   .10

Drinks Consumed in a Two-Hour Period

12 oz. beer (4.5% alcohol by volume)

1/2 beer

1/4 beer

FIGURE 2.3 *Alcohol Consumption and Blood Alcohol Levels*
GAO

of persons aged 12 or older (more than 148 million persons) in the United States reported having smoked cigarettes during their lifetime (SAMHSA 2002).

Addiction to nicotine is one of the most difficult addictions to overcome. "Nicotine, as any smoker or any physician who's treated a smoker can tell you, is one of the most virulent of all addictions" (Gold 1995). The relapse rate is extremely high. Only 3 percent of the 20 million smokers in the United States who try to quit each year are successful. See Table 2.3 for some of the clinical aspects of smoking-related disease.

Smoking has a history of being associated with a particular image, dating back to the Marlboro man and Virginia Slims. The tobacco industry, with $48 billion in annual revenues, is a powerful lobby. Despite the U.S. Surgeon General's 1988 report that nicotine is an addictive substance similar to cocaine or opiates, smoking has leveled off at about 25 percent of the population. The American Society of Addiction Medicine estimates that no less than 40 million U.S. adults are active smokers. Many of the 3 million teenagers who currently smoke on a regular basis will become adult smokers.

TABLE 2.3

Clinical Opportunities to Talk About Smoking with Patients

Symptoms

Cough
Sputum production
Shortness of breath

Tests

Electrocardiography
Pulmonary function tests
Total leukocyte counts
Blood pressure measurements
Hematocrit
Auscultation of heart and lungs = blood lipid studies
Blood coagulation studies
Serum alpha$_1$ antiprotease determinations
Pregnancy tests
Carboxyhemoglobin determinations

Diagnosis of Disease and Risk Factors

Coronary heart disease
Peripheral vascular disease
Angina pectoris
Hypertension
Emphysema
Chronic bronchitis
Pneumonia
Asthma
Acute bronchitis
Recurrent respiratory infection
Diabetes mellitus
Hypercholesterolemia
Peptic ulcer
Allergy

Drug Prescriptions

Drug-tobacco-smoke interactions
Pharmacological aids to smoking cessation

Source: *Clinical Opportunities for Smoking Intervention: A Guide for the Busy Physician.* U.S. Department of Health and Human Services, Public Health Service, National Institutes of Health, 1986.

Eight out of every 10 alcoholics are smokers. Ironically, the founders of Alcoholics Anonymous, Bill Wilson and Dr. Bob, both were able through mutual support to overcome their alcoholism and maintain sobriety but died from smoking cigarettes. Bill Wilson died of emphysema and Dr. Bob of oral pharyngeal cancer. Alcoholics account for 25 percent of the population of smokers, and many of those in recovery from alcoholism will die of smoking-related illnesses. This creates a challenge for most chemical dependency treatment programs: If they save their clients from alcoholism but don't get them to stop smoking, their clients can still die prematurely.

The risks of smoking are numerous. Prevention approaches with young people, education and treatment for those already addicted to smoking and nicotine, increasing the tax on cigarettes, and fighting the alcohol lobby when it misrepresents the harmful effects of cigarette smoking are just a few of the approaches to reduce adolescent cigarette smoking.

A number of genetic, familial, psychological, environmental, socioeconomic, and community factors contribute to risk for developing alcohol/drug problems. There are also factors that decrease the risk of substance abuse and addiction.

✖ Risk Factors for Problems with Alcohol/ Drugs

Denial of Family Problems—Parental Alcoholism and Addiction

The longer a family denies its alcohol/drug problem, the more vulnerable the family members become to experiencing the destructive consequences of substance abuse. Early assessment of alcohol/drug problems and dysfunctional behavior may prevent a problem from getting out of control. Parental alcoholism and drug addiction make the children in that family four to eight times more likely to develop problems with alcohol/drugs. Children who grow up in families that exhibit dysfunctional behaviors such as physical and emotional abuse, sexual violation, and other traumas are at a greater risk for developing problems with alcohol/drugs.

Public media are beginning to address the issues of child abuse, sexual violation, and other abuses by parents. However, increased public awareness and multimedia programs need to be further developed to address these issues, as well as information on early assessment and referral for treatment.

Before addressing these systemic problems, one must recognize that systems are often threatened by change, are resistant to change, or change too slowly. The pressures of public opinion and the influence of vested interests may cause systems not to respond to the need for change or to respond inappropriately in trying to solve the problem.

Academic Failure—a Risk Factor

Alcohol/drug problems may occur when there is academic failure. Particularly in late elementary grades, early antisocial and other problem behaviors may correlate with academic failure. Frequently, these children fail to develop the skills necessary to learn, integrate concepts, and succeed in school. Many have learning disabilities, emotional problems, and attention-deficit disorders. Parents often deny these emotional and learning disabilities until the children are much older. The school system may also fail to adequately address these problems, resulting in educational failure for these children. Failure at school causes children to disregard school as a viable option for success in the real world. Alcohol and drugs are often the choice for these young people. Discouraged by their failure in school, the additional shame of being labeled poor learners (e.g., stupid) leads to rebellious behaviors and alcohol/drug use.

Some children do well during adolescence, some barely escape alcohol/drug problems, some develop addictions, and some die in alcohol/drug–related accidents and overdoses.

Hawkins, Catalano, and Miller (1992) identified 17 risk factors for adolescents and young adults:

1. Laws and norms
2. Availability of alcohol and drugs
3. Extreme economic deprivation
4. Neighborhood disorganization
5. Physiological factors
   a. Biochemical
   b. Genetic
6. Family drug behavior
7. Family management practices
8. Family conflict
9. Low bonding to family
10. Early and persistent problem behavior
11. Academic failure
    a. Intelligence
    b. School failure
12. Low commitment to school
13. Peer rejection in elementary grades
14. Association with drug-using peers
15. Alienation and rebelliousness
16. Attitude favorable to drug use
17. Early onset of drug use

More information on these risk factors and prevention strategies can be found in Chapter 8.

✵ Systemic Problems

Emphasis on the Supply Side and Neglect of the Demand Side of the Drug Problem in the United States

Approximately 70 percent or more of the federal money available to fight the drug problem is being spent on programs and agencies that focus on reducing the supply of drugs in the United States. Despite these efforts, there appears to be no real reduction in the availability of drugs. The lucrative profits are such a strong incentive at every level of the illegal drug trade that government efforts to decrease drug trafficking have not been successful.

As a result of this strong emphasis on the supply side, funding has been neglected for demand-side programs of drug prevention, intervention, and treatment. The problem has escalated to such levels that respected government officials and other prominent individuals are considering the legalization of illicit drugs. In 1988, Mayor Kurt Schmoke of Baltimore, Maryland, asked for a "national debate on the question of decriminalizing marijuana." Schmoke's suggestion was not well received by supply-siders in the war on drugs, because it dramatically highlighted the ineffectiveness of the supply-side approach. Even considering legalizing drugs clearly points to the frustration of a segment of the American society with the lack of progress being made by the supply-side approach.

Most publicly funded agencies are seeing their funding base diminishing, caseloads increasing, and severity of their patients needs increasing. The March 1990 survey by the National Association of State Alcohol and Drug Abuse Directors indicated that publicly financed programs had long waiting lists for both inpatient and outpatient treatment services. The average waiting time for publicly funded outpatient alcohol/drug treatment was 22 days. The average waiting time for publicly funded inpatient alcohol/drug treatment was 45 days. Nationally, more than 65,000 people are waiting to enter public alcohol/drug treatment programs. Once the alcoholic/addict is ready for treatment and breaks through denial, there is such a long waiting list that relapse is inevitable. This costs taxpayers additional money in increased crime and public health care costs.

The same survey reported that, in 1988, states outspent the federal government in supporting chemical dependency treatment programs. Only 23 percent of the $2.1 billion spent on state-supported treatment programs comes from the federal government. In the 1991 federal budget, the $700 million in treatment grants represented only an 11 percent increase, despite backlogs in treatment services and dramatic funding needs to expand alcohol/drug treatment services.

There is a gap between the demand for substance-abuse treatment and its availability. The 1996 National Household Survey on Drug Abuse estimated that 5.3 million people, age 12 and over, needed drug treatment but only 37 percent of that number received it in the same year (NIDA 1997).

In 1997, the U.S. Bureau of the Census reported that 16 percent (43,448,000) of U.S. residents did not have health insurance, making it very difficult for large numbers of people who need alcohol/drug treatment to receive it because they lack the resources to pay for it.

Money alone cannot necessarily solve the problem. However, it can alleviate delays in providing treatment for those desperately seeking and needing treatment.

Funding for innovative programs addressing the needs of the inner-city crack addict and programs for the prevention of addiction in pregnant women are high priorities. Funding is also needed for alcohol/drug prevention programs for high-risk youth in their communities, with a special early focus on kindergarten to sixth grade. To make a major impact, longitudinal prevention projects with funding for several years are needed. Innovative yet realistic methods of funding are also necessary to attract the support of big business.

Neglect of the Alcohol/Drug Treatment Needs of People of Color

Historically, there has been prejudice and oppression of people of color, a scapegoating of minorities, and a neglect of substance-abuse problems in the inner city. Legislation on drug policy was often based more on racial scapegoating prejudices than on a concern for the harmful impact of drugs on people. "People's attitudes toward a specific drug became inseparable from their feelings about that group of people with which the drug's use was associated" (White 1976). For instance, in 1875, the goal of suppressing opium smoking and opium dens had little to do with the control of opium but more to do with the fear of interracial contact and a fear of interracial mixing of the Chinese with American women and the white working class. The Chinese question dominated California politics in the 1870s. The tremendous racial and class conflicts resulted in many racial riots, the lynching and killing of Chinese, and the burning of their dwellings in numerous West Coast cities. The California Working Man's Party was organized under the cry "The Chinese must go!"

The association between opium and the Chinese into the 1900s was part of the national legislation to prohibit opium smoking and opium dens, even though, at the time, opium was a primary ingredient in most over-the-counter medications and elixirs for physical ailments (White 1976).

The same held true for the association between cocaine and African Americans during the late 1800s and early 1900s. Hamilton Wright, a State Department official considered by many as the father of American narcotics laws, went before Congress in 1910 and gave the following warning about cocaine.

> It has been authoritatively stated that cocaine is often the direct incentive to the crime of rape by the Negroes of the South and other sections of the country.
>
> Once the Negro has reached the stage of being a "dope taker" [dope here referring to cocaine] . . . he is a constant menace to his community until he is eliminated. . . . Sexual desires are increased and perverted, peaceful Negroes become quarrelsome, and timid Negroes develop a degree of "Dutch courage." . . . Many of these officers in the South have increased the caliber of their guns for the express purpose of stopping the cocaine fiend when he runs amuck. (Williams 1914/1976)

These racial associations with drugs were documented in a *New York Times* article that reflected anti-Semitic feelings of the time: "There is little doubt that every Jew Peddler in the South carries the stuff [cocaine]."

This historical association of drugs with minority groups includes these associations:

- Opium with the Chinese
- Cocaine with African Americans
- Alcohol with urban Catholic immigrants
- Heroin with urban immigrants, African Americans
- Marijuana and PCP with Latinos

The underlying assumption was that minorities were not able to control or tolerate the use of alcohol and drugs because they were inherently lazy and physically, emotionally, and morally/ethically weak. Of course, it was thought, most self-respecting white men could control their alcohol/drug use. This prejudice and association of drugs with minority subgroups caused politicians and others to stir up negative emotions to gain support for antidrug legislation.

Unfortunately, as long as drugs were confined to minority populations, funding and treatment resources were limited. It wasn't until the 1960s, when white middle- and upper-class young adults and college students were using marijuana, hallucinogens, and other drugs, that the modern drug war began.

Until we resolve the more dramatic issues of socioeconomic inequities, racial prejudice and the oppression of minorities, inequities in pay and occupational opportunities, and other related issues, the inner city will continue to be a breeding ground for the abuse of alcohol/drugs.

Academic Failure and the Failure of the U.S. Educational System to Motivate and Educate Young People to Strive for Productive Lives

In 1959, the former U.S.S.R.'s launching of the first manned spacecraft caught the United States by surprise. As a result, the United States took up the challenge for space by rededicating energy and resources to the study of science and math as well as the general education of our young people. Perhaps the current failure of the U.S. educational system and the high incidence of alcohol/drug use by young people will be the impetus to implement reform and innovation in school systems, much like that of the 1960s.

The U.S. educational system has become so neglected that the rates of academic failure and dropout are continually rising. The academic standards for students who do graduate are inferior. The ripple effect of this lowering of academic standards is also seen in colleges and education in general. Illiteracy has increased, and the quest for knowledge and general personal and intellectual improvement is not emphasized or valued by the average American citizen. This complacency in education affects standards in American business and industry. The worker who has no motivation for personal improvement also is not motivated to do high-quality, productive work on the job. The quality and pride in American workmanship are also decreased, resulting in inferior goods and services and a general public attitude that accepts these standards. The industries that employ individuals with good educational backgrounds and positive self-motivating attitudes tend to experience fewer of these problems.

The current failure of the U.S. educational system results from a variety of problems. The biggest problems are poor administration, teacher burnout, lack of adequate funding, and a bureaucratic system that promotes complacency.

The factor that contributes the most to teacher burnout is lack of support from the principal and school board. Innovation is threatening to some school administrations, and the fear of parents' complaints and litigation often results in a political administration that is more concerned with how parents and the school board may respond than the effective development and education of the child.

Another factor is the lack of incentives—other than the genuine desire to work with young people—for teachers to invest themselves in their profession. The teacher who repeats the same lesson plan over and over without making any investment in the job receives the same salary as the teacher who is attentive, is involved, and spends time and energy in educating students.

The combination of inadequate pay, lack of support from the administration, and no financial incentives or other motivations has resulted in dedicated and talented teachers' leaving the educational system. This puts students in the hands of teachers who lack the talent or motivation to help them overcome academic failure and a poor sense of self.

Reforms such as site-based management, parent involvement, shared decision making, accountability, and alternative schools have been successful in turning school systems around. We need to apply these principles in educational reform to provide children the opportunity for academic and personal success. The development of our children as a natural resource is essential in developing a future generation strong enough not to become dependent on or addicted to alcohol/drugs.

Socioeconomic Inequities That Undermine the American Dream

The inequities in socioeconomic opportunities have created bitterness, racial conflict, and a general rebelliousness and hopelessness, which fuel the desire to use alcohol/drugs. The American Dream is a nightmare for those who are unable to develop feelings of competency and pride in their lives.

The reality is that hard work and dedication can be rewarded with the attainment of each person's American Dream. Many successful people have refused to be limited by the prejudice of others to the color of their skin, their sex, their religious or ethnic background, or their lack of membership in the inner circles of our society. Many individuals positively strive to reach their full potential by overcoming the prejudices of others and work to correct these inequities when they have an opportunity to change them. Other individuals become so embittered by socioeconomic injustices that they give up, become alienated from society, and lack a personal commitment to strive in life. They use alcohol/drugs to numb and shut down these feelings of embitterment, anger, and pain. Instead of working through these issues and resolving the conflict, they give in to a bitter hopelessness that makes their lives feel meaningless.

Elizabeth Schnoor, in her book *Within Our Reach: Breaking the Cycle of Disadvantage* (1988), identifies poverty as the greatest risk factor for chemical dependency and other destructive behaviors. Violent crime, school-age childbearing, and school failure are outcomes that need "early interventions to prevent rotten outcomes," and "high-risk families need high-intensity services." Changes in economic policy, health care reform, and welfare reform can help in "breaking the cycle of disadvantage."

American society needs to acknowledge and address these issues of disparity in opportunity. Other factors contributing to the alcohol/drug problem are the breakdown of the neighborhood, changes in the traditional nuclear and extended family system, limited support systems, stress, and trauma.

✇ The Major Perspectives on Alcohol/ Drug Use

In *Drugs Demystified,* Helen Nowlis (1975) described four major perspectives on drug use: (1) the moral-legal perspective, (2) the medical-health perspective, (3) the psychosocial perspective, and (4) the social-cultural perspective.

The Moral-Legal Perspective

The moral-legal perspective is primarily the viewpoint of law enforcement and the criminal justice system. The major focus of this perspective is to keep specific drugs away from people and people away from specific drugs. This approach reduces the availability of drugs and uses punishment as a deterrent in addressing the supply side of drugs, not the demand side.

The agencies in this perspective have not been able to significantly diminish the availability of drugs. Although they are doing their best with limited resources, these agencies are unable to substantially affect the price of drugs by reducing their availability. The criminal justice system is a deterrent for some people, but few people stop using or dealing drugs because they fear criminal-justice interventions. The antisocial personality of the people caught by the system makes rehabilitation difficult. The weak rehabilitative components of the criminal-justice system have resulted in minimal changes in the attitudes of those convicted or caught by the system.

The moral-legal perspective is the one emphasized by most politicians, yet this perspective alone cannot be effective. Unless we address the demand side, the moral-legal perspective is ineffective. With so many buyers in the marketplace, sellers are motivated to deal, despite the risks.

The moral-legal perspective also encodes specific value judgments about drugs and alcohol. These are often expressed in the licit-versus-illicit debate, personal biases about punishment for illegal use, and moral/ethical views regarding the use of alcohol and other drugs.

The Medical-Health Perspective

The medical-health perspective is held by physicians, nurses, and the medical and health treatment fields. In this perspective, alcohol and drug use is a public health problem. Treatment focuses on the physical damage related to alcohol/drug use, abuse, and dependence.

The medical-health perspective assumes that people seek good health. The perspective is also based on the assumption that health information influences attitudes and behaviors. However, information alone does not change attitudes about the use of alcohol/drugs.

The Psychosocial Perspective

The psychosocial perspective is a common viewpoint shared by a variety of agencies that specialize in addressing the demand side of alcohol/drugs. The services these agencies provide include these:

- Recovery from substance dependence
- Intervention and treatment services
- Early intervention approaches with adolescents
- Prevention services for young children, adolescents, adults, and seniors

The goals of this perspective are to prevent, intervene in, and treat alcohol/drug problems. Inadequate funding for chemical dependency treatment programs and alcohol/drug prevention programs has made it difficult for many alcohol/drug users to obtain treatment services and for agencies to maintain prevention programs long enough to see conclusive results. (See Chapter 8.)

The Social-Cultural Perspective

The social-cultural perspective is held by most social agencies and institutions. The basic goal of this perspective is to adapt the environment to meet the individual's needs. The underlying assumption of this perspective is that alcohol/drug use is due to the frustration and hopelessness of people's lives. If users had any hope that they could attain the American Dream, they would be motivated to achieve and establish a constructive place in society.

Unfortunately, most social agencies are impersonal, bureaucratic, and rigid in dealing with their clients' needs. Such agencies are poorly funded and therefore poorly staffed; their employees are overworked, underappreciated, and underpaid. As a result, the agencies are reluctant to change, change too slowly, or may even lack a mechanism to change.

Edward Brecher, renowned author of *Licit and Illicit Drugs* (1992), believes we should "stop viewing the drug problem as primarily a national problem to be solved on a national scale. In fact, . . . the drug problem is a collection of local problems." By supporting neighborhood and community efforts, we could provide an environment that could prevent the development of alcohol/drug problems.

The Fifth Perspective—Your Perspective

What is your perspective on alcohol/drugs? Complete the following Fifth Perspective Worksheet to clarify your perspective on alcohol/drugs.

Moral-Legal Perspective

1. Should drugs be legalized? Explain.
2. Is the supply-side approach to the drug problem effective? Explain.
3. Is alcoholism/drug addiction a defense for irresponsible or criminal behavior? Explain.

Medical-Health Perspective

1. Is alcoholism/drug addiction a disease? Explain.
2. Describe the physician's role in making a patient aware of problems with alcohol/drugs.
3. Do people need more information about the health risks of alcohol/drug use? Does this information change attitudes? Explain.

Psychosocial Perspective

1. What role does parenting play in the development of alcohol/drug problems?
2. Is it important for the entire family system to be involved in alcohol/drug treatment? Explain.
3. How can alcohol/drug treatment be more effective?

Personal Perspective

Circle *true* or *false* and explain the reasoning supporting your answer to each question.

1. Illicit drugs are not necessary, and drug use is harmful.
   True
   False

2. Illicit drugs can play a role in enhancing life experiences.
    True
    False
3. Alcohol is a drug with great potential for abuse.
    True
    False
4. My family history does not make me at risk for developing problems with alcohol/drugs.
    True
    False
5. If a family member or close friend had an alcohol/drug problem, I could suggest that the person either get help or participate in an intervention.
    True
    False
6. Persons with alcohol/drug problems have to break through their own denial.
    True
    False
7. Alcoholism and drug addiction are family diseases.
    True
    False
8. Parent modeling of alcohol/drug use is an important influence on a child's use of alcohol/drugs.
    True
    False
    Other personal views

A Perspective of Hope

Perhaps the problems that spawn alcohol/drug abuse and addiction seem too difficult to overcome. The negative impact of these problems frequently gives rise to feelings of hopelessness that we can never adequately resolve these issues. However, there have been positive and dramatic success: millions of Americans are in recovery from alcoholism and drug addiction. Family members are changing their own codependent and enabling behavior in relationships. Adult children of alcoholics are overcoming the trauma of their childhoods. Most important, families are successfully developing more functional and healthy systems for the next generation of youngsters. Their children will be less vulnerable to the familial problems of alcohol/drug dependence and addiction.

There is something to be said for thinking small. Initially, this might sound like strange advice. We each must think about our own small contribution to solving problems that seem large and insurmountable. Each of us needs to first think about our own behavior and our own family and address growth and positive development in those areas. Then we can begin to address these issues in our neighborhoods, communities, workplaces, and other interpersonal interactions. My hope is that we can each, in our own small ways, address the issue of alcohol/drug dependence and other issues in our society by focusing on our own and our children's functional growth and development.

References

Abbey, Antonia. 2002. Alcohol-related sexual assault: A common problem among college students. *Journal on Alcohol Studies* 14: 118–127.

Brecher, Edward M. 1992. *Licit and illicit drugs.* Boston: Little, Brown.

Easton, Caroline J., Suzanne Swan, and Rahita Sinha. 2000. Prevalence of family violence in clients entering substance abuse treatment. *Journal of Substance Abuse Treatment* 18: 23–28.

Gold, M. 1995. *Tobacco.* New York: Plenum Medical.

Hawkins, J. David, Richard E. Catalono, and Janet Y. Miller. 1992. Risk and protective factors for alcohol and other drug problems in adolescence and early adulthood: Implications for substance abuse prevention. *Psychological Bulletin* 112(1): 64–105.

Keeling, Richard. 2002. Binge drinking and the college environment. *Journal of American College Health* 50(5): 197–201.

National Institute for Alcohol Abuse and Alcoholism [NIAAA]. 2001. *Alcohol alert,* no. 52 (April).

National Institute on Drug Abuse [NIDA]. 2002. *NHSDA report.* (May 31).

Nowlis, Helen. 1975. *Drugs demystified.* Paris: UNESCO Press.

O'Malley, Patrick, and Lloyd Johnston. 2002. Epidemiology of alcohol and other drug use among American college students. *Journal of Studies on Alcohol* 14: 91–100.

Presley, Cheryl, Phillip Meilman, and Jami Leichliter. 2002. College factors that influence drinking. *Journal of Studies on Alcohol* 14: 82–89.

Schorr, Lisbeth B., and Daniel Schorr. 1988. *Within our reach: Breaking the cycle of disadvantage.* New York: Anchor/Doubleday.

Straus, R., and S. D. Bacon. 1953. *Drinking in college.* New Haven, Conn.: Yale University Press.

Swan, Gary E., and David J. Balfour, eds. 2002. *Nicotine Tobacco Research* 4(2).

U.S. Surgeon General. 1988. *The health consequences of smoking: Nicotine addiction.* Rockville, Md.: U.S. Dept. Health and Human Services.

White, William. 1976. Chemical prohibition. In *Facts about drug abuse: Participant manual.* Rockville, MD: National Institute on Drug Abuse.

Williams, Edward H. 1914/1976. [Editorial from *Medical Record Newspaper,* 1914.] In *Facts about drug abuse: Participant manual.* Rockville, Md.: National Institute on Drug Abuse.

Ziemelis, Andris, Ronald Bucknam, and Abdulaziz Elfessi. 2002. Prevention efforts underlying decreases in binge drinking at institutions of higher learning. *Journal of American College Health* 50(5): 238–252.

Drug-Specific Information
Drugs on the Street Where You Live

Chapter in Review

Alcohol and other drugs are found in each
neighborhood and community in our society,
and every family is vulnerable to the
problems associated with alcohol/drugs. The
following terms, commonly used in the
chemical dependency field, are defined in
this chapter.
- *Physical dependence*
- *Withdrawal*
- *Psychological dependence*
- *Metabolism, absorption, excretion*
- *Routes of administration*
- *Set, setting*
- *Tolerance, cross-tolerance*
- *Synergism, antagonism*
- *Toxicity*

The "Drug Update" section presents information
on MDMA (Ecstasy), Oxycontin, Rohypnol,
nicotine, crystal methamphetamine, LSD,
heroin, marijuana, and inhalants.

The behavioral definition of addiction includes the
compulsive use of a chemical; an obsession
with the drug; loss of control or inability to
stop using; and continued use despite known
adverse consequences. A drug is a nonfood
substance that affects the structure and
function of the body.

Drugs are classified as either nonpsychoactive or
psychoactive. Nonpsychoactive drugs are the
substances that in normal doses do not
directly affect the brain. Psychoactive drugs
affect brain functions, mood, and behavior
and are subdivided primarily on the basis of
physiological and psychological effects.

The major psychoactive drug categories are the
following:
1. Narcotic analgesics—painkillers and
   designer drugs (e.g., Fetanyl)
2. Central nervous system
   depressants–sedative hypnotics (alcohol,
   tranquilizers, and barbiturates)
3. Central nervous system stimulants—
   amphetamines, cocaine, nicotine, and
   caffeine
4. Hallucinogens
5. *Cannabis sativa*—marijuana and hashish
6. Inhalants—volatile solvents
7. PCP

Each of these psychoactive drugs has specific
major effects, hazards, withdrawal
symptoms, and problems.

The substances that athletes use to enhance athletic
performance include caffeine, chewing
tobacco, amphetamines, and steroids. Steroid
use by athletes, especially young people, can
be a major tragedy.

Every neighborhood and community is affected
in some way by problems with alcohol/drugs.
No house, farm, tenement, high-rise, or alleyway is
immune from alcohol/drugs. Many streets of inner
cities are infected with crack cocaine, and other
streets are contaminated by heroin. Perhaps families
on your own block have problems with alcohol, cocaine, hallucinogens, or marijuana. Perhaps families
who live down the street are mixing highly explosive chemicals to produce methamphetamine. Even

in rural areas, children might be inhaling the fumes of gasoline to get high, growing marijuana in secluded areas, or harvesting hallucinogenic mushrooms. Every family in every community is vulnerable to the problems associated with alcohol and drugs.

✖ Drugs in Our Society

The 1960s and 1970s were truly the birth of the modern drug revolution. Marijuana, hallucinogens (especially LSD), and other drugs became a major part of the hippie movement of that time. It was a time when young people rebelled against their parents' traditional values by using drugs, dressing differently, growing their hair long, espousing open love, and listening to rock 'n' roll. Protests against civil rights violations, the war in Vietnam, and the traditional values of our political system further became the cause for young people.

In the 1980s, a new drug became the rage—a drug that was thought to produce only psychological dependence. However, over the next 10 years this drug would cause us to dramatically change our definition of addiction and our whole outlook on drug abuse. That drug is cocaine. Cocaine was soon being used intravenously and smoked in the form of *freebase cocaine.* Comedian Richard Pryor set himself on fire while smoking freebase cocaine, and John Belushi killed himself when he overdosed by injecting cocaine and heroin ("speedballing"). Both of these unfortunate tragedies brought cocaine to the forefront. A dramatic and tragic victim of cocaine was Len Bias. Bias was a talented college basketball player who had been drafted by the Boston Celtics. The Boston fans were elated at the prospect of Bias and Larry Bird being on the same team. Unfortunately, on the evening he was drafted by the Celtics, Bias celebrated with freebase cocaine and died.

Soon cocaine was being converted to *crack cocaine.* Crack addicts in the inner cities became a major addict population that quickly challenged our treatment and criminal-justice system. Babies born to mothers who were addicted to crack cocaine were another casualty of this new drug.

It is fair to say that cocaine changed our entire outlook about addiction. Even individuals who thought that drugs were rather benign and produced only psychological dependence could not ignore the high addiction potential of cocaine. This short-acting drug created addicts very quickly, with dramatic and disastrous effects on their lives. It also affected people from all socioeconomic levels.

Another group of drugs that came to our attention in the mid 1980s was synthetically produced drugs. In an attempt to subvert existing controlled substance laws, new drugs were created by underground chemists. These new drugs were chemically different (by a molecule or two) from those banned by existing drug laws.

Donald Wesson defined designer drugs as "substances wherein the psychoactive properties of a scheduled drug have been retained, but the molecular structure has been altered in order to avoid prosecution under the Controlled Substance Act." The potency and volume of production of these drugs challenged our perception of illicit drug manufacturing. There was no need for the large production and distribution networks like those used for cocaine and marijuana. There was no harvest of the drug. Instead, one chemist with the basic raw materials could produce enough of the drug to supply the entire United States.

In the early 1990s, another new drug brought to public attention was *ice.* Ice is a transparent, sheetlike crystalline structure that is a purified form of the drug methamphetamine hydrochloride. In the early 1990s, ice was imported to the mainland United States by eastern drug cartels operating out of Oahu, Hawaii. In January 1990, authorities busted the operation of an ice factory in northern California. At that time, the National Institute on Drug Abuse reported the use of ice in cities such as Atlanta, Dallas, Los Angeles, Phoenix, San Diego, and Seattle. Attempts to develop ice on the East Coast did not pan out. Much as crack is to cocaine, ice is to methamphetamine. Ice is a smokable and more powerful form of methamphetamine hydrochloride. Smoking ice allows more rapid absorption into the blood via the lungs. Unlike the extremely short-acting high of freebase and crack cocaine, the ice high can last from 7 to 30 hours. Dr. David Smith, of the Haight Ashbury Free Clinic, has noted, "Ice did not replace crack, it widened the group of people who use drugs."

MDMA (Ecstasy)

✖ Drug Update— In the New Millennium

In this fifth edition, we are putting MDMA at the top of our drug update because of the increase in MDMA use by young people. MDMA is better known as Ecstasy, XTC, X, Rave, or Adam. Although MDMA was first synthesized and patented in 1914 as an appetite suppressant, it became popular in the 1980s with college students. Prior to July 1985, when it became illegal to sell MDMA, or Ecstasy, the drug was legally sold in bars in Texas catering to college students. A major factor that contributed to MDMA's emergence in the rest of the country was publicity—associated with the drug being blatantly sold in bars and then with its being scheduled as a controlled substance. In 1985, *Newsweek, Time, Life,* and other magazines sensationalized the euphoric, therapeutic, and aphrodisiac qualities of the drug. MDMA is related to both mescaline and amphetamines and could be best described as a "mood-enhancing stimulant." It is often perceived as "mild speed," and users often claim that it increases empathy and communication, which is why it is also called the "hug drug." A subculture has evolved around the drug, with resultant Ecstasy and rave parties, which are often clandestine (although most young adults seem to have no problem knowing where they are), changing location as often as every weekend.

Even though it is often referred to as hallucinogenic, it rarely produces delusions. MDMA is most frequently taken orally, with reports of a variety of psychological effects, including the following:

- Positive mood change
- Dramatic drop in defense mechanisms
- Increased empathy for others
- Increased self-esteem and elevated mood

Combined with the stimulant effect, these also may produce an increase in communication, intimacy, and enhanced pleasure of touching, yet MDMA inhibits orgasm and interferes with erection.

Negative effects include overdose potential, extreme fatigue with too much use, dilated pupils, dry mouth and throat, tension in the lower jaw, grinding of the teeth, and too much stimulation.

Although users tend to perceive MDMA as harmless, there are reports of cases of acute and chronic paranoia associated with usage, and even panic reactions requiring emergency care. As with other central nervous stimulants, a rise in blood pressure accompanies its use; this is of no consequence to most otherwise healthy young adults but can have a potentially deadly effect on someone with an underlying cardiac problem or a congenital abnormality.

There often appears to be a hangover effect, consisting of muscle aches, especially of the jaw and facial muscles (clenching of the teeth is common); generalized

TABLE 3.1

Effects of MDMA

Minor Adverse Effects (relatively common and generally short-lived reactions, which occur shortly after taking a dose)

Mydriasis (dilated pupils)

Photophobia (discomfort when looking at bright lights)

Headache

Anorexia (diminished appetite), nausea, dry mouth, abdominal cramps, diarrhea

Sweating, tachypnea (rapid breathing), tachycardia (rapid heart rate), palpitations, tremor

Bruxism (grinding of teeth)

Trismus (uncomfortable rigidity of the jaw muscles)

Gait disturbance, ataxia (difficulty walking)

Serious Acute Adverse Effects (uncommon reactions)

Hallucinations, severe anxiety, agitation, panic attacks, paranoia

Hypertension (increased blood pressure)

Cardiac arrhythmias (irregular heart rhythms)

Severe central chest pain (probably due to intercostal muscle spasm)

Severe abdominal cramps

Urinary retention (due to alpha-adrenergic stimulation of bladder neck)

Adverse Effects Only in Certain Circumstances

Overexertion, dehydration, collapse

Hyperpyrexia (increased body temperature)

Convulsions (seizures)

Rhabdomyolysis (muscle breakdown)

Disseminated intravascular coagulation (blood clots throughout the body)

Cerebrovascular accident (stroke), intracerebral hemorrhage

Acute renal failure

Polydipsia (excessive drinking), low sodium levels, and stupor

Road traffic accidents

Facial dermatosis (pimples)

Delayed Reactions to Exposure

Jaundice, hepatotoxicity

Tooth wear

Possible congenital anomalies

Poor concentration and attention, memory impairment, depression

Sleep disturbance

Weight loss, exhaustion

Source: Holland 2001.

fatigue; decreased concentration; and insomnia. Tolerance to the mood- and mind-altering effect does develop, with subsequent increase in the "unwanted" side effects. See Table 3.1 for a summary of the effects of MDMA.

Oxycontin Abuse: A Prescription Addiction

Oxycontin is a semisynthetic opiod analgesic prescribed for chronic pain. It is often prescribed for cancer patients with chronic, long-lasting pain, or for other related chronic pain. It is effective and beneficial for chronic pain sufferers because it is a long-acting medication that is time-released over 12 hours, so patients need to take it only twice a day.

The active ingredient in Oxycontin is oxycodone. Oxycontin contains a much larger amount of oxycodone than other prescription opiate pain medications—between 10 and 150 milligrams of oxycodone in each time-released tablet.

Oxycontin abusers are seeking a quick, powerful rush. They crush the Oxycontin tablets and inject or snort the powder, or mix it in water and drink it. This disarms the timed-release mechanism, resulting in a quick, powerful high.

By prescription, Oxycontin costs about $4 for a 40-milligram pill. On the street, the cost escalates to $20 to $40 for a 40-milligram pill. As a result, many pharmacies are being robbed for Oxycontin, and many prescriptions are being forged to obtain Oxycontin ("CSAT Advisory," 2001).

Rohypnol

Rohypnol is also known as narcozep, rohipnols, and roiphol. It is the brand name for flunotrazepam, a sleeping pill legally manufactured and prescribed for use in Europe, Mexico, South America, and the Asias. It is from the benzodiazepine class (e.g., Valium, Xanax, Restoril) and is not available on the formulary of drugs that may be legally prescribed in the United States. All rohypnols in the United States are therefore illegally purchased. Common street names are rohies, ropies, roofies, wheels, and row-shapys.

Like other benzodiazepines, when taken alone, Rohypnol is unlikely to cause problems. But if combined even with a small amount of alcohol, the intoxication effects may be extreme, leading to severely impaired judgment and motor skills. Individuals given such a combination often "come to" anywhere from 8 to 24 hours later, with no memory of any events that transpired after the time they ingested the drugs (blackouts).

Teens and young adults often follow the abuse pattern of taking the drug in combination with alcohol, as an "alcohol extender." There is a synergistic effect that increases the impairment of memory and judgment. It may also be used by drug addicts to "boost the high" or to "parachute down" from a cocaine binge. Rohypnols have been widely implicated in date rape, in which the female victims are seduced or tricked into ingesting the drug plus alcohol. The disinhibition effect, as well as amnesia for the subsequent events, are why they have been given the appellation "leg splitters."

The federal government has begun the process of classifying this drug as a category 1 substance, putting it into the same category as narcotics. This would bring with it severe penalties for dealing and possession of the drug.

Nicotine—Cigar Use

The annual number of new cigar users rose in the 1990s from 2 million users in 1990 to nearly 5 million in 1998. In 2000, cigar use was higher among young adults than among other age groups (NIDA 2001).

There is an increased risk of esophageal, lung, oral, and laryngeal cancer among cigar smokers. The popularity of cigars with young people may prove to be a big problem in years to come.

Crystal Methamphetamine

The United States is currently experiencing an upward cycle of stimulant abuse, with a dramatic increase in the availability and use of crystal methamphetamine, in a potency, purity, and accessibility unlike any previous time in our history. This is a substance that does not occur in nature and thus must be synthesized in a laboratory.

Street names for this drug include speed, crank, crystal, ice, meth, chalk, chicken powder, peanut butter-crank, go-fast, crystal meth, shabu-shabu, glass, go qip, chris, and christy, depending on the geographical area, the dealer, and the physical form, crystal versus powder.

The name *ice* has been used by dealers to represent methamphetamine as well as other substances, including methamphetamine mixed with heroin, cocaine or other adulterants, quarts, and rock salt.

Part of this alarming trend is ascribed to the takeover of the manufacture and distribution of speed, formerly the province of outlaw fringe individuals, by Mexican nationals, who already had a strong, well-organized distribution network. This has resulted in a much purer, significantly more potent, and lower-priced drug, precipitating a sharp increase in the number of users, including much younger users.

Methamphetamine enters the brain more rapidly than any other CNS stimulant, rapidly producing a "rush" of euphoria when injected or smoked. Many people who try methamphetamine go on to compulsive abuse of the drug. Typically, small doses can have a profound effect, including stimulated movement and increased speech, feelings of excitement and euphoria, and decreased appetite. A significant rise in pulse rate and blood pressure occurs, as well as a sensation often described by users as "my heart pounding out of my chest." This may progress to irregularities in heart rhythm, a dramatic rise in body temperature, convulsions, cardiovascular collapse, and death.

Populations Using Methamphetamine

- Traditionally associated with white, male, blue-collar workers, methamphetamine is now reportedly being used by diverse groups in all regions of the country.
- Use is increasing among men who have sex with men and use other drugs, making this population more vulnerable to contracting and spreading sexually transmitted diseases, especially HIV/AIDS.
- Young adults who attend "raves" or private clubs are increasingly using methamphetamine.

- Notable increases are occurring among homeless and runaway youth.
- Increasing use of methamphetamine is reported among male and female commercial sex workers who also trade sex for drugs and among members of motorcycle gangs. Also, people in occupations that demand long hours, mental alertness, and physical endurance (such as long-haul truckers) have been using this drug at increased rates. (National Institute on Drug Abuse 1998)

You Can Identify Methamphetamine Users By . . .

- Signs of agitation, excited speech, decreased appetites, and increased physical activity levels. Other common symptoms include dilated pupils, high blood pressure, irregular heartbeat, chest pain, shortness of breath, nausea and vomiting, diarrhea, and elevated body temperature.
- Occasional episodes of sudden and violent behavior, intense paranoia, visual and auditory hallucinations, and bouts of insomnia
- A tendency to compulsively clean and groom and repetitively sort and disassemble objects, such as cars and other mechanical devices. (National Institute on Drug Abuse 1998)

Chronic use leads to a state of paranoia, with individuals displaying behaviors strikingly resembling those of someone experiencing an acute episode of paranoid schizophrenia. Tolerance develops quickly, and chronic users must increase their dose, which, in turn, leads to magnification of the side effects and may lead to permanent brain damage.

In addition to the physical symptoms, the chronic user will experience a profound depression, with low energy levels, anhedonia (the total inability to experience any pleasurable feelings), and such a profound craving for the drug, remembering when the drug "worked" for them, that the cycle is often repeated many times, often with tragic results.

Ice, the smokable form of methamphetamine, is of extremely high purity—greater than 90 percent—and can lead to "runs" of 4 to 5 days without any sleep and often without food or even fluids. Then a "crash" of 4 days or so occurs, before the user begins another "run."

The drug, regardless of form, is often used concurrently with alcohol, either to blunt some of the stimulant effect or to help the user "come down" after a protracted period of use. The use of other depressant psychoactive substances leads to a poly-drug use pattern that can be extremely dangerous.

LSD

"Designer acid," also know as "cocktail acid," is emerging on the drug scene. This hallucinogen is less potent, shorter acting, and milder than the acid from the 1960s. It is therefore easier to conceal the use of this hallucinogen by young people. It has begun to make its way into the party scene, and one can "drop acid" in the afternoon, party for 6 to 8 hours, and then safely return home and sleep off the residual effects.

Brand names help identify the stronger, more potent preparations, such as Mr.

Natural, muscle man, and yin yang, with some brands sporting the "dead head" logo (from the psychedelic band the Grateful Dead), and even a "Mr. Bill" caricature of our thirty-ninth president, President Bill Clinton.

Heroin

The 1990s saw a significant increase in the use of heroin. The number of hard-core users, estimated by the National Institute of Drug Abuse (NIDA), has remained fairly constant over the past 25 years, at 750,000 to 1 million. However, the past several years have seen a disturbing number of individuals using heroin who are dramatically unlike the stereotypical heroin addict. The profile now contains well-educated, often female individuals, frequently employed in white-collar and even professional capacities. The age of users is also alarming, considering reports of use in high schools and even middle schools.

The reasons for this trend are many. For one, heroin use has assumed the trappings of glamour, often associated with the "arts," fashion, and entertainment world. It is now much purer, and thus more potent, which enables it to be inhaled, either through smoking it, "chasing the dragon," or snorting it in its powder form. The very fact that it does not have to be injected makes it more attractive by alleviating the aversion most people have to needles (i.e., needle phobia, stigma, risk of AIDS virus). There is also the widespread misbelief, and rationalization, that if one smokes or snorts heroin it will be nonaddicting.

To add to its "attractiveness," it is also relatively inexpensive, especially compared with crack cocaine. A bag of heroin containing enough to get the user high for 6 to 8 hours may be purchased for as little as $3 in New York City and will be of significant purity and potency, whereas a $10 bag of heroin purchased on the streets in 1980 was about 4 percent pure. Today it is not uncommon for a sample to be 65 percent pure, or even higher.

Another factor is that the drug is more easily obtained. The neophyte user is no longer forced to venture into dangerous neighborhoods to purchase the drug. It may be as easy as paging the dealer, who then delivers it, or it may be available on certain street corners in middle-class or industrial neighborhoods or even at the workplace.

One of the more insidious aspects of the drug is that, unlike cocaine and even alcohol, heroin use may exist for a significant period of time before its use is suspected. Individuals may be fairly high and functioning for quite a while, and, if they are careful, it may take months before they have to increase their dose and risk getting toxic. By the time it becomes obvious, the problem has progressed to the point where medical treatment and appropriate intervention is most often necessary to treat the addiction.

Heroin-related emergency department visits doubled from 33,900 in 1990 to 70,500 in 1996. In 1993, more than 3,805 deaths nationwide were related to heroin. "Both urban and suburban emergency departments treat patients with heroin overdoses daily and hospitalize 3 to 7 percent of these patients for related complications" (Sporer 2000).

Heroin use can no longer be confined along geographic, economic, or social lines. It is in "Heartland USA," as well as in suburbia and in the urban centers of the nation. It is found among the unemployed and disadvantaged, blue-collar workers, professional workers, the economically advantaged, and even homemakers.

Marijuana

So-called hybrid superweeds, known in some areas of the country as tastybun or purple tar, are 10 times more potent than the marijuana available in the 1960s or 1970s. This marijuana is often smoked in the form of "blunts," which are cheap, hollowed-out cigars filled with this powerful drug.

Inhalants

In addition to glue, paint, room deodorizers (e.g., Glade), butane, and even propane, there are commercial products that are often inhaled to get high. This includes ethyl chloride and nitrous oxide, which are known as "whippets," found in whipped cream canisters. It is estimated that there are 10,000 common household products that contain ingredients that can be abused.

✖ Definitions of Terms

Physical Dependence

Physical dependence is the altered state that develops when a person cannot stop taking a certain drug without suffering from withdrawal.

Withdrawal

Withdrawal symptoms are physical symptoms resulting from stopping the use of a drug (see Table 3.2). These vary according to the specific drug, the amount used, and the length of time over which it has been used. Because the body has actually adapted metabolically to the presence of the drug, when it is withdrawn (or even tapered off too rapidly), the reactions may vary from mild, flulike symptoms for a person coming off of opiates to a severe, potentially life-threatening situation when withdrawing from alcohol or other sedative hypnotics.

Psychological Dependence (Formerly Habituation)

A user with a profound emotional or mental need for the repetitive use of a drug or a class of drugs is **psychologically dependent.** The user becomes so preoccupied with taking the drug to achieve the optimal level of functioning or to maintain a sense of well-being that it becomes extremely difficult to abstain. Psychological dependence is a subjective state that is almost impossible to quantify; therefore, it is of limited usefulness in establishing a diagnosis of chemical dependency.

Routes of Administration

The route of administration is the method by which the alcohol/drug is ingested. Ingestion may be oral, through the skin, by injection, by smoking, or through other orifices (e.g., suppositories). The most rapid reaction occurs after inhalation while

TABLE 3.2

Diagnostic Criteria for Drug Withdrawal

Opioid	Alcohol	Cocaine	Nicotine
Dysphoric mood	Autonomic hyperactivity	Dysphoric mood	Dysphoric or depressed mood
Nausea or vomiting	Hand tremor	Fatigue	Insomnia
Muscle aches	Insomnia	Unpleasant dreams	Irritability
Lacrimation	Nausea or vomiting	Insomnia or hypersomnia	Anxiety
Rhinorrhea	Hallucinations	Increased appetite	Difficulty concentrating
Pupillary dilation	Illusions	Psychomotor retardation or agitation	Restlessness
Piloerection	Psychomotor agitation		Decreased heart rate
Sweating	Anxiety		Increased appetite
Diarrhea	Seizures		Weight gain
Yawning			
Fever			
Insomnia			

Source: Data are from the *Diagnostic and Statistical Manual of Mental Disorders* (4th ed.); American Psychiatric Association, 1994.

smoking a drug; injection is the next most rapid route. Oral administration and absorption through the skin are the slowest routes.

Set and Setting

Set refers to the user's state of mind at the time of use. *Setting* refers to the physical environment or environmental factors surrounding alcohol/drug use.

Tolerance

Tolerance to a drug develops when the individual requires increasingly larger doses to achieve the desired optimal effect. In other words, users require larger doses to achieve the same high produced previously by a smaller dose of the same drug.

Cross-Tolerance

Cross-tolerance is a diminished or reduced response to the effect of a psychoactive drug. This response is due to prior use of other psychoactive drugs, usually in the same drug category.

Synergism

In a synergistic process, one chemical enhances, or adds power to, the effect of another. The combined effect of two or more drugs is greater, therefore, than the effect of each agent added together (e.g., 1 + 1 = 3 or more).

Antagonism

The opposite of synergism, antagonism occurs when the combined effect of two drugs is less than the sum of the drugs' effects acting separately (e.g., 1 + 1 = less than 2). For example, the depressant effects of alcohol are counteracted by the stimulant effects of cocaine.

Historically, there has been a wide range of definitions of addiction—for example:

A chronic, progressive and potentially fatal disease. It is characterized by
tolerance, psychological and physical dependence, pathogenic organ
changes, all of which are the direct or indirect consequence of the alcohol
ingested. (National Council on Alcoholism)
An illness characterized by preoccupation with alcohol and loss of control over its
consequences, which usually leads to intoxication if drinking is begun; by
chronicity; by progression; and by the tendency to relapse. Typically
associated with physical disability and impaired emotional, occupational,
and/or social adjustments as a direct consequence. (American Medical
Association, 1957)

⚔ Definition
of Addiction

As described throughout this textbook, the current definition of addiction used in the alcohol/drug field is the one developed by David Smith. An expanded version of that definition of addiction follows:

1. Compulsion and obsession
   a. The compulsive use of the chemical despite its no longer having the desired effect
   b. The fear of being without the substance
   c. The compulsion to substitute other drugs if that particular substance is unavailable
   d. Thoughts about the drug as a dominant theme or integral part of one's life
2. Loss of control or inability to stop
   a. The inability to limit the amount of use
   b. The inability to refuse the substance if available
   c. The inability to stop using the substance for three months or longer
   d. Binge patterns of use
3. Continued use despite known adverse consequences
   a. Medical complications
   b. Psychiatric complications ranging from mood swings and anxiety to depression, panic disorders, and paranoid-schizophrenic reactions or other psychoses

      c. Social consequences, the deterioration of family and other significant relationships, work status, and legal complications

A simple way of remembering this behavioral definition is the 3*C*s mnemonic:

- **C**ompulsion
- **C**ontrol
- Continued use despite negative **C**onsequences

      A more diagnostic definition of substance abuse and dependence can be found in Chapter 4.

✄ Classification of Drugs

Drug may be most simply defined as a nonfood substance intended to affect the structure and function of the body, most often to diagnose, cure, mitigate, treat, or prevent disease.

      There are many ways to classify drugs, such as by chemical structure or specific effects on particular organ systems. Most frequently, drugs are classified as nonpsychoactive and psychoactive. **Nonpsychoactive drugs** are substances that in normal doses do not directly affect the brain, such as vitamins, antibiotics, and topical skin preparations. **Psychoactive drugs** affect brain functions, mood, and behavior and are subdivided primarily on the basis of physiological and psychological effects. The psychoactive drug classification includes the following:

1. Narcotic analgesics: painkillers and designer drugs (fentanyl)
2. Central nervous system depressants: sedative hypnotics, alcohol, tranquilizers, and barbiturates
3. Central nervous system stimulants: amphetamines, cocaine, nicotine, and caffeine
4. Hallucinogens
5. *Cannabis sativa:* marijuana and hashish
6. Inhalants: volatile solvents
7. Phencyclidine (PCP)

Narcotic Analgesics
Definition
The term *narcotic* comes from the Greek word *narkosis,* which means to numb or to be in a stupor. *Analgesia* means to relieve pain, without producing unconsciousness.

      The narcotic analgesics (morphine, codeine, and heroin) come from the poppy plant (*Papaver somniferum*). (See Table 3.3.) The narcotic analgesics category also includes synthetic and semisynthetic drugs that have morphinelike action, such as meperidine (Demerol), methadone, Dilaudid, and Percodan.

      The term *narcotic* was often incorrectly applied to a wide variety of drugs, including marijuana, alcohol, and cocaine. This was the result of a legal classification system rather than a medical classification. The emotional overtone of *narcotic* was frequently misapplied to those drugs considered dangerous by legislators and policymakers.

      The term *narcotic* has a variety of meanings. Its scientific meaning is drugs related botanically to the opium poppy and pharmacologically to opium, morphine,

TABLE 3.3

Narcotic Analgesics Classification

Natural Opioids	Synthetic	Semisynthetic	Antagonists
Morphine	Demerol	Dilaudid	Narcan
Codeine	Meperidine	Percodan	Naloxone
Opium		Talwin	

and heroin. Its medical meaning is synthetic drugs having morphinelike effects on a user. Its legal meaning is anything the legislature of a state wants to classify. Its public meaning is anything the general public wants to label as belonging to a particular drug category. In some states, this includes all drugs having morphinelike action. Elsewhere the term may also be applied to drugs chemically unrelated to narcotics (e.g., cocaine and marijuana).

Additional analgesics are nonnarcotic and satisfy other functions, such as reducing fever (antipyretic) and reducing inflammation (anti-inflammatory). Other nonnarcotic analgesics include aspirin, phenacetin, and Darvon. Nonsteroidal anti-inflammatory drugs (NSAIDs) include Naprosyn and Motrin.

Heroin

It is estimated that there are 2.1 million lifetime heroin users (people who used the drug throughout their adult life, with or without intermittent periods of abstinence, then return to use) in the United States (NIDA 1995), and this is a conservative estimate.

Common street names for heroin include big bag, big H, blanco, bomb, boy, brother, brown, brown rocks, brown sugar, caballo, cat, chich, Chinese red, Chinese white, chiva, crap, dogie, doojee, dope, duji, dust, eighth, flea powder, garbage, good stuff, H, hard stuff, harry, H-caps, henry, him, horse, hombre, jones, joy powder, junk, Mexican mud, mojo, muzzle, pack, poison, powder, pure, red chicken, red rock, rock, scag, schmeck, smack, stuff, tecata, thing, white boy, white junk, and white stuff.

Brief History of the Narcotic Analgesics

The opiates have been used for medicinal purposes and pleasure since prehistoric times. Opium eating has been known in Asia for thousands of years. A brief history follows:

1806: Friedrich Wilhelm Adam Serturner, a German chemist, isolated morphine from opium.
1832: Codeine was isolated.
1845: Alexander Wood invented the hypodermic syringe.
1861–65: Approximately 45,000 Civil War soldiers were addicted to morphine.
1874: Alder Wright, a London chemist, first synthesized heroin from morphine.
1875: A San Francisco ordinance prohibited the smoking of opium in public houses and opium dens.
1906: Pure Food and Drug Act required all medicines containing opiates and certain other drugs to list them on the labels.

1914: Harrison Narcotics Act required licensure of drug manufacturers, importers, pharmacists, and physicians marketing or prescribing narcotics. Patent medicine manufacturers were exempt from the act, provided that their products did not contain more than two grains of opium, or one-eighth grain of heroin per ounce.

1942–43: During World War II, a German chemist, Aschenbrenner, synthesized methadone and named it after Adolph Hitler, Dolophine.

1970s: Most addicted soldiers returning from Vietnam withdrew from heroin on the trip back to the United States or shortly thereafter. The anticipated need for heroin treatment was not realized.

1978: Scientists discovered endorphins; these proteins play an important role in the body's pain suppression system.

Chemists first isolated morphine in the early nineteenth century. During the Civil War, doctors widely used morphine in injectable form. Addiction to morphine was very common at that time, resulting in a significant addict population. Fortunately, society attached no stigma to the soldiers' addiction to morphine; it was commonly referred to as "soldiers' disease." Most soldiers withdrew from morphine on their own or under medical supervision, and there was minimal social impact.

Around the 1870s, manufacturers added tincture of opium to many patent medicines sold over the counter for treatment of diarrhea in infants and children. When first introduced at the end of the nineteenth century, heroin was thought to cure opium dependence and morphinism.

Routes of Administration

Users may inject narcotics either intravenously, subcutaneously (under the surface of the skin—known as skin popping), or deep within the muscle. They can also snort narcotics intranasally, smoke it, or absorb it into their bodies via the mucous membrane of the mouth or rectum (using suppositories). The route of administration determines how quickly the drug affects the brain: a drug that is smoked reaches the brain in 5 seconds. A drug injected intravenously reaches the brain 14 seconds later. A drug taken by mouth doesn't hit the brain until 30 to 45 minutes later.

The intensity of the drug effect and the complications are also influenced by the route of administration. Intravenous use can lead to infection, local abscesses, disseminated infections (HIV, hepatitis B, pulmonary emboli), and local damage to the lungs and lining of the nose.

Major Effects

1. Pain relief (analgesia)
2. Euphoria (sense of well-being)
3. Cough suppressant (antitussive)
4. Respiratory depression
5. Sedation or drowsiness
6. Constriction of the pupils (pinpoint pupils)
7. Nausea and vomiting
8. Itching
9. Decrease in gastrointestinal activity (constipation)

Hazards

Even while using low to moderate doses, users face many hazards related to the circumstances of illicit use, such as drug impurities, infection, and the consequences of the addict lifestyle. By using dirty and shared needles, they contract infections (AIDS, hepatitis, and tetanus) and all other blood-borne infections (septicemia) leading to endocarditis, and liver, brain, and skin abscesses.

Other hazards include allergic (anaphylactic) reactions to the narcotic or substances used to cut or dilute the narcotic. Overdosing causes cardiac arrest, lung reaction, and the narcotic's direct actions on the brain, leading to coma, shock, respiratory arrest, and death.

Tolerance

Tolerance develops to a rapid degree with the effects of analgesia, respiratory depression, sedation, and feelings of euphoria. In effect, users must take more and more of the narcotic to get the original effect.

The rate of tolerance depends on the pattern of use, route of administration, and physical aspects of each individual. Even though some addicts build to phenomenally high doses, inevitably there is always a final dose that can produce death from respiratory depression.

Tolerance often returns to normal after withdrawal. Many narcotic addicts have fatally overdosed by returning to their normal and customary doses after detoxification.

Cross-tolerance exists between even chemically dissimilar opioids.

Withdrawal

Withdrawal symptoms and their severity depend on the specifics of the drug being used. With low doses of intermittent narcotic use, withdrawal symptoms may be negligible or perhaps resemble mild, flulike symptoms. Anyone who has ever been seasick can identify with these feelings. Withdrawal symptoms include the following:

- Appetite suppression
- Nausea and vomiting
- Dilated pupils
- Gooseflesh, or increased pylomotor activity—the skin resembles a plucked turkey, hence the expression "going cold turkey"
- Restlessness
- Intestinal spasms
- Abdominal pain
- Muscle spasms
- Kicking movements—hence the expression "kicking the habit"
- Occasional diarrhea
- Increased heart rate and blood pressure
- Chills alternating with flushing and sweating
- Irritability
- Insomnia
- Violent yawning
- Severe sneezing and runny nose (rhinorhea)

- Crying and tearing, nasal inflammation
- Depressive mood and tremor

The peak intensity of withdrawal occurs at 48 to 72 hours (2 to 3 days) for heroin, but for methadone the peak withdrawal is from 5 to 7 days.

Despite these symptoms, the management of withdrawal from opiates is far less dangerous than the management of alcohol withdrawal. The effects of the withdrawal are not life threatening but may need medical attention. The medical conditions worthy of attention may be excessive weight loss, dehydration, body chemistry disturbances, and stress on the cardiovascular system. Without treatment, symptoms usually disappear in 7 to 10 days for heroin but may last 2 to 3 weeks for methadone (see Table 3.2).

Opiates and Pregnancy

Chronic use of opiates, especially heroin, results in a variety of obstetrical compromises. Because withdrawal in an addicted mother may lead to spontaneous miscarriage, the consensus of the medical community to date is to stabilize the heroin-addicted mother on methadone during the pregnancy. However, these babies tend to be born prematurely, with a lower birth weight. Born addicted, these babies may display withdrawal symptoms and have significant neonatal difficulties, with lifelong negative effects on psychomotor development.

Central Nervous System Depressants

Most central nervous system (CNS) depressants are sedative hypnotics. These include alcohol, barbiturates, and tranquilizers.

Alcohol

Alcohol acts as a depressant on the central nervous system. Once absorbed, it is distributed throughout the body, enters the brain easily, and is uniformly found in all body fluids. In pregnant women, alcohol crosses the placental barrier into the fetus.

A blood alcohol level of 0.05 percent or higher produces some driving impairment. In all U.S. states, anyone driving with a 0.10 percent blood alcohol level is driving under the influence. Alcohol is metabolized at a relatively constant rate, which depends primarily on the body weight of the drinker. A 150-pound man metabolizes approximately three-quarters to one ounce of alcohol in an hour.

Brief History of Alcohol

1500 B.C.: Book of the Dead mentioned "hek," a form of beer made from grain.

2225 B.C.: The Code of Hammurabi, Assyria, involved rules for the keeping of beer and wine shops and taverns.

400 B.C.: Plato wrote rules for the leader of the "symposia" to try to control the excessive drinking that went on. This was probably an ancient version of the "designated driver" (of course, back then it was the chariot driver).

"I keep forgetting. Is alcohol a depressant or a stimulant?"

Alcohol is a CNS depressant.

© 1980 Richard Guindon. Reprinted by permission.

These alcoholic beverages contain equal amounts of alcohol.

Michael Siluk.

Eighth century: Numerous taverns and beer houses were established in Britain.

Sixteenth century: Through the distillation process, Irish settlers manufactured and distributed "usquebach," or whiskey.

1660: Distilleries were licensed and the popularity of gin became widespread.

1770s: British brought beer and alcohol to the Colonial Americans.

1777: After the American Revolution, there was an increase in rum consumption as a new American freedom, when prior to the revolution there was some success in regulating taverns. Corn whiskey became popular after the Louisiana Purchase added new American corn-growing territories.

Late 1700s: Dr. Benjamin Rush, champion of the temperance movement and author of *An Inquiry into the Effects of Ardent Spirits,* inspired the nineteenth-century American temperance movement.

1917: Alcohol Prohibition came about with the 18th Amendment to the Constitution.

1920s: The Roaring Twenties brought bootlegging, bathtub gin, homemade beer, and speakeasies.

1932: The 21st Amendment to the Constitution repealed the highly unpopular 18th Amendment.

1970–present: Numerous alcohol products have been developed and marketed, especially to young people (e.g., malt liquors, wine coolers, a variety of beers).

Estimates of Alcoholism   Other than tobacco products containing nicotine, beverage alcohol (ethanol) is the most widely used psychoactive drug known to humanity. In 1994, approximately 113 million persons age 12 and over had used alcohol in the past month, which was about 54 percent of the total population age 12 and older.

About 13 million Americans (6.2 percent of the population) were heavy drinkers (NIDA 1995).

Major Effects   The range of physical reactions to varying doses of alcohol is vast. The effects depend on the amount consumed, the circumstances of consumption (set and setting), the drinker's body size, and the experience of the drinker. Someone unaccustomed to alcohol use is more likely to show signs of impairment than a conditioned drinker who has learned to compensate for impaired behavior. One or two alcoholic drinks may induce talkativeness in one individual, along with slight flushing, and reduce the drinker's inhibitions, so he or she appears more expansive and more animated, perhaps grandiose at times. The same amount of alcohol in another individual may induce drowsiness and lethargy.

Alcohol in even moderate doses generally reduces one's performance in tasks that require physical coordination or mental agility, such as driving a car. Larger doses can alter perception and cause staggering, blurred vision, and the manifestations of drunkenness. However, one person may become emotional or amorous, while another becomes aggressive and hostile. Extremely high doses—typical during binges—can knock out a drinker, even kill the person, if the central nervous system is depressed to the point that body functions, such as breathing, cease altogether.

Alcohol is a toxic drug with irritating as well as sedative properties. It can have a negative effect on every tissue in the human body, as shown in the following:

1. Brain
   a. Amnesia—most commonly called blackouts—causes partial, or sometimes temporary, loss of memory, often following binge patterns of alcohol use. Blackouts can occur even after low-dose alcohol consumption, or first-time alcohol consumption by someone who has a family history of alcoholism. Blackouts may be a significant early indicator of a diagnosis of alcoholism.
   b. Permanent loss of memory and mental confusion, as in Wernicke-Korsakoff's syndrome
   c. Damage to the cerebellum, affecting balance and coordination
2. Peripheral nerves
   a. Usually in the legs and sometimes other extremities, alcoholics experience pain, loss of sensation, and general weakness.
   b. Optic nerves are damaged, causing blurred or dimmed vision.
3. Gastrointestinal tract
   a. Gastritis and esophagitis, irritation of the lining of the esophagus and stomach, causing mild to severe pain; may aggravate an ulcer
   b. Peptic ulcer at the outlet of the stomach (duodenal)
   c. Fatty liver, hepatitis, or cirrhosis (a scarring of the liver that destroys the tissue and is a leading cause of death from alcohol)
   d. Pancreatitis, in which muscle spasms block the duct from the pancreas, causes the acidic juices to back up and start digesting the pancreas. This is often very painful and can also cause death.
4. Heart and blood vessels
   a. Heart muscle becomes weaker, and heart expands because it is working harder. Alcohol complicates problems with heart disease.

    b. Peripheral blood vessels are dilated by alcohol. Initially, this causes a sensation of warmth, followed by serious heat loss in the cold. The old habit of drinking alcohol to fend off the cold actually makes the person more susceptible to the cold.

    c. High blood pressure is often associated with alcoholism, but the relationship is not clearly established.

  5. Lungs: emphysema occurs most frequently in the alcoholic who also smokes. Alcohol seems to have a direct toxic effect on the cells lining the alveoli, or small air sacs in the lungs, as the alcohol is excreted into the air.

Sobering Up   Contrary to much public opinion, steam baths, vigorous exercise, black coffee, and other sobering-up agents have no effect on the rate at which alcohol is metabolized. Time is the only thing that works.

Tolerance   Tolerance to most of the immediate effects of alcohol develops with frequent use. Regular heavy drinkers may be able to consume two or three times as much alcohol as novice drinkers. Heavy drinkers have to drink more and more to achieve the desired effect.

Stage 1 Withdrawal Symptoms   Withdrawal from alcohol usually begins 6 to 12 hours after the last drink and may even begin in the presence of significant blood alcohol levels. Table 3.4 lists the Stage 1 withdrawal symptoms. These symptoms, in varying degrees, may last anywhere from 3 to 5 days and are relieved by drinking more alcohol.

Stage 2 Withdrawal Symptoms   The onset of Stage 2 withdrawal symptoms is usually within 24 hours after the last drink but may occur as long as 3 days later. Stage 2 consists of the symptoms in Stage 1, plus hallucinations. These may be visual, auditory, tactile, olfactory (smell), or mixed. Although the visual hallucinations usually predominate, olfactory hallucinations are a particularly more ominous sign and may be accompanied by seizures. The delirium tremens—disorientation to person, place, or time—also can be life threatening; this is a true medical emergency, with a 15 percent mortality rate if untreated.

Related Illnesses   Alcoholics have twice the chance of experiencing premature deaths as nonalcoholic persons. Liver disease of varying types is one of the most

TABLE 3.4

Stage 1 Alcohol Withdrawal Symptoms

1. Psychomotor agitation
2. Anxiety
3. Insomnia
4. Appetite suppression
5. Gastrointestinal disturbances
6. Elevated heart rate, blood pressure, sweating, and tremors

prominent manifestations of alcoholism. Among young males 20 to 40 years of age, liver cirrhosis is the third fastest growing cause of death, after heart disease and lung cancer. Alcoholics also show higher than normal rates of peptic ulcers, pneumonia, cancer of the upper digestive and respiratory tracts, heart and artery disease, tuberculosis, and suicide.

Many heavy drinkers also suffer vitamin deficiencies, gastritis, sexual impotence, and infections. The more serious alcohol-related neurological disorders include peripheral neuritis (loss of sensation), Korsakoff's psychosis (loss of memory), and Wernicke's encephalopathy (mental confusion).

Fetal Alcohol Syndrome   Alcohol use and abuse by pregnant women is the third leading cause of birth defects, exceeded only by Down syndrome and spina bifida. The four basic abnormalities characteristic of fetal alcohol syndrome (FAS) are as follows:

1. Distorted facial features. A baby born with FAS has short fissures in the eyelids, a small or underdeveloped upper lip with thinned vermilion, and a diminished philtrum, the line running between the upper lip and nose.
2. Prenatal onset growth deficiency. Babies with FAS are usually two standard deviations below normal in weight and height; they exhibit little or no indication of growth spurts to catch up after birth.
3. Reduced central nervous system performance. As a result, babies with FAS have mild to moderate mental retardation; microcephaly, or disproportionately small heads; poor coordination; irritability in infancy; and hyperactivity in childhood.
4. Increased frequency of major abnormalities. Such disorders range from gross cardiovascular abnormalities and congenital heart disease to abnormal and malformed limbs.

Alcohol use during the first trimester is often responsible for stillbirths. Research further supports the position that even small doses of alcohol affect the development of the fetus, especially in the first trimester. The only safe dose of alcohol during pregnancy is no alcohol at all.

Antabuse   Some alcoholics have extreme difficulty in abstaining from alcohol. Usually, they choose Antabuse (disulfiram) when other methods to stop drinking have failed. At early stages of recovery, alcoholics may use Antabuse as a deterrent to drinking alcohol, but it must not be viewed as the only modality. (See Chapter 11.)

Alcohol is metabolized by a liver enzyme (aldehyde dehydrogenose) to form acetaldehyde. Normally, acetaldehyde is rapidly metabolized by another enzyme, which breaks it into inert substances, eventually becoming carbon dioxide and water. Antabuse interferes with the enzyme that breaks down acetaldehyde. A person taking Antabuse and drinking alcohol would have a sharp increase in acetaldehyde, resulting in extreme feelings of discomfort, which include nausea and vomiting, flushing, sweating, palpitations, increased heart rate, breathing difficulty, and anxiety. Blood pressure may first rise and then fall, making the person appear to be in shock. Feelings of drowsiness may occur later. People rarely die from an alcohol-Antabuse reaction, but they feel so sick they think they will die. Nevertheless, some people continue to drink alcohol while on Antabuse.

Barbiturates

Barbiturates also belong to the sedative-hypnotic class of drugs and are widely prescribed to decrease central nervous system activity (e.g., induce sleep, relax the nervous system). Barbiturates and barbiturate-like drugs seem to affect the cortex of the brain or those areas related to sleep more than other sedative hypnotics.

Medical Uses   In low doses of 25 to 50 milligrams, the short- or intermediate-acting compounds such as amobarbital (Amytal), pentobarbital (Nembutal), secobarbital (Seconal), and butabarbital (Butisol) treat or prevent acute convulsions associated with tetanus; epilepsy; and an overdose of stimulants such as strychnine, nicotine, or cocaine and the withdrawal symptoms associated with alcoholism and other sedative drug dependence. (See Table 3.5.)

For years, doctors prescribed barbiturates in the treatment of asthma, premenstrual tension, motion sickness, nausea and vomiting, peptic ulcer and other gastrointestinal disturbances, hyperthyroidism, high blood pressure, and other cardiovascular diseases. Now doctors can prescribe many newer drugs, which have fewer side effects and less potential for abuse.

Estimates of Use and Addiction   After minor tranquilizers, barbiturates are prescribed more than any other psychoactive drug in the United States. Most individuals are introduced to barbiturates by physicians, who prescribe them as mild tranquilizers or sleeping pills.

Many individuals find barbiturates make coping with life easier. As tolerance to the tranquilizing and sedating effects set in, individuals increase their doses, often without their physicians' knowledge. Teenagers and young adults take enough barbiturates orally to produce highs the same way as alcohol might be taken. The sources of the supply for these young people are often the black market, the family medicine cabinet, and sometimes manipulation of otherwise legitimate prescriptions.

T A B L E   3 . 5

Classification of Barbiturates and Their Street Names

Short-Acting

Amobarbital (Amytal)—known as blues, blue angels, bluebirds, blue devils, blue bullets

Pentobarbital (Nembutal)—known as yellows, yellow jackets, yellow bullets, nembies
Butabarbital (Butisol)

Intermediate-Acting

Phenobarbital (Luminal, Eskabarb)—know as phennies

Secobarbital (Seconal)—known as reds, pinks, red birds, red bullets, red dolls, seccies, F-40s

Long-Acting

Pento-secobarbital (Tuinal)—known as trees, tootsies, double trouble, gorilla pills, rainbows

Illicit use of barbiturates has been on the decline for the past several years in North America. Because they are still prescribed so often for a variety of medical conditions, however, their pharmaceutical use remains widespread, as is their abuse by those who have obtained legitimate prescriptions.

Routes of Administration   Usually taken orally, barbiturates are readily absorbed by the stomach and small intestine. Absorption into the bloodstream can be rapid, especially on an empty stomach. Most barbiturates are white powders, odorless but with a slightly bitter taste. Most often packed in capsules and tablets of varying colors, they are also available as liquids, injectable solutions, and suppositories.

Major Effects   The short-term effects of barbiturates are very similar to those of alcohol. At low doses, barbiturates tend to induce relaxation, a sense of well-being, and drowsiness. At higher doses, the drug reduces the individual's ability to react quickly and to perform skilled, precise tasks. Often there is a feeling of sedation, and the individual may alternate between feelings of euphoria and hostility and aggressiveness. This is very similar to the high-dose reactions under the influence of alcohol.

At still higher doses, the symptoms may be similar to those of drunkenness, with confusion and difficulty communicating. The person may fall into a stupor or sleep. If the dose is high enough, it may impair the respiratory function so severely that the individual stops breathing and dies.

Barbiturates and Sleep   Barbiturates are generally considered by the public as sleep medication. However, long-term barbiturate use can interfere with the rapid eye movement (REM) phase of sleep. REM sleep is associated with an essential feature of healthy sleep—dreaming. Normal functioning is further disturbed with the disruption of REM sleep. When the individual stops taking barbiturates, there is often a rebound effect and more REM sleep occurs. But the dreaming is more intense and frequently turns into a nightmare. The user interprets this as poor sleeping and again takes sleeping pills, often escalating the dose, and a vicious cycle is put into play.

Barbiturates and Pregnancy   Barbiturates should never be taken during pregnancy, unless advised by a physician, because they could cause birth defects. Also, the baby may be born addicted to barbiturates and have potentially dangerous withdrawal symptoms.

Tolerance   Barbiturates used repeatedly over a long period can induce tolerance and physical and psychological dependence. Tolerance to the euphoric effects of the drug develops quickly in many users, so larger and larger amounts of the drug must be taken to achieve the same high.

The lethal dose is usually only 10 to 15 times the therapeutic dose, so the margin of safety is low. As tolerance develops, the difference between the amount needed to get high may be only one or two pills away from an overdose; such an amount is also potentially lethal in combination with alcohol use.

TABLE 3.6

Barbiturate Withdrawal

The withdrawal symptoms may include
1. Physical weakness
2. Dizziness
3. Anxiety
4. Tremors
5. Sleeplessness
6. Nausea
7. Abdominal cramps and vomiting

From the third to seventh day of withdrawal, the user may experience
1. Delirium
2. Delusions
3. Hallucinations

Withdrawal   Table 3.6 lists typical symptoms of barbiturate withdrawal; these and other symptoms may last for days or even months. Anyone greatly addicted to barbiturates also runs a risk of having a grand mal seizure. Grand mal seizures can occur up to two weeks after the barbiturates are withdrawn and can be fatal. This is why it is essential that barbiturate addicts withdraw under a doctor's supervision, preferably in a medical facility.

Overdose Signs and Symptoms   The signs and symptoms of an overdose include the following:

1. Mood alteration ranging from depression to euphoria
2. Sedation or drowsiness proceeding to stupor and coma with increasing doses. Paradoxical excitement rather than drowsiness may occur, especially in the young or the old.
3. Confusion and disorientation
4. Slurred speech (dysarthria)
5. Staggering gait (ataxia), indicating that motor coordination is impaired
6. Nystagmus, or involuntary rapid eye movement from side to side
7. Pupils constricting a little at first; later as the level of unconsciousness deepens, they dilate
8. Respiratory depression, with a decrease in the oxygen supply to the brain; this can cause death

Barbiturates Used with Other Drugs   Barbiturates are often used in conjunction with stimulants. Amphetamine users often use barbiturates to come down after a prolonged period of amphetamine use. Barbiturates are also used by heroin addicts when their drug of choice is not available.

Barbiturates plus other central nervous system depressants can have a synergistic effect when taken together. People who drink alcohol and use barbiturates run the risk of accidental overdose. Overdoses on barbiturates plus alcohol are more common than on barbiturates alone.

Methaqualone   Methaqualone is one of several nonbarbiturates that have barbiturate-like effects (see Table 3.7). Methaqualone was introduced to the American medical market in the mid-1960s for the treatment of insomnia and anxiety. It was originally believed to have none of the abuse potential of short-acting barbiturates. It was alleged to be a safe, nonaddictive sedative; however, this drug has an extremely high abuse potential.

The popularity of methaqualone grew swiftly, given its enthusiastic medical use and street use. Among its most enthusiastic users were college students in the 1970s. Since then, methaqualone has spread not only to high school and college campuses throughout the United States but also into the adult population. Methaqualone use has also become popular among methadone maintenance patients because of the additive high the drug produces in combination with methadone.

Some street names for methaqualone are sopors, ludes, and love drug.

Principally, younger age groups use this illicit drug, with the heaviest concentration of use between high school age and people in their mid 30s. The cost of illicit methaqualone ranges from $4 to $8 per tablet.

Methaqualone is usually taken orally in pill form. Since 1984, pharmaceutical companies can no longer legally produce methaqualone in the United States. The drug is most often found on the street in bootlegged forms, which look real but may or may not contain actual methaqualone.

Following its ingestion, methaqualone is readily absorbed from the gastrointestinal tract. Once transported into the blood plasma, it is distributed in body fat, the liver, and brain tissue.

Relatively low doses (75 milligrams four times a day) produce sedation; larger doses of 150 to 300 milligrams lead to sleep. Those who use the drug to get high often take far larger doses, sometimes 600 to 900 milligrams and much more if they have been using the drug steadily enough to develop a tolerance.

TABLE 3.7

Nonbarbiturates with Barbiturate-like Action

- Chloral hyudrate (Noctec)—known as Mickey Finn, or knockout drops when used with alcohol
- Methaqualone (Quaalude, Sopor)
- Flurazepam (Dalmane)
- Glutethimide (Doriden)—known as goofers
- Ethchlorvynol (Placidyl)
- Methyprylon (Noludar)
- Paraldehyde

Users describe the sensation produced by methaqualone as "a peaceful calm, a rush, a drunk." Some describe it as a love drug due to methaqualone's alcohol-like symptoms (e.g., loss of motor and muscle control, loss of inhibitions), although, just as with alcohol, actual sexual performance is reduced.

Basically, intoxication with methaqualone is similar to intoxication with barbiturates or alcohol and subjects the individual to similar risks: death by overdose and accidents due to confusion and impaired motor coordination.

Methaqualone has induced headaches, hangovers, fatigue, dizziness, drowsiness, torpor (extreme sluggishness, apathy, dullness), menstrual disturbances, dry mouth, nosebleeds, diarrhea, skin eruptions, lack of appetite, numbness, and pain in the extremities. Researchers have found that a coma occurs following 2.4 grams of Quaalude. Eight to 20 grams have produced severe toxicity and death.

Methaqualone overdoses are less often associated with cardiac and respiratory depression than are overdoses of the oral barbiturates. However, shock and respiratory arrests may occasionally occur. Methaqualone overdose can also result in delirium, restlessness, hypertonia (excessive tension), and muscle spasms leading to convulsions.

As with barbiturates, tolerance to the intoxicating effects of methaqualone develops more rapidly than does tolerance to the lethal dose. Withdrawal from methaqualone dependence carries approximately the same risks as withdrawal from the short-acting barbiturates and can be quite severe for a large addiction.

Japanese researchers have provided a good deal of the information about methaqualone's addiction potential. In Japan, where this drug was once available over the counter, it was widely abused by young people (Tamura 1989). During 1963 to 1966, a survey of drug addicts in Japan found that 176 out of 411 (41.8 percent) were addicted to methaqualone. Withdrawal convulsions occurred in 7 percent of the methaqualone addicts and 9 percent developed delirium tremens symptoms. Subsequent studies in England and in the United States have documented cases of physical dependence as manifested by a withdrawal syndrome. The symptoms include insomnia, abdominal cramps, headaches, anorexia, and nightmares.

Research conducted in Philadelphia and at the Haight-Ashbury Clinic in San Francisco has also documented the high abuse potential and dependence-producing properties of methaqualone, as well as its cross-tolerance with the short-acting barbiturates.

Tranquilizers

Minor tranquilizers are drugs that act primarily as antianxiety agents (Table 3.8). They reduce anxiety and tension. Major tranquilizers—drugs that are used over the long term in the treatment of mental illnesses, such as schizophrenia—are antipsychotic agents (Table 3.9).

All of the antipsychotic drugs can produce Parkinson-like signs and symptoms with tremor, rigidity, and shuffling gait. To counteract these side effects, one of the following anti-Parkinsonism drugs is often prescribed along with the antipsychotic drug: Artane, Cogentin, Kemadrin, or Benadryl.

Because the major tranquilizers do not produce pleasant psychological effects, they are rarely used nonmedically and have no illicit attraction. The focus of this section is on the minor tranquilizers, which do have an abuse and dependence potential.

TABLE 3.8

Classification of Minor Tranquilizers (Antianxiety Agents)

Benzodiazepines	Meprobamate	Sedating Antihistamines
Valium (diazepam)	Equanil	Atarax, Vistaril (hydroxyzine)
Librium (chlordiazepoxide)	Miltown	Benadryl (diphenhydramine)
Serax (oxazepam)		Sleep-Eze, Sominex, Nytol
Tranxene (chlorazepate)		
Ativan (lorazepam)		
Xanax (alprazolam)		
Halcion (triazolam)		

TABLE 3.9

Classification of Major Tranquilizers (Antipsychotic Agents)

Phenothiazines	Butyrophenones	Thioxanthenes	Other
Thorazine (chlorpromazine)	Haldol (haloperidol)	Navane (thiothixene)	Serpasil (reserpine)
Mellaril (thioridazine)		Taractan (chlorprothixene)	Moban (molindone hydrochloride)
Stelazine (trifluoperazine)			
Compazine (prochlorperazine)			Loxitane
Trilafon (perphenazine)			
Prolixin (fluphenazine)			

Medical Uses   Doctors prescribe the minor tranquilizers mainly for treatment of tension, insomnia, behavioral excitement, and anxiety. Some treat convulsive disorders, symptoms of barbiturate-alcohol dependence, and the anxiety and panic that sometimes result from the use of hallucinogenic drugs. Although fairly high doses are necessary, some minor tranquilizers are also effective muscle relaxants (e.g., Valium may be used in injectable form for this purpose).

Estimates of Use   Most Americans are introduced to minor tranquilizers by physicians, and most use them according to prescription, but there are large numbers who do not stay within the physician's guidelines. Recent statistics show that the prescribing of tranquilizers is on a downward trend, and some authorities believe this trend may continue.

Routes of Administration   Most minor tranquilizers are usually taken orally as tablets, capsules, or liquids. Occasionally, they are injected for both medical and nonmedical purposes.

Major Effects   With normal therapeutic doses, individuals usually feel well, feel relaxed, and may lose some of their inhibitions. They feel a lessening of anxiety, tension, and agitation.

As the dosage is increased, patients usually feel more sedated and may have a sensation of floating. Many individuals at this dosage level experience some depression of nervous and muscular activity, mental confusion, and physical unsteadiness. High doses may produce the following:

- Drowsiness
- Loss of muscle coordination
- Lethargy
- Disorientation and confusion
- Low blood pressure
- Memory impairment
- Rage reactions
- Moodiness and personality alterations
- Symptoms resembling drunkenness

Obviously, the ability to drive a car under high-dose levels is also impaired. Other side effects may include skin rashes, nausea, loss of sex drive, and menstrual and ovulatory irregularities.

The margin of safety of minor tranquilizers is so wide that death rarely results from use of these drugs alone, with the lethal dose being 100 or more times the effective dose. Where death has occurred, it has often been due to an interaction between the tranquilizer and other drugs, such as alcohol.

Tolerance   With regular use, tolerance can develop to most of the effects of these sedatives. This means that the user has to take increased doses to get the desired effect.

Dependence and Withdrawal   Even though physical dependence and withdrawal can occur with most tranquilizers, these effects are infrequent in relation to the large number of people who take these drugs. On a therapeutic dosage level, addiction may still occur. Escalation of the amount and frequency of the dose without a doctor's orders increases the chance of physical dependence.

Withdrawal from a large habit may involve anxiety states, apprehension, tremors, insomnia, rapid pulse, fever, loss of appetite, nausea, vomiting, stomach cramps, sweating, fainting, and other symptoms. Withdrawal from high-dose tranquilizer dependence is often done gradually as the individual is tapered off of the medication. A quick withdrawal can produce life-threatening withdrawal symptoms.

Addiction Potential with Alcoholics/Addicts   Physicians should not prescribe minor tranquilizers for patients who are addiction-prone. Pharmaceutical manufacturers warn physicians through medical journal ads and the *Physicians Desk Reference* that tranquilizers are capable of abuse and dependence, especially when prescribed to addiction-prone individuals. Many patients deny or are unaware of their problems with alcohol and/or drugs, however, and fail to report this to their physicians. A thorough assessment for alcohol/drug problems is necessary before prescribing minor tranquilizers. "Non-medical use of benzodiazepines in the general population is rare and of little or no consequence; on the other hand, benzodiazepines are used with some frequency among populations with histories of drug abuse" (Woods et al. 1988).

Central Nervous System Stimulants
Amphetamines

Overview   Amphetamines are central nervous system stimulants (Table 3.10). Until recently they were widely prescribed by physicians for conditions such as obesity, depression, and narcolepsy (uncontrolled fits of sleep). For certain kinds of hyperactive behavior in children, Ritalin is most commonly prescribed.

Doctors also prescribe amphetamines for Parkinson's disease, epilepsy, nausea during pregnancy, bed-wetting, asthma, sedative overdoses, and hypotensive states associated with anesthesia. Because amphetamines relieve sleepiness and fatigue, they are widely used nonmedically by students cramming for exams, long-distance truck drivers, nightshift workers, and individuals seeking general stimulation.

In the mid 1960s, a phenomenon new to North America emerged: intravenous use of massive doses of amphetamines (usually methamphetamines) by chronic abusers, or speed freaks. This abuse pattern had been common in Japan and some parts of Europe following World War II, when stockpiles of amphetamines used by the military were diverted to more general use.

As a result of amphetamines' abuse potential, physicians have sharply restricted their use. Now they prescribe amphetamines primarily for narcolepsy, hyperkinetic syndrome in children, certain mental conditions, and short-term weight control. David Smith and Donald Wesson (1988) note that in 1972, when the U.S. government put federal control over stimulants in the same category as narcotic control, legitimate production of stimulants was reduced by 80 percent.

Street Names for Amphetamines   Common street names are A, AMT, bam, beans, bennies, black beauties, black mollies, brain ticklers, brownies, bumblebees, cartwheels, chalk, chicken powder, crank, Christmas trees, crossroads, cross tops, crystal, dexies, diet pills, dolls, double cross, eye openers, fives, footballs, forwards,

TABLE 3.10

Classification of Stimulants

Amphetamines	Cocaine (Benzoylmethylecognine)	Other Stimulants
Benzedrine (amphetamine)		Ritalin (methylphenidate)
Dexedrine (dextroamphetamine)		Preludin (phenmetrazine)
		Tenuate (diethylpropion)
Methedrine, Desoxyn (methamphetamine)		INH (isoniazid)
		Coffee, colas, tea (caffeine)
		Tobacco (nicotine)

hearts, jam, jellybeans, leapers, lid poppers, lightning, meth, pep pills, purple hearts, rippers, sparkle plenties, sparklers, speed, splash, sweets, tens, thrusters, truck drivers, turnabouts, uppers, uppie, ups, wake-ups, water, and white crosses.

Estimates of Use   The Domestic Council Drug Abuse Task Force estimates that close to 500,000 American adults are now using stimulant drugs (primarily amphetamines) regularly and nonmedically. A new and emerging population of methamphetamine users is developing in adolescents and young adults (15 to 30 years of age) (National Institute on Drug Abuse 1989).

Routes of Administration   Amphetamines are available in a variety of forms; tablets and capsules are the most common. Amphetamines are usually taken orally or injected intravenously.

Methamphetamine (speed) is usually in powder or crystal form and is made illicitly. The solid form of methamphetamine with the street name ice was first cooked up in Hawaii. Ice is smoked much like freebase or crack cocaine.

Major Effects   Typical therapeutic doses of amphetamines stimulate the central nervous system, increase blood pressure, widen the pupils, increase respiration rate, depress the appetite, relieve sleepiness, and decrease fatigue and boredom. Other effects include increased awareness and alertness, slight euphoria, elevation of mood and self-confidence (although the ability to perform complex tasks is usually diminished), increased talkativeness and excitement, reduced nausea and gastrointestinal upset, and dry mouth.

Adverse Effects   In some individuals, even a moderate dose of amphetamines can have adverse effects, such as agitation, an inability to concentrate, anxiety, confusion, blurred vision, tremors, and heart palpitations. Higher doses of amphetamines can produce quite severe adverse reactions, which include the following:

- Tremors, palpitations
- Dilated pupils (mydriasis)
- Sweating and flushing, abdominal cramps, nausea
- Tachycardia (rapid heartbeat), heart abnormalities
- Hypertension (later hypotension), circulatory collapse
- Anxiety, agitation, and panic
- Aggression and violent behavior often associated with paranoia
- Rapid breathing, respiratory collapse
- Hallucination (visual and auditory), delirium
- Extremely high fevers
- Convulsions and seizures

Although death reports from amphetamine use are rare, some individuals who are unusually sensitive to these drugs have died as a result of burst blood vessels in the brain, heart failure, or high fever. Amphetamine psychosis, a mental disturbance similar to paranoid schizophrenia, is sometimes associated with high-dose amphetamine use, but many of its symptoms have been observed with moderate dose levels.

Injecting amphetamines causes other complications: unsterile and shared needles cause problems with tetanus, AIDS, abscesses, and hepatitis. The injection of insoluble particles in street speed also causes many problems.

Dependence and Withdrawal   Abruptly stopping amphetamines after chronic heavy use is often followed by symptoms such as fatigue, brain wave abnormalities, prolonged sleep, voracious appetite, stomach cramps, muscle pains, lethargy, and severe emotional depression. Some of these symptoms seem just as dramatic as withdrawal symptoms from depressant drugs.

Withdrawing amphetamines from chronic users does not seem as physically distressing as withdrawal from depressant drugs. There is little evidence of any physical dependence on moderate doses of amphetamines, but researchers frequently report psychological dependence on even low doses.

Prolonged use of amphetamines leads to a broad range of illnesses. Chronic users suffer dehydration, weight loss, and vitamin deficiency. Their reduced resistance to disease allows sores, nonhealing ulcers, and chronic chest infections. Users have a higher than normal rate of liver and cardiovascular disease, hypertensive disorders, and psychiatric problems.

Coca leaves and cocaine.
DEA/Department of Justice.

Bootlegged Amphetamines   The newer, tighter regulations imposed on the legitimate prescribing of amphetamines have caused the widespread bootlegging of amphetamines and substitution of other substances to mimic the amphetamine high. The most common substitutes include ephedrine—a mild stimulant found in some over-the-counter asthma remedies—and phenylpropanolamine, or PPA, the ingredients in most legal diet capsules. The moderate to large amounts of caffeine in most illicit amphetamines sometimes account for the bulk of the ingredients.

Cocaine

Cocaine is a central nervous system stimulant that has gained great popularity in a variety of drug forms. At first, cocaine was expensive; only the wealthy could afford it. Today, crack cocaine is used by every socioeconomic class, making it the scourge of humanity.

Brief History of Cocaine

2500 B.C.: Coca leaves were found in burial sites in Peru.

500 B.C.: In Columbia, South America, large stone monolithic idols possessed puffed-out cheeks, representative of a coca chewer.

Tenth century: Incans started to use the plant referred to as "Mama Coca," and the coca tree was pictured as a beautiful woman.

Eighteenth century: The Spanish took coca leaves back to Europe. However, there was general disinterest in coca by Europeans. One can speculate that the sample of coca leaves taken from South America lost their potency during the trip.

1786: Lamarck named the species of the coca plant *Erythroxylum coca.*

1844: Conflicting reports stated that either Albert Nieman or Gaedecke isolated cocaine.

1878: W. H. Bentley espoused cocaine as a cure for morphine addiction.

1883: Aschenbrandt prescribed the use of cocaine to counteract the battle fatigue of the Bavarian troops.

1883: Sigmund Freud wrote *Über Coca* praising the medicinal effects of cocaine.

1887: Sigmund Freud recognized cocaine addiction and wrote a book titled *Fear of and Craving for Cocaine.*

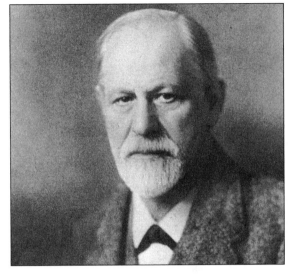

Sigmund Freud.

Cocaine is obtained from the leaves of *Erythroxylum coca,* a bush grown in parts of South America. Mountain Indians of Peru and Bolivia have chewed coca leaves as a social ritual for more than a thousand years.

The coca leaf was taken to Europe in the nineteenth century and became quite popular in certain circles. Sigmund Freud, the father of psychoanalysis, used cocaine extensively. In 1883, he recommended cocaine for treatment of morphine addiction, alcohol dependence, asthma, digestive disorders, and depression and fatigue. Freud frequently recommended the drug for what was then called neurasthenia (i.e., nervous anxiety). Freud soon realized cocaine was addictive; in 1887, he wrote *Fear of and Craving for Cocaine,* describing dependence on cocaine.

One of the most popular soft drinks of all time, Coca-Cola, originally contained extracts of the coca leaf. Coca was also present in wines such as Vin Mariani, a wine that was extremely popular with the pope and the royal families in Italy and other countries. Today, a little more than 100 years after the cocaine problems

This late-nineteenth-century ad for Mariani wine, which contained cocaine, portrays the beverage as a panacea for all ills.

Bettmann Archive.

of the 1880s, we have another cocaine problem caused by coca products that are far more addicting than those of the past. Cocaine was also used as a topical anesthetic (e.g., in eye surgery) and as a local vasoconstrictor.

Street Names for Cocaine There are several street names for cocaine: Bernice, bernieds, big C, blow, bombita, bouncing powder, burese, C, charles, charlie, coke, cola, corrine, dream, dust, flake, fly, girl, gold dust, heaven, heaven dust, her, ice (not to be confused with the form of methamphetamine), incentive, jay, joy powder, lady, lady snow, nose candy, nose powder, paradise, poison, powder, rock, schoolboy, snow, star dust, sugar, white, white lady, white powder, and white stuff.

Estimates of Use In 1994, an estimated 1.4 million Americans were cocaine users. This represents 0.7 percent of the population aged 12 and older, while the estimated number of crack users was about one-half million (NIDA, 1995).

Routes of Administration Cocaine can be inhaled, injected, or smoked. Cocaine hydrochloride is snorted or injected, while crack cocaine is smoked.

Freebase cocaine is another smokable form of cocaine. Heating up cocaine hydrochloride with a volatile solvent (usually ether) and a base (baby laxative) results in cocaine free of its hydrochloride base, with by-products of water and salt.

Cocaine HCl + ether + base + heat = pure cocaine + NaCl (salt) + H_2O (water)

Because this cocaine is extremely pure, the volatile point, or the temperature at which cocaine burns, is raised. This allows freebase cocaine to be smoked without burning it. Simply burning cocaine does not produce a high. Freebase cocaine smoke goes from the lungs to the brain in 6 seconds, resulting in an immediate and intense high. This high lasts only 40 to 50 seconds and requires repeated doses, making it extremely expensive to maintain a habit. Crack cocaine is formed by combining cocaine with baking soda; this overrides the hydrochloride acid and allows the crack to be smoked. Crack is sold in small rocks at lower prices to lower economic populations.

Major Effects The cocaine user experiences 15 to 30 minutes of excitation and euphoria, tends to talk a lot, and feels energetic and self-confident. The effect of cocaine often gives the individual a supreme feeling of well-being, control, and enjoyment of activities that may previously have been mundane. At early stages of use, men report feeling a stimulation of sexuality. Cocaine is very short-acting because it has an extremely short half-life; after the euphoria, psychological depression, nervousness, fatigue, and irritability set in. (See Table 3.11.)

Adverse Effects With heavy regular use, depression and anxiety can be so severe that the user continues to snort, smoke, or inject cocaine every 20 minutes or so for several hours to avoid the onset of depression. This pattern may develop into binges—or 24 to 48 hours of cocaine use.

Another method to take the edge off cocaine is to inject heroin with cocaine (speedballing). This form of cocaine use was implicated in the death of comedian and actor John Belushi. Addicts frequently turn to the sedative hypnotics (alcohol, tranquilizers, and barbiturates) to counteract the downside after using cocaine. This pat-

---

TABLE 3.11

Cocaine Clinical Syndromes

Cocaine Euphoria	Cocaine Dysphoria	Cocaine Schizophreniform Psychosis
Euphoria	Sadness	Anhedonia (inability to feel pleasure from what would have normally given pleasure)
Affective Lability	Melancholia	
Increased intellectual function	Apathy	Disorientation
Hyperalertness	Inability to concentrate	Hallucinations
Hyperactivity	Painful delusions	Concern with minutia
Anorexia	Anorexia	Stereotyped behavior
Insomnia	Insomnia	Paranoid delusions (parasitosis)
Hypersexuality		Insomnia
Proneness to violence		Proneness to violence

---

tern of sedative hypnotic use may also cause a dependence on drugs in this classification. Acute toxicity can occur from any method of cocaine use. In the past, cocaine was thought of as a rather benign drug. Today, we know that cocaine-related deaths are more common than once thought. Cases of sudden death from cocaine use are increasing. Large doses of cocaine may cause shallow breathing, fever, restlessness, anxiety, and confusion. Even small doses of cocaine can cause a slowing of the heart rate. Cocaine use can also result in arrythmia and heart attack. High doses also have an impact on the motor systems in the brain and spinal cord, resulting in tremors and convulsive movements. Long-term chronic snorting of large amounts of cocaine can destroy tissue in the nose. Nausea, vomiting, and abdominal pains can occur. Death from cocaine overdose is usually due to convulsions, respiratory arrest, and/or the Casey Jones reaction, a condition during which the body acts like a runaway train exceeding its own metabolic limits. People have done and seen some bizarre things under the influence of cocaine. Case studies in Chapter 5 describe these in more detail.

Tolerance and Withdrawal   According to our behavioral definition of addiction, cocaine is the most addicting drug known today, especially freebase cocaine. However, a physical tolerance to cocaine does not develop. When cocaine is used, the dopamine neurotransmitters are blocked from reuptake, stranding them in the synaptic clefts. This causes a cessation of stimulant response. However, this is not a classical tolerance reaction. This was one of the factors that led to the tragic miscalculation that cocaine was not an addicting drug. Its intense high and the user's need to avoid the crash or depression makes cocaine highly addicting and contributes to the binge patterns of cocaine use. Cocaine is one of the few chemicals (other than amphetamines and other stimulants) that exist outside of the body and stimulate catecholamine. Catecholamines are responsible for extraordinarily intense reactions to stressful situations (e.g., a father lifts a car to release his child pinned beneath it). The Casey Jones reaction previously mentioned is directly related to this catecholamine-enhancing property of cocaine. Once this reaction is set in motion, it usually results in death. Some people die from nontoxic doses of cocaine due to a phenomenon known as the kindling effect.

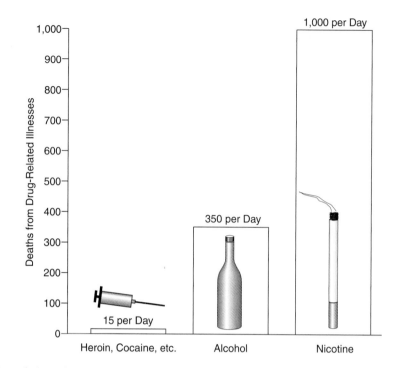

This graph shows the number of deaths from drug-related illnesses for illicit drugs (heroin, cocaine, etc.) and licit drugs (alcohol and nicotine).

The brain is primed for, sensitized to, the effect of cocaine, so that one additional dose may trigger firing or discharge, leading to sudden death.

Cocaine Additives   Cocaine purchased on the illicit market is very seldom, if ever, pure by the time it reaches the consumer. As it makes its way from the original source down to the illicit market, the drug's purity is cut with various substances. These additives include mannitol (a mild baby laxative), lactose (milk sugar), or the psychoactive drugs procaine (Novocain), Lidocaine (Xylocaine), benzocaine, tetracaine, and amphetamine. Some individuals have allergic reactions to these substances.

Tobacco

Tobacco is the most widely abused drug. Despite warnings regarding the health hazards, approximately one-fifth of adults in the United States continue to use tobacco products; tobacco use is the single leading cause of preventable death in this country (U.S. Surgeon General 1988). In comparing deaths related to alcohol and other drugs, smoking tobacco contributes to far more deaths.

Diseases Related to Smoking Tobacco

1. Heart disease (coronary heart disease, increased artherosclerotic disease). Smoking elevates low-density lipoproteins (LDL, or bad cholesterol), while reducing high-density lipoproteins (HDL, or good cholesterol).

2. Peripheral vascular disease
3. Cerebrovascular disease
4. Cancer (lung cancer; cancer of the larynx, mouth, esophagus; contributing factor in urinary cancer, kidney cancer, and pancreatic cancer)
5. Chronic obstructive lung disease and colds (chronic bronchitis and emphysema)

Health Consequences

- More women die from lung cancer than breast cancer each year.
- Twenty to 25 percent of female smokers don't stop during pregnancy.
- Over three-fourths of smokers start during the developmental teenage years.
- One out of every five high school seniors smoke cigarettes on a daily basis.
- Chewing tobacco (smokeless tobacco) is the leading cause of oral cancer.
- Approximately 75 to 80 percent of recovering alcoholics smoke cigarettes.

In recent years, there has been a decrease in use of tobacco products by the general public, yet the use of tobacco, especially by young people, makes them a significant population at-risk for the development of smoking-related diseases.

Hallucinogens
Definition

The term *hallucinogen* is derived from the Latin word *hallucinari,* which means "to dream or to wander in the mind." Other terms describing hallucinogens are *psychedelic* ("alters consciousness"), *psychotomimetic* ("mimics psychosis"), and *psychotogenic* ("produces psychosis").

Hallucinogens are capable of altering time and space perception; of changing feelings of self-awareness and emotion; of changing one's sense of body image; and of increasing sensitivity to textures and shapes, sounds, and taste. In addition, these drugs bring visions of luminescence, flashes of light, kaleidoscopic patterns, and landscapes. They can also induce hallucinations and feelings of enlightenment and spiritual or religious awakening.

In the past, any substance whose function is to change the habitual way of perceiving and orienting oneself toward one's physical, psychological, and social environment was considered a hallucinogen. As a result, many drugs such as marijuana, PCP, and even cocaine are inappropriately classified as hallucinogens because that is the category they seem to fit best.

In the 1960s, Timothy Leary advocated LSD as a means of "turning on, tuning in, and dropping out" of mainstream lifestyles and thinking. Of the many natural and synthetic hallucinogens, LSD is the most potent by weight and the most thoroughly researched.

Other hallucinogens include mescaline, which is derived from the dried buttons or heads of the peyote cactus; peyote buttons, which can be eaten or made into a tea; and psilocybin, which is found in a wide range of American and Mexican mushrooms. Some street names for peyote are bad seed, big chief, buttons, cactus, P, peyotl, and topi. Common street names for mescaline include beans, big chief, buttons, cactus, cactus buttons, mesc, mescal, and moon topi. (See Table 3.12.)

Panther mushroom.

DEA/Dept. of Justice.

Psilocybe mushroom.

Peyote cactus.

LSD blotter paper.

LSD

Common street names for LSD are acid, barrels, beast, Big D, blotter, blue acid, blue cheer, blue heaven, blue mist, brown dots, California sunshine, cap, chocolate chips, contact lens, cubes, cupcakes, D, deeda, domes, dots, electric Kool-Aid, flash, ghost, hawk, haze, L, lysergic, mellow yellows, microdots, orange cubes, paper acid, peace, pearly gates, pellets, pink owsley, purple haze, sacrament, strawberries, strawberry fields, sugar, sugar cubes, sunshine, tabs, ticket twenty-five, wedges, white lightning, window pane, and yellow.

TABLE 3.12

Classification of Hallucinogens

LSD-25 (lysergic acid diethylamide)
Dimethyltryptamine (DMT)
Psilocybin (mushrooms)
Psilocin
Bufotenine
Harmine
Mescaline (active part of peyote cactus)
Diethytryptamine (DET)
Dipropryltryptamine (DPT)
Dimethoxymethamphetamine (DOM/STP)
Methylenedioxyamphetamine (MDA)
Belladonna alkaloids (atropine, scopoliamine, and stramonium are found in many
  medicines for asthma and stomach cramps)
Nutmeg (myristicin)

Brief History of LSD and Other Hallucinogens

1000 B.C. or earlier: Hallucinogenic mushrooms were used in religious and tribal
  use.
700 B.C.: Hallucinogenic mandrake root was referred to by the Assyrians and
  mentioned in the Bible as a fertility substance.
38: Datura was used by the early Incas and other Indians of South America. Peyote
  cactus (mescaline) was used by Incas and later by Native Americans.
1899: Oklahoma was the first state to outlaw the use of peyote.
April 16, 1943: Albert Hoffman, a chemist who discovered aspirin, working at
  Sandoz Laboratories in Basel, Switzerland, discovered LSD-25 and
  experienced the first LSD-25 trip.
Until mid 1960s: LSD was used in experiments in mental hospitals and
  laboratories to explore the treatment of mental disorders and as a means of
  studying psychotic behavior.
1960: Timothy Leary, Ph.D., a research professor in the Department of Social and
  Human Relations at Harvard University, reported in 1960 a "full-blown
  conversion experience" after eating psilocybin mushrooms. He and Richard
  Alpert, Ph.D. (today known as lecturer Ram Dass), distributed psilocybin.
1961: Leary and Alpert distributed LSD.
1963: Leary and Alpert were dismissed from Harvard, giving them tremendous
  publicity. They coined the famous phrase "Turn on, tune in, and drop out."
1965: At an LSD conference, Sidney Cohen summarized the research on LSD use
  with psychiatric patients and other experiments.
1969: The Woodstock Festival took place in Woodstock, New York.

1960s and 1970s: LSD was extremely popular on the streets, especially among young people and college students.

1992–93: An increase in the trend of LSD use by young people became evident.

Estimates of Use

In comparison with the use of hallucinogens in the late 1960s, today's use rate is smaller. But, contrary to media reports, that use has not all but died out. These drugs continue to be taken by millions of people in the United States each year. LSD is the most commonly used hallucinogen. In 1994, the rate of LSD use was 1.0 percent for persons 18 to 25 years old and 0.5 percent for youth (NIDA 1995). LSD is easily manufactured, and hallucinogenic mushrooms grow wild in many states, as do many plants with hallucinogenic or toxic-hallucinogenic properties. (See the section "Drug Update" earlier in this chapter.)

Routes of Administration

Hallucinogens are usually ingested orally, but they may be smoked, snorted, or injected. Because such small amounts are required at any one time (25 to 150 millionths of a gram), LSD is often impregnated in sugar pills, blotter paper, or small gelatin squares. The nasty taste of some hallucinogens requires mixing them with other substances to counteract their taste. Teas and broths are a common method of ingesting hallucinogens.

Major Effects

The effects of hallucinogens are influenced by the personality of the user, the expectations of use, the user's general experience with drugs, the mind set of the individual, and, most important, the setting. The right group of trusting friends, a comfortable, soothing environment (e.g., dim lights and soft music), and someone experienced with hallucinogens are described as integral in developing a good hallucinogenic trip.

As a result of all these variables, users of hallucinogens report a wide range of reactions. Some individuals feel an insight and expanded consciousness, while others report a discomfort and fear of losing control that is quite disturbing. Generally, low to moderate doses of hallucinogens produce mood and perceptual alterations. LSD and other hallucinogens can produce profound effects on the user's thinking, self-awareness, and emotions. Hallucinogens distort time and space perception and induce hallucinations.

Adverse Effects

Hallucinogenic experiences can sometimes add to existing neuroses, or character disorders, and can produce transient waves of mild anxiety, paranoia, or severe panic. Flashbacks (recurrences of negative hallucinogenic experiences) usually occur within a year or less from the previous use of hallucinogens. However, the incidence of flashbacks occurring is relatively small. Flashbacks can occur in individuals who have used hallucinogens excessively and in the occasional or first-time user.

Accidents are very common under the influence of hallucinogens. The high degree of suggestibility and perceptual distortions and hallucinations often lead to accidents. Such accidents include walking through a plate glass window; jumping from a roof due to the coaxing of a friend (high degree of suggestibility); and suffering accidental falls, drownings, and car accidents.

Tolerance and Dependence

Researchers have observed psychological dependence in long-term LSD users but have rarely reported dependence as a consequence of other hallucinogenic use. Hallucinogenic trips can be of long duration, compared with other drug use. Users tend to trip for from 4 to 6 hours to 12 to 24 hours. Following these trips, users are usually quite tired. This often necessitates periods of getting back to normal functioning before again using hallucinogens. Because of this pattern of occasional or intermittent use of hallucinogens, physical dependence is unlikely under most conditions. Tolerance has been shown to develop to some of the psychological and physiological effects of LSD. Quite frequently, there is cross-tolerance to other hallucinogens. For example, an individual who has recently been taking LSD generally shows a reduced response to mescaline and psilocybin.

Cannabis Sativa

Cannabis refers to any product of the plant *Cannabis sativa,* which grows in most parts of the world. In North America, the most commonly used products derived from this plant are marijuana and hashish. Marijuana is the unprocessed, dried leaves, flowers, seeds, and stems of the plant. Hashish is a more potent product processed from the resin of this herb. Researchers have obtained more than 300 cannabis products (cannabinoids) from cannabis. They have isolated and synthesized the most active ingredient in marijuana. This product, tetrahydrocannabinol (THC), is the psychoactive compound found in the greatest amount in the plant; it is thought to produce most of the high.

Marijuana plant.

Street Names

Common street names for marijuana include Acapulco gold, ace, African black, aunt mary, baby, bale, bomb, boo, brick, broccoli, bush, Canadian black, charge, Colombian, doobie, dry high, fatty, fingers, flowers, gage, ganga, gauge, giggleweed, grass, green, grefa, greta, grifa, grillo, grunt, hay, hemp, herb, homegrown, Indian hay, Indian hemp, J, jane, jay smoke, joint, joy stick, juanita, kick sticks, kif, killer, killer weed, kilter, loco, mary, maryann, maryjane, mary warner, mary weaver, meserole (messerole), Mexican brown, Mexican green, Mexican locoweed, MJ, mooca, moota, mooters, mootie, mota, mother, mu, muggles, muta, number, Panama gold, Panama red, panatella, pin, pode, pot, ragweed, rainy day woman, red dirt, reefer, roach, root, sassafras, sinsemilla, smoke, snop, stick, sweet lucy, tea, Texas tea, twist, weed, wheat, yerba, and Zacatecas purple. Street names for hashish include black hash, black Russian, blond hash, canned sativa, hash, Lebanese, and mahjuema.

Brief History of Marijuana

2737 B.C.: The earliest reference to marijuana by a Chinese treatise on pharmacology was attributed to Emperor Shen Nung.

Second century B.C.: The Scythians, a warlike and mobile Middle Eastern tribe, spread cannabis into Egypt and then northward to Russia and Europe. They had a ritual of throwing hemp seeds on heated stones and inhaling the vapors (funeral rite).

650 B.C.: The use of cannabis was mentioned in Persia and Assyria.

400 B.C.: The use of cannabis was mentioned in Rome.

1545: The first record of a marijuana plant in the New World occurred when Spanish traders introduced marijuana to Chile.

1611: Sir Walter Raleigh was ordered by the British to grow hemp in his Virginia colony. Hemp was much needed for the strong shipbuilding industry of the time.

1765: George Washington grew marijuana hemp and is said to have experimented with the medicinal or intoxicating potency of the plants.

1804–44: Jacques-Joseph Moreau of France used marijuana in the treatment of melancolia, hypomania, and other forms of mental disorder.

1839: W. B. O'Shaughnessy, a young chemistry professor, used marijuana for medicinal use as an anticonvulsant and an appetite stimulant.

1846: A group of French writers formed the "Club des Hachichias," meeting in Paris once a month, where they often smoked marijuana. The meetings were attended by Victor Hugo, Baudelaire, Dumas, Gautier, and De Nerval.

Early 1900s: It is believed that the drug and use of the word *marijuana* were introduced to the United States by migrant Mexican laborers.

1937: Henry Anslinger, commissioner of the Bureau of Narcotics, campaigned on the dangers of marijuana.

1937: The federal government developed the Marijuana Tax Act and used taxes to outlaw the drug.

October 1969: A Gallup Poll estimated that 10 million Americans, half of them under 21 years of age, have smoked marijuana.

1970: The Controlled Substance Act, supported by the American Medical Association, reported that marijuana had no potential medicinal use, ignoring years of medical evidence to the contrary.

Estimates of Use

Marijuana is the most widely used of all illicit drugs. By various estimates, 35 to 50 million Americans have tried this drug, and 12 to 18 million are regular users of two or more joints per week (National Institute on Drug Abuse 1989).

Medical Uses

Cannabis, primarily in the form of synthetic THC, has been under scientific investigation in recent years to ascertain its potential therapeutic uses. One approved therapeutic use is as an antiemetic (antivomiting) agent for the nausea and vomiting associated with chemotherapy treatment for cancer patients. It is also medically used to relieve the intraocular pressure accompanying glaucoma. Both of these medical uses are the most well researched. Other potential medical uses of marijuana researched thus far include spasm relief, asthma relief, anxiety reduction, and relief of alcohol withdrawal symptoms. Studies in these areas have not been as prolific, or as conclusive, as those regarding chemotherapy and glaucoma (Solomons and Neppve 1989).

As of 2001, thirty-four states had statutes on the books allowing marijuana, typically in the form of THC, to be used in medical research and/or medical treatment as a part of a clinical investigation. The number of states that have actually implemented these procedures is much smaller. The political and moral/ethical emotionality of our times may further hinder these investigations into the effectiveness of marijuana in medical research. For this reason, other synthetically produced cannabis derivatives are also under investigation.

Routes of Administration

Marijuana can be smoked in hand-rolled cigarettes or joints. Today's higher- potency marijuana is usually smoked in a pipe—most frequently, a water pipe. This allows the most intense high with the least waste of the marijuana.

Generally, hashish has a much higher THC content, though it varies widely in potency. Hashish can be crumbled and rolled into a cigarette for smoking; often, it is mixed with a lower-grade marijuana or tobacco. In this country, hashish is normally smoked in a water pipe.

Marijuana and hashish can also be eaten in cookies, brownies, and other food or made into a tea. In this form, the high lasts longer, since it is slowed down by the digestive processes.

Cannabis resin is not water soluble, so the drug cannot be injected. The few who have tried using it this way usually experienced violent convulsions.

Major Effects

The effects of cannabis depend on the potency of the drug, the method of use, and the experience and expectations of the user regarding what will happen. For low-dose periodic use, the common effects of marijuana use are these:

- Intensification of thoughts and feelings
- Feelings of exhilaration, relaxation, giddiness
- Minor increase in heart rate
- Drowsiness, dry mouth and throat, bloodshot eyes

TABLE 3.13

Aspects of Life Experience Adult Daily Users Most Frequently Described as Positively Affected by Marijuana

- Ability to relax and enjoy life
- Enjoyment of food
- Ability to overcome worry and anxiety
- Ability to sleep well.
- Ability to avoid feeling bored
- Enjoyment of sex
- Understanding of others
- Creativity
- Ability to avoid feeling angry
- Ability to enjoy varied activities
- Self-understanding
- Overall happiness
- Ability to avoid feeling depressed
- Ability to be tolerant and considerate of others

Source: Herbert Hendin et al., *Living High: Daily Marijuana Use by Adults,* Copyright © 1987 Human Sciences Press. Reprinted by permission of Insight Books, New York, NY.

- Impaired short-term memory
- Altered states of time and space
- Dilated pupils

For a list of experiences that adult users tend to describe as positively affected by marijuana use, see Table 3.13.

Increased Potency of Marijuana

You might remember hearing about types of marijuana such as Acapulco gold, Maui Wowi, or Panama red. Most of the potent marijuana in the 1960s was imported from these places. Today, homegrown marijuana is the staple of American pot smokers. The more than 22 million pot smokers in the United States prefer the high-potency sinsemilla grown in hidden caches throughout the United States. Humboldt County in California is an example of this homegrown cultivation. The California gold rush still goes on there in the form of marijuana crops, despite increased eradication efforts.

In the 1960s, the THC content of marijuana was 1 to 2 percent in potency. Most users would smoke half a joint to get high. Two or three joints passed among friends could get everyone high. Today, the THC content of marijuana averages 6 percent. One hit is enough to keep an individual loaded. Today, hashish is 10 percent THC, and hash oil is 20 percent THC. This increase in the potency of marijuana means we are looking at a new drug with new problems. The research of the past with marijuana in the 1 to 2 percent THC level does not apply to marijuana now in use.

Subjective effects of cannabis intoxication have been reported in hundreds of different ways. Common reports include happiness, warmth, conviviality, camaraderie, and the ability to enjoy music and art better than when sober. Reactions to marijuana depend a great deal on the attitude of the user and the compatibility of the surroundings (set and setting). Cannabis is sometimes classified as a mild hallucinogen. With the increase in potency of marijuana, this classification may be warranted.

Adverse Effects

The long-term effects of chronic cannabis use are at the heart of the current medical debate on this drug. Strong psychological dependence does develop in many regular users of marijuana, as evidenced by a need for cannabis use every day to perform certain tasks, to relax and unwind, or to sleep. The individual's life begins to revolve around the use of marijuana as a primary activity. The user tends to use marijuana more frequently throughout the day and evening.

Withdrawal symptoms after steady use may include irritability, decreased appetite, restlessness, sleep disturbances, sweating, nausea, or diarrhea. Hangovers the next morning are not uncommon. However, unlike the alcohol hangover, which causes headaches and sensitive optic nerves, the cannabis hangover is more likely to be light-headedness characterized by the inability to gather thoughts. When the drug is ingested, the effect can linger on for an entire day, along with nausea, body aches, and other symptoms.

Despite the lack of classic withdrawal symptoms, some patterns of marijuana use fit the behavioral definition of addiction. Researchers have well established the fact that chronic marijuana use can cause physical dependence by identifying full-blown withdrawal symptoms in the newborn babies of marijuana-dependent mothers. Treatment for the addiction to marijuana requires the support of an outpatient treatment counselor knowledgeable about alcohol/drug recovery and marijuana dependence. Marijuana Anonymous groups have also developed to meet the rising incidence of dependence on marijuana.

Anxiety and panic reactions are common with chronic marijuana use. Many individuals who have used marijuana to self-medicate affective disorders, such as depression and bipolar disorder, can experience severe anxiety and panic reactions. Individuals experiencing psychologically negative reactions may require temporary hospitalization so they don't get out of control and hurt themselves or others.

Damage to the Respiratory System

The tars in cannabis smoke are 50 percent greater by weight than tobacco tars and 70 percent higher in cancer-producing substances. Considering that marijuana is deeply inhaled and the smoke is held in the lungs, instead of passively inhaled, as in cigarette smoking, the cancer-causing risk is increased by marijuana smoking.

Long-term, heavy smoking of cannabis is associated with bronchial problems, sore throat, and chronic coughing. These conditions may be more severe in chronic hashish users. In addition, those who smoke tobacco as well as cannabis products have an added risk of bronchial problems and cancer.

Immune System Effects

Research suggests that cannabis, particularly when used regularly, tends to suppress the body's immune response and ability to combat infections (Cohen 1986). Marijuana temporarily arrests the maturation of developing t-cells, which protect the body from colds and other bacterial infections. This increases the chances of illness due to either bacteria or viruses. The most prominent indication of this effect is the higher incidence of bronchial infections, coughing, bronchitis, and pneumonia noted among chronic, heavy marijuana users.

Reproductive System Effects
Chronic use of cannabis decreases sperm motility and serum testosterone in men and interferes with the menstrual cycle in women, thus affecting fertility. Most of these effects are reversed after marijuana use is discontinued. Marijuana is suspected to be harmful to the fetuses in pregnant women; research with rhesus monkeys has shown pregnancy problems such as stillbirth and spontaneous abortion. Reduced birth weight is also a characteristic of surviving fetuses.

Brain System Effects
Considerable debate continues over the effects of cannabis on the brain. A certain percentage of users develop lethargy, apathy, and disorientation, which persist long after chronic use has been discontinued. Fortunately, these effects appear to wear off gradually. Some researchers claim that long-term changes occur in some brain wave patterns; these claims are being investigated further.

Impairment of Maturation Process
Most researchers agree that cannabis use, during the primary developmental years of 11 to 15, in particular, interferes with physical and mental maturation processes and impedes emotional development. Research describes an amotivational syndrome with symptoms of apathy, lethargy, and a general lack of involvement and motivation in growth and developmental activities.

Marijuana and Driving
Cannabis intoxication and chronic marijuana use impair short-term memory, alter the user's sense of time and space, and impair overall coordination and motor functioning. The ability to track other vehicles is also impaired and is a major problem in driving a car. Tracking involves judging time, distance, and the speed of other cars. Skills such as merging into traffic, making U-turns, and performing other driving tasks require tracking skills. Adding another drug, such as alcohol, only makes the situation worse. Many persons insist that their driving performance is improved under the influence of marijuana. This is due to their increased sensitivity to enjoying driving, not to a realistic evaluation of driving ability.

Smoking marijuana also makes it very dangerous to operate machinery and other equipment, since perception and timing are off, and the drug may also produce fatigue and drowsiness.

A study of airplane pilots reported that, after smoking marijuana, performance was impaired up to two to three days later, despite the pilots' thinking that they did extremely well on simulated tests (Rohr 1989). Other problems include (1) true allergic reactions to cannabis for a small minority of users; (2) gastrointestinal disturbances and weight loss among a small percentage of heavy users; and (3) difficulty in medical control of some diabetic users.

TABLE 3.14

Classification of Inhalants

A wide variety of names apply to inhaled substances. Many liquids also contain alcohol and petroleum distillates.

Naphtha	Fluorocarbon propellants
Benzene	Nitrous oxide
Acetone	Amyl nitrite, butyl nitrite
Toluene	Anesthetic gases (e.g., ether, chloroform)
Carbon tetrachloride	Gasoline

Inhalants

From time to time, the phenomenon of inhalant use is brought to public attention. In the 1960s, there was an epidemic of glue sniffing. Nowadays, there is still a consistent use of various solvents, aerosols, and other gases that people inhale to get high. For young people, people of color, and minorities who do not have the money to buy drugs, inhalant use is more prevalent. And, in certain locations, the problem is much more serious because of the number of young people who use inhalants to get high, yet this is hardly a modern-day phenomenon. Table 3.14 lists some common inhalants.

Brief History

Some inhalants and anesthetics, such as nitrous oxide, ether, and chloroform, were used recreationally in the nineteenth century, especially during times of liquor scarcity. This occurred in Europe, Great Britain, and North America, where ether inhalation parties were common among students and physicians.

In the 1960s, the inhalation of volatile substances such as plastic model glue, nail polish removers, and aerosol sprays occurred frequently among adolescents. A wave of antiglue-sniffing publicity at the time resulted in many local and state laws prohibiting minors from buying such substances. In spite of these laws, inhalant vapors and sprays continue to be used to this day, partially because of the widespread application of such products in household use and partially because of ineffective legislation and enforcement.

In the 1970s and 1980s, paint became the primary inhalant of abuse. Users sprayed cans of paint, preferably gold and silver, into rags which they stuffed under their noses to inhale the fumes. These huffers (paint inhalers) were often inner-city Latinos and other young people of color. Native American youth have an extremely high incidence of gasoline inhalant use. In 1994, the 12- to 17-year-old age group had the highest rate of current inhalant use—1.6 percent (NIDA 1995).

Route of Administration

Inhalation is accomplished in any number of ways, depending on the ingenuity of the user. Inhaling fumes can be accomplished by placing the substance on a rag;

placing or spraying the substance in a plastic bag; or, in the case of some pressurized gases, filling up a balloon, then waiting for the frozen vapor to warm up (if necessary) before inhaling. Users also sometimes go into a food market, smash the bottom of whipped cream cans, and squirt the gas from the broken containers into the backs of their throats. This aerosol freon gives them a cheap high.

Absorption of gases and volatile liquids is efficient and rapid. Absorption into tissues begins with the nasal mucous membranes. The major absorption site is the lungs, where substances enter the bloodstream. From the lungs, substances are distributed directly to the brain and other organ systems. They also enter fatty tissue.

Available Forms of Inhalants

Glue, model cement, fingernail polish removers, various cosmetics, various cleaning solvents, gasoline, paint, paint thinners, lighter fluids, antifreeze, aerosol cans, and white correction fluids can all be inhaled.

Major Effects

Users report a feeling of well-being, a reduction of inhibitions, and an elevated mood. In many respects, the effects are similar to those produced by alcohol and other sedatives. Higher doses often produce laughing and giddiness, feelings of floating, dizziness, time and space distortions, and illusions. (See Table 3.15.) Some substances induce psychedelic effects. An inhalant's effects may last anywhere from 5 minutes to an hour, depending on the substance and the dose.

Many people do not understand why anyone would actively seek a high from inhalants. They forget how young children often twirl to feel the effect of dizziness and how children, adolescents, and even adults are exhilarated by the rides at amusement parks, especially the rides that give them feelings of vertigo. These effects are altered states of consciousness that are reinforcing to many individuals. Such is the case with inhalant abusers. Other reasons for using inhalants include (1) recreation (fun, mood elevation, the high); (2) peer group influence ("it was what everyone was doing"); (3) cost effectiveness (a quicker and cheaper high); and (4) easy availability.

TABLE 3.15

Signs and Symptoms of Inhalant Use

1. Slurred speech
2. Odor of the substance being used
3. Mental disorientation or confusion
4. Headaches, dizziness, and weakness
5. Muscle spasms in the neck, chest, or lower extremities
6. Euphoria, exaggerated feeling of well-being
7. Loss of balance and ataxia (uncoordinated walk)
8. Nystagmus (eye movement from side to side)

Tolerance and Dependence

When use of volatile substances continues for a long time and becomes heavy, tolerance may develop. Physical dependence with withdrawal symptoms has also occurred among some chronic users. These withdrawal symptoms include hallucinations, headaches, chills, delirium tremens, and stomach cramps. Hangovers lasting several days have also occurred.

There is cross-tolerance between some solvents and central nervous system depressants. For example, skid row alcoholics inhale hydrocarbon vapors from kerosene or spray paint when they run out of liquor. These solvents forestall withdrawal symptoms from the alcohol, especially delirium tremens.

Alcohol and barbiturates potentiate some of the adverse effects of certain solvents. Consequently, users risk unconsciousness or even heart failure if they add the effects of alcohol to the effects of volatile solvents.

Acute Adverse Effects

Acute use of solvents often brings on confusion, drunkenness, slurred speech, numbness, runny nose, tears, headache, and muscular incoordination. Frequently, there is nausea and vomiting. Due to impaired judgment from solvent use, users often feel confusion, panic, irritation, tension, and hyperactivity and become physically aggressive.

In cases of high dosage, the general sedative-anesthetic effects take over, resulting in drowsiness, stupor, respiratory depression, and unconsciousness. Extremely heavy use can inhibit breathing and bring on death.

Many of these substances are capable of sensitizing the heart to adrenaline. Since the early 1960s, heart failure due to this effect has been suspected in hundreds of users. This has been referred to as sudden sniffing death syndrome (SSD).

Some deaths have been directly attributed to solvent use. Most of them are due to suffocation when the users faint from inhalation and their noses and mouths remain covered by the plastic bags or when they suffocate in their own vomit. Additional acute adverse effects depend on the specific products and their chemical makeup.

Long-Term Effects

Some temporary abnormalities take place in liver and kidney function and bone marrow activity; gastritis, hepatitis, jaundice, blood abnormalities, and peptic ulcers also occur.

Chronic users have exhibited slow-healing ulcers around their mouths and noses. Other effects are loss of appetite, weight loss, and nutritional disorders. Brain damage also results from regular solvent use; most of the time, this has been reversible (without permanent effect) once the use was stopped. Reports of chromosome damage and blood abnormalities as a result of solvent inhaling have not yet been conclusively proven and remain under study (Ashton 1990).

With so many different kinds of solvents and hydrocarbons with chemically different structures, it is impossible to predict the long-term effects of the inhalation of all possible substances. Recent information suggests that some substances, such as toluene, may actually be less harmful than previously believed. On the other hand, long-term use of other substances, such as n-hexane, which is commonly found in some plastic cements, gasoline, various adhesives, and rubber cements, may cause permanent damage to the muscles. Because spray paint, aerosols, glues, and other such substances often contain a half-dozen or more ingredients in combination, re-searchers have had a great deal of difficulty ascertaining the exact damage potential for humans (Ashton 1990).

Phencyclidine (PCP).

Phencyclidine

Phencyclidine (PCP) is a drug that cannot be classified properly as a hallucinogen, a stimulant, or a depressant, causing it to be listed in a separate drug category. Originally, PCP was developed in the 1950s as a sedative, general anesthetic, and analgesic. In clinical testing, it worked fine as a painkiller, although subjects often developed visual disturbances, severe agitation, and other unpleasant side effects. These side effects caused its discontinued use with humans. Until 1978, phencyclidine was sold as a veterinary medication for immobilizing primates and other large animals. Its use as an illicit drug began in the mid 1960s.

Street Names for PCP
Common street names for PCP are angel dust, animal trank, aurora borealis, DOA, dust, elephant, hog, peace, peace pill, rocket fuel, supergrass, and tic tac.

Estimates of Use
The geographic patterns of PCP use are haphazard. It has long been popular on the West Coast and in certain large cities; recently, the geographical pattern of use has become more widespread.

    The majority of users are young, approximately 12 to 18 years of age, though there is use by young children and adults. (PCP users inadvertently exposed infants to PCP when they stored their drugs in empty milk bottles.) Few users have been involved for as long as 10 years, probably due to negative effects, resulting in discontinuance or a switch to another intoxicant (Thombs 1989).

Routes of Administration
PCP is a white, crystalline powder, soluble in water. Most commonly smoked or ingested, it may occasionally be injected. As tablets or capsules, PCP commonly comes in various sizes and colors. When PCP is smoked, users sprinkle the drug over mint leaves, marijuana, tobacco, or other substances, or they spray PCP liquid onto the substance to be smoked. One popular method is to dip cigarettes into liquid PCP. Given all these possibilities, this drug may appear as a drug or be disguised to look like any number of other substances.

Major Effects
With a moderate or low dose, PCP produces a state of euphoria lasting three to five hours when smoked or five to eight hours when eaten. Reactions to the drug vary

greatly; much depends on the personality of the user and the circumstances surrounding the use (set and setting). Users who have bought this drug thinking it was THC have sworn that the high was like a heavy marijuana intoxication. When PCP is misrepresented as a hallucinogen, users report LSD experiences. Users who believe they are getting PCP, however, seldom have these convictions.

The most common reactions from moderate to low doses are auditory, visual, time, and other sensory disturbances. The most consistent effect is deadening of the extremities. Due to the drug's anesthetic properties, users lose control of their muscles. Depending on the individual, the overall reaction may vary anywhere from hyperactivity to complete immobility. The drug, though not a true hallucinogen, may mimic hallucinogenic drugs in some ways. It has been described by one authority as a *delusionogen,* a term that may more accurately describe its effect on the user.

Intoxication by PCP produces an experience of tranquilization, euphoria, inebriation, dissociation, and usually tactile and auditory hallucinations. The most common effects are changes in body imagery, perceptual distortions, and feelings of apathy and estrangement. The experience often includes drowsiness, inability to verbalize, and feelings of nothingness or emptiness. Reports of difficulty in thinking, poor concentration, and preoccupation with death are frequent.

Adverse Effects

As with most other drugs, for some users occasional recreational or social use of small amounts of PCP does not cause undesirable side effects. However, this situation is likely to change when users take or smoke larger doses or smaller amounts consistently day after day. Users often smoke or ingest other drugs in addition to PCP, causing many unusual reactions.

Accidents

With high doses of PCP, accidents are common. Because PCP produces a loss of feeling, users frequently report cuts, bruises, and torn muscles and ligaments. The dissociative effects of PCP may make users believe these injuries are happening to someone else at the time.

In the heyday of PCP use in southern California in the 1960s, high doses resulted in many drownings. In those drownings, the individuals under the influence of PCP became disoriented; once underwater, they did not know which way was up. Drownings also result when users are so anesthetized that they forget to breathe; friends who are also stoned may not realize what is taking place (Thombs 1989).

Violence

Higher or consistent doses of PCP have also led to incidents of violence. These vary widely, but many are characterized by the user's inability to feel pain. The result is a situation where the user feels extraordinary strength and immunity to pain. Police have reported high-dose PCP users breaking out of steel handcuffs, failing to stop an attack even though shot several times, coming forward and attacking police, or bleeding to death because of an inability to feel the injury inflicted during an attack. Despite several hundred reports of incidents like these, in relation to the millions who use this drug, they are considered rare.

More common adverse reactions include the following:

- Paranoia
- Severe agitation
- A severe withdrawn or isolated feeling
- Bizarre delusions
- Increases in heart rate, blood pressure
- Sweating, salivation, and flushing of the skin (these increase according to the dose)
- Nystagmus (jerky eye movements) and other reactions

PCP is unsafe to use during pregnancy, though the exact potential for damage to the fetus is unknown. PCP may also interfere with the hormones governing normal growth and development in the adolescent user. The principal proven negative effects on youthful users, however, relate to a decreased learning capacity, difficulty in concentration, poor grades, and poor social adjustment.

Unpredictable episodes of panic may occur. Latent psychopathology may be unmasked or triggered either by acute doses or by patterns of chronic use, as evidenced by episodes of violence, paranoia, and so forth. With prolonged regular PCP use, the effects can linger after the intoxication has worn off, necessitating therapy or rehabilitation. Flashbacks are also reported from prolonged PCP use. With very large doses, convulsions or coma may occur.

Several PCP deaths have been due to the direct effects of the drug. Other deaths have been attributed to PCP combined with other drugs, particularly central nervous system depressants. As mentioned earlier, deaths are more frequently due to accidental causes while under the influence.

Tolerance and Dependence

PCP does not appear to be physically addictive, even though some tolerance does develop in regular users. When used orally, PCP is most often used only occasionally. When smoked, it is very often used more frequently and can create a very strong psychological dependence. Few data substantiate a withdrawal syndrome with PCP, though the drug often produces aftereffects lasting many months after use is discontinued. One of these aftereffects is depression, which can last up to a year; if untreated, it can lead to relapse and suicide.

✖ Athletes and Drugs

Athletes have been using drugs to enhance their performance since ancient times. The use of drugs by athletes is almost as old as the Olympic games themselves.

In the marathon event of the 1904 Olympic games in St. Louis, Missouri, the winning runner was American Thomas Hicks, who was aided by a heady cocktail of brandy and strychnine (a stimulant at low doses, a poison at high doses). Today, more than 50 psychomotor stimulant drugs are banned from use during an Olympic competition.

Caffeine

Comedian George Carlin once described coffee as "the low end of the speed spectrum." The International Olympic Committee found that this joke contains a grain of truth. After high concentrations of caffeine were found in several competitors' urine during the 1976 summer Olympic games, studies were conducted to see if caffeine affects athletic performance.

Controlled studies involved both athletes and nonathletes using cycle ergometers. Results showed that the caffeine present in two and a half cups of coffee is sufficient to increase endurance, as measured by maximal oxygen consumption when cycling to exhaustion. A further study involving five young athletes concluded that small doses of caffeine significantly increase the power of leg muscle contractions. The enhancement, however, is limited to endurance athletes. Caffeine does not significantly improve performance during maximal short-term bursts of exercise (Lombardo 1990).

Based on this information and other reports, the International Olympic Committee banned caffeine in amounts greater than 12 ug-ml. An average of four cups of coffee could produce this level.

Caffeine is also produced synthetically, used in some pain-killing preparations, and sold over the counter in diet preparations and caffeine tablets.

The adverse effects of caffeine are mainly dose-related. Depending on the individual's sensitivity, symptoms may include headaches, tremors, nausea, and irregular heartbeat, especially in the 200- to 500-milligram dose range.

A particular effect that may have significance to athletes is the increase in urine output. This might not only increase the number of involuntary bathroom stops during an endurance event but also have potential implications for the athletes' hydration status.

Caffeinism is now a recognized entity. People have gone to emergency rooms complaining of heart palpitations, restlessness, anxiety, insomnia, and myriad other symptoms directly attributable to their high caffeine intake. People who consume significant amounts of coffee daily and then taper off too rapidly suffer from caffeine abstinence syndrome. Withdrawal symptoms include headaches, drowsiness, lethargy, irritability, and depression.

The relationship between caffeine consumption and athletic performance has been studied extensively. Although small doses of caffeine increase endurance, there are adverse effects (e.g., dehydration) on athletic performance.

Chewing Tobacco

Epidemiologically, the percentage of smokers among athletes in the United States has declined, along with the decreasing trend in the general population. The use of chewing tobacco, however, remains inordinately high among athletes. Part of this can certainly be ascribed to new marketing and promotion campaigns by the tobacco companies, as well as the almost mythic, traditional relationship of "chewing" tobacco to the great American pastime of baseball. Ironically, the original baseball cards advertised tobacco. Long ago, politicians recognized the health hazards and declared chewing and spitting tobacco illegal in most places—except the baseball park.

From 1978 to 1985, celebrity athletes promoted chewing tobacco. Free supply programs and heavy advertising at sporting events stimulated the sale of chewing tobacco. As a result, chewing tobacco saw a 55 percent rise in sales at a time when cigarette sales dropped off. In 1970, men 55 and older were the heaviest users of chewing tobacco. By

America's favorite pastime: baseball. Players still chew tobacco.

Bettmann Archive.

1985, males under the age of 20 displaced them. Smokeless tobacco, a marketing label for chewing tobacco, is used by kindergarten children in Arkansas and Alaska; in Texas, reportedly, up to one-third of varsity football and baseball players use smokeless tobacco (Lombardo 1985).

Many people have been misled into thinking that smokeless tobacco is a safe alternative to smoking. The surgeon general's *Report on the Health Consequences of Smokeless Tobacco Use* concluded that smokeless tobacco is causally related to oral cancer and gum recession, that it can lead to dependence on nicotine, and that it is not a safe alternative to cigarettes (U.S. Surgeon General 1988).

Nonetheless, some athletes use nicotine products for their perceived stimulating effect before their events, while others paradoxically use the tobacco for its calming effect. Still others state they use nicotine for its effect on the satiety center ("I'll gain weight if I stop smoking"). Some just use tobacco products for personal rather than performance reasons.

Regarding the widely held misconception that smokeless tobacco enhances performance, it is critical to make known that nicotine does not heighten energy or strength. In reality, the user who smokes, chews, or snorts nicotine is simply experiencing elevation in heart rate and blood pressure. The perceived relaxation is actually relief from the craving associated with nicotine withdrawal.

Clearly, young people will continue chewing smokeless tobacco unless professional athletes, coaches, and managers act as role models and point out the negative effects of all tobacco products.

Amphetamines

The first widespread abuse of drugs in professional sports occurred in the late 1960s and early 1970s, when professional football players used amphetamines. Mandell (1979) reported this as a so-called Sunday syndrome of amphetamine use to enhance performance. However, athletes in many other sports—notably, those involved in endurance events—also have used amphetamines.

Amphetamines have an appetite-suppression effect attractive to a variety of athletes for whom making and keeping a required weight is essential (e.g., jockeys, gymnasts, wrestlers, and boxers). Numerous studies have attempted to document the effects of amphetamines on performance. Some have looked at psychomotor tasks, others have examined certain variables related to overall performance, and still others have studied athletic performance (Derlet and Heischober 1990).

Smith and Beecher (1959) reported that approximately 75 percent of trained swimmers, weight lifters, and runners showed improvements in performance after administration of amphetamines. However, Karpovich (1969) found improvement in only 3 of 20 athletes, and 1 athlete actually performed more poorly. A review in 1981, using criteria based on knee-extension strength and running to exhaustion, showed that performance usually improved by only a small percentage. However, in highly competitive sports, even a 1 percent improvement can mean the difference between victory and defeat.

Most people also would probably agree that the alertness of the fatigued person, whether an athlete, a truck driver, a student, or a subject of an experiment, increases with the use of amphetamines. However, Chandler and Blair concluded in

1980 that "amphetamines do not prevent fatigue but rather mask the effects of fatigue and interfere with the body's fatigue-alarm system which could lead to disastrous results, especially under extreme environmental conditions."

Deaths caused by amphetamine use have involved cerebral vascular accidents (strokes) secondary to hemorrhages in the brain, acute heart failure with arrhythmias, and hyperthermia. The elevation of body temperature, if not fatal, can combine with heat exhaustion and circulatory collapse to cause heat stroke, because amphetamines obscure the athlete's normally protective physiologic fatigue level.

By diminishing pain thresholds, amphetamines allow athletes to continue to compete despite injury, thus potentially causing more tissue damage to the injured areas. Finally, there is an added potential for injury to others in contact sports because of the increase in aggressiveness caused by amphetamine use.

Steroids

All of the previously described drugs used in sports and athletics can be labeled *ergogenic* because they are performance-enhancing substances. By far, the most controversial ergogenic drug used by many athletes—especially young, developing boys and girls—is steroids.

Brief History

Steroids were developed in the 1930s for the treatment of anemia and a variety of diseases that wasted away muscles. Physicians have also used steroids to treat cancer, burn victims, intestinal problems, asthma, and emaciation. After World War II, steroid use restored body tissue to victims of starvation. The increased aggressiveness caused by steroid use was one of the benefits sought by German soldiers in World War II.

In 1988, Canadian sprinter Ben Johnson lost the gold medals he won in the Olympic games because he tested positive for steroids. Today, steroid use is not only a problem with world-class Olympic athletes but also with teenagers. Steroid use became the adolescent rage of the 1990s. Studies indicate that 6 to 10 percent of high school boys will use steroids by graduation, as will 1 percent of girls. Unfortunately, two-thirds of these young people will start to use steroids prior to the age of 16. Most young people who use steroids do so to enhance their performance in sports, yet a surprisingly large percentage (25 percent) use steroids for appearance. The skinny boy on the beach who gets sand kicked in his face no longer chooses the old Charles Atlas weight-training program to bulk up. Instead, steroid use with weight training and diet create the hulking bodies that young men desire. Beefing up and strengthening their bodies give these young people added self-confidence because they feel attractive (Hough 1988).

Steroids are illegal without a prescription. Federal officials estimate the illicit steroid market at $400 million.

Terminology

Androgenic steroids, which include testosterone, primarily develop and maintain male sex characteristics. So-called **anabolic** steroids are synthetic derivatives of testosterone developed in an attempt to minimize testosterone's androgenic or masculinizing effects on the individual while promoting protein synthesis and muscular growth.

Because none of these compounds is purely anabolic or purely androgenic in their effects, and since athletes usually stack, or use the steroids in combination, technically the more correct designation is "anabolic-androgenic steroids (A-AS)" rather than just anabolic steroids (AS).

Major Effects

Many of the early studies regarding the effectiveness of steroids produced conflicting results. More recent studies have clearly indicated significant increases in strength as a result of steroid use. The American College of Sports Medicine in its position statement on steroids in 1989 concluded that "gains in strength can occur through a variety of mechanisms in the highly trained athlete who takes steroids."

Increases in lean body mass do occur in A-AS steroid use. In the past, this was thought to be the result of water retention. It is now clear that there is an actual increase in muscle tissue and enhancement of muscle contractility. In addition, some reports cite an increase in actual bone density. However, most of these changes do not increase strength unless their use is combined with high-intensity weight training and a properly balanced diet.

Anabolic-androgenic steroids also increase the ability to perform high-intensity training sessions. In part, this is due to increased protein metabolism as well as the inhibition of the metabolic (breaking down) effects of corticosteroids, which are released in increased amounts whenever the body is stressed. The result is that the body requires less recuperation time between intensive workouts to repair itself. However, most studies have also shown that aerobic capacity is not affected or improved at all with steroid use.

Adverse Effects

The problem with steroids is that they do not act exclusively on one muscle or tissue group. Therefore, they stimulate all muscles and tissues, making the individual at risk for other adverse effects. The body's homeostasis is disrupted with the use of steroids, causing a variety of physical problems. "Heart disease will probably be the most widely noted side effect with anabolic steroid abuse. Blood pressure elevates significantly when an individual takes anabolic steroids due to the retained fluid and increased blood volume. . . . High Density Lipoproteins (HDL-C) that aid the body in removing cholesterol, and are important to cardiac longevity, are drastically reduced with the use of androgens" (American Osteopathic Academy of Sports Medicine 1989).

For adolescents, the drug can cause stunted growth and the premature closing of growth plates. Other problems resulting from steroid abuse by men include the following:

- Liver and kidney damage
- Breast development
- Acne, baldness

- Cysts
- Shrinking of the testicles and sterility
- Reduced sex drive
- Headaches, nausea, and dizziness

For women the drug can cause the following:

- Infertility
- Clitoral enlargement
- Breast atrophy
- Menstrual irregularities
- Male pattern baldness and voice change

More and more evidence is accruing that the most significant effect of A-AS use may be psychiatric. Psychological reactions such as extreme aggressiveness, mood swings, depression, and delusions are reported in some individuals. Signs and symptoms similar to drug and alcohol dependence (e.g., loss of control; continued use despite known adverse consequences, tolerance, and withdrawal) suggest that both physical and psychological dependence can occur with A-AS use.

Other Drugs/Alcohol in Sports

The pressures of professional athletic competition and the accompanying lifestyle can create a situation in which athletes seek both relief and the enhancement of performance by using alcohol or other drugs. Many high school, college, and even professional athletes are ill prepared for these pressures.

The widespread use of cocaine, marijuana, alcohol, amphetamines, and other drugs in professional sports came to the attention of the general public in the drug scandals of the past three decades. This was an indicator of the high level of denial and enabling behavior by players, coaches, and management. Today, teams are making more concerted efforts at education, assessment, and treatment. They have programs that help athletes develop the skills to deal with the pressures. However, alcohol/drug problems are still enabled and/or denied at many levels of athletic competition. Additional efforts are needed to resolve the issue of alcohol/drug abuse and addiction at all levels of athletic endeavor.

References

American Osteopathic Academy of Sports Medicine. 1989.

American Psychiatric Association. 1994. *Diagnostic and statistical manual of mental disorders.* 4th ed. Washington, D.C.: Author.

Ashton, C. H. 1990. Solvent abuse: Little progress after 20 years. *British Medical Journal* 300: 135–38.

Chandler, J. V., and S. N. Blair. 1980. The effect of amphetamines on selected physiological components related to athletic success. *Medicine and Science in Sports and Exercise* 12:65–69.

Cohen, S. 1986. Marijuana research: Selected recent findings. *Drug and Alcohol Newsletter, Vista Hill Foundation* 15(1).

CSAT advisory: Breaking news for the treatment field: Oxycontin. 2001. *Prescription Drug Abuse* 1(1).

Derlet, R., and B. Heischober. 1990. Methamphetamine: Stimulant of the 1990s. *Western Journal of Medicine* (December): 153(6): 625–28.

Holland, Julie, ed. 2001. *Ecstasy: The complete guide: A comprehensive look at the risks and benefits of MDMA.* Rochester, VT.: Park Street Press.

Hough, D. 1988. Anabolic steroids and ergogenic aids. *Academy of Family Practice* 41: 1157–64.

Karpovich, P. V. 1969. Effect of amphetamine sulfate on athletic performance. *Journal of American Medical Association* 170.

Lombardo, J. 1990. Stimulants and athletic performance. Amphetamine and caffeine. *Physician and Sports Medicine* 4: 1157–64.

Mandell, A. J. 1979. The Sunday syndrome: A unique pattern of amphetamine abuse indigenous to American professional football. *Clinical Toxicology* 15(2): 225–232.

National Institute on Drug Abuse [NIDA]. 1989. *Drug use among American high school students, college students, and other young adults. National trends through 1988.* Rockville, MD: Author.

National Institute on Drug Abuse [NIDA]. 1995. *1994 National Household Survey on Drug Abuse.* Advance Report No. 10. Washington, D.C.: Author.

National Institute on Drug Abuse [NIDA]. 1998. *Community drug alert bulletin.* Rockville, MD: Author.

National Institute on Drug Abuse [NIDA]. 2001. *The National Household Survey on Drug Abuse: Cigar use.* Washington, D.C.: Author.

Rohr, V. 1989. Withdrawal sequelae to cannabis use. *International Journal of the Addictions* 24: 627–31.

Smith, David, and Donald Wesson. 1988. *Treating cocaine dependence.* Center City, MN: Hazeldon Foundation.

Smith, G. M., and H. G. Beecher. 1959. Amphetamine sulfate and athletic performance. *Journal of American Medical Association* 170(5): 542–557.

Solomons, K., and V. M. Neppe. 1989. Review article: Cannabis: Its clinical effects. *South American Medical Journal* 78: 476–481.

Sporer, Karl A. 2000. Acute heroin overdose. In *Heroin overdose: Research and interventions.* San Francisco: Linden Center.

Tamura, M. 1989. Japan: Stimulant epidemics, past and present. *Bulletin on Narcotics* 1: 83–93.

Thombs, D. 1989. A review of PCP abuse, trends, and perceptions. *Public Health Reports* 104(4): 325–28.

U.S. Surgeon General. 1988. *The health consequences of smoking: Nicotine addiction.* Rockville, MD: U.S. Dept. Health and Human Services.

Woods, James H., et al. 1988. Use and abuse of benzodiazepines. *Journal of the American Medical Association* 260(23): 3476–3480.

Screening and Assessment of Alcohol/Drug Problems

❖ Chapter in Review

The behavioral definition of addiction is expressed by the 3Cs mnemonic defined in this chapter as:
1. Compulsion
2. Control (inability)
3. Continued use despite negative Consequences.

The stages of drug use are non-use, initial contact, experimentation, integrated use, excessive (continuous and periodic) use, and addiction. There are different types of alcoholics, as outlined by Jellinek.

The *Diagnostic and Statistical Manual of Mental Disorders* (APA 2000) establishes standards for assessing mental disorders and substance-related disorders. The major substance-related disorders are substance dependence, substance abuse, substance-induced withdrawal, and substance-induced intoxication. All four of these disorders are described by their diagnostic criteria.

The topics of relapse, family disease, adolescent alcohol/drug assessment are also described. Assessment involves not only taking a good alcohol/drug history, but also assessing the individual's vulnerability to alcohol/drugs, the consequences of alcohol/drug use, and the person's suicide potential.

Denial is the major defense, due to users' minimization and rationalization of their level of involvement with alcohol/drugs.

A variety of alcohol/drug screening inventories are available for review in this chapter.

The most difficult assessment question is differentiating those individuals who fall in the gray area between occasional, or nonproblematic, use of alcohol/drugs and those who use excessively and/or have an alcohol/drug problem. Assessment is also complicated by the fact that people strongly deny problems with alcohol and drugs. Individual, family, and societal perceptions of alcohol/drugs are distorted by this denial system.

This chapter defines addiction and describes the stages of alcohol/drug use (Figure 4.1) and stages of recovery. The major goal of this chapter is to help the reader develop a more focused perception of chemical dependency.

❖ Definition of Addiction

In the early 1980s, the rise in cocaine use challenged the basic framework of our definition of alcohol/drug addiction. Cocaine was previously thought to be a drug that incurred psychological dependence with no physical dependence. At that time, we defined addiction as a physical dependence measured by a significant and noticeable medical withdrawal symptom. Although cocaine had no significant medically noticeable withdrawal symptoms, users reported a severe addiction to it. David

The names and circumstances of case studies in this chapter have been changed to maintain anonymity.

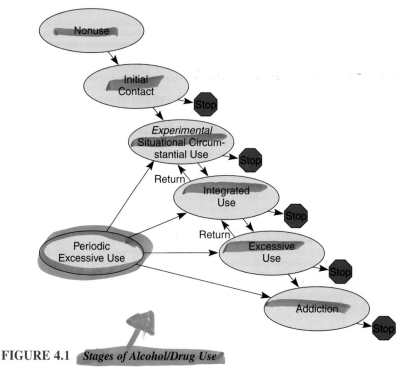

FIGURE 4.1   *Stages of Alcohol/Drug Use*

Richard Fields Ph.D. 1986, revised, 1988.

Smith (Smith and Wesson 1988) was aware of this discrepancy and proposed a more behavioral definition of addiction. Because this definition is more functional, counselors in the fields of chemical dependency treatment and addictionology use it. In fact, counselors can apply this behavioral definition of addiction to a wide variety of types of disorders, including eating, gambling, sex, workaholism, television, smoking, video games, spending/consumerism, and other activities.

Alcoholism and drug addiction are best described metaphorically as "the dragon in the corner, eating its own tail."

The three basic components of the behavioral definition of addiction are the three Cs—*compulsion, control,* and *consequences.*

1. **Obsessive-compulsive behavior** with alcohol/drugs. Users think about alcohol and drugs in a vicious negative cycle; their obsessive concern and preoccupation follow an incessant use of alcohol/drugs in a continuous pattern and compulsive lifestyle.
2. **Inability to stop** using the substances. Users cannot stop using alcohol/drugs for at least three months and/or make feeble attempts to cut back in a stop-then-start pattern. They are unable to refuse readily available drugs.
3. **Continued use despite adverse consequences.** Users are caught up in their addictions, illustrating the pervasive defense mechanisms of denial (rationalization and minimization). Eventually, the alcoholic/addict suffers family, social and interpersonal, economic, and spiritual bankruptcy.

Defining addiction is a challenge; however, defining the stages and patterns of alcohol/drug use that precede addiction is even more challenging.

❄ Stages of Alcohol and Drug Use

Nonuse of Alcohol/Drugs by Children

The most successful preventive approach is not to use drugs and alcohol, especially at early ages. Not smoking cigarettes at early ages highly correlates with not developing addictions later in life. Children are less likely to develop chemical dependencies later in life, if parents

1. Do not model alcohol/drug use and encourage a healthy approach to life
2. Encourage children to participate in activities that enhance the development of a strong sense of self
3. Promote positive alternative activities to alcohol/drug use (see prevention chapter)
4. Are sensitive to what children feel while parents are setting appropriate boundaries
5. Provide structure, discipline, and consistency
6. Develop a climate of discussion, which facilitates an effective exploration of values and the development of coping skills in goal setting, decision making, and conflict resolution

Parents can establish nonuse of drugs and alcohol by teaching children to make positive lifestyle choices that they can maintain throughout adult life. Although the drive or desire to alter one's consciousness is innate, learning to alter one's consciousness with alternatives other than chemicals is a developmental task of childhood. Children can be encouraged to be more active in choosing things to do that change their mood and develop their sense of self, instead of choosing a passive solution, the use of alcohol/drugs.

Nonuse of Alcohol/Drugs by Adolescents

Some young people are able to use alcohol and drugs and not suffer any significant problems. For others, especially those who have family histories of alcoholism and drug addiction, such a trial could be the beginning of a lifelong pattern of addiction.

To help their at-risk adolescents, parents should

1. Establish clear, consistent guidelines and rules regarding alcohol/drugs
2. Model nonuse of alcohol/drugs
3. Establish clear, consistent communication of the hazards and potential harm of alcohol/drugs, especially at early ages of adolescence
4. Encourage the development of alternative activities to alleviate feelings of boredom, depression, and isolation and to promote the development of a strong sense of self
5. Promote active involvement in school, athletics, social situations, church, and other activities
6. Encourage active development of skills and talents
7. Promote trust and establish healthy boundaries in relationships

8. Support adolescents in their perseverance through their developmental tasks of identity and individuation

Initial Contact with Alcohol/Drugs

The initial contact stage is defined as the first time one tries alcohol/drugs. Usually, this stage is thought to be relatively harmless, yet there are potential hazards from initial contact, such as the following:

- Anaphylactic (allergic) reactions, which can cause death
- Toxic and lethal doses
- Loss of control and emotional overreactions
- Physical and psychological problems
- Accidents and/or dangerous situations

The three major components of alcohol and drug use are the individual, the drug, and the set and setting in which the drug is taken. Set and setting often determine the individual's reaction to alcohol/drugs.

As mentioned in an earlier chapter, **set** refers to the psychological and emotional frame of mind of a person when using alcohol/drugs. Those who are relaxed, comfortable, and secure in the knowledge that they can handle possibly losing control usually have less trouble with the initial use of alcohol/drugs. Individuals who have a set that can be described as anxious, extremely nervous, or overly concerned with maintaining control are more prone to a negative drug reaction. If a person is not emotionally stable and/or has psychiatric problems, alcohol/drug use can exacerbate those problems. (See Chapter 10.) This is especially true for hallucinogens and marijuana. Set can also be influenced by the person's mood or emotional state at the time of alcohol/drug use. The individual who has just received some bad news or has had a negative experience might be feeling down or depressed; this may result in a negative set and a negative experience with alcohol/drugs. Significant trauma, shame, and embarrassment can also contribute to a negative experience with alcohol/drugs.

Setting involves not only the physical environment but also the social and interpersonal environment. Negative drug reactions may be the result of being in an uncomfortable setting, with unknown people who are not trusted.

Alcohol/Drug Use—A Progressive Disease

Certainly, the beginning of alcohol/drug use starts with initial contact. Because alcohol/drug use is a progressive disease, individuals get more involved as they progress through the stages. A positive initial contact usually leads to the next stage of drug use—experimentation. Experimentation may lead to the subsequent stages, which end in addiction. Richard Rawson (1989) has written about his outpatient treatment of cocaine addicts. He describes the progressive themes at various stages of cocaine addiction, as shown in Table 4.1. These descriptions can easily be adapted to alcohol and other drugs and illustrate the progressive nature of addiction.

As was stated earlier, a positive initial contact may be the beginning of a progressive cycle to addiction. This is especially true for those who grew up in alcoholic/addict and/or dysfunctional family systems.

TABLE 4.1

Phases of Cocaine Addiction

Initial contact	"Isn't this a great drug?"
Experimentation	"It's sure expensive, but it's worth it."
Excessive use	"I really should cut down."
Addiction	"I know I have to stop, but I can't."

Source: Rawson 1989.

Experimentation

Experimentation is the stage of using alcohol/drugs in different situations and circumstances. People explore and experiment with a drug, testing their own capacity to use alcohol/drugs in different situations and circumstances. Users learn about alcohol/drugs by experimenting with various doses, frequencies of use, methods of ingestion, and sometimes combinations (polydrug use). Each individual's reaction to a drug is also affected by physiological, psychological, and emotional factors. Some factors include not eating prior to use, fatigue, and levels of physical and emotional well-being. During experimentation, individuals change and adjust the drug, the set, and the setting and then determine their reaction.

Experimenters use drugs during this stage in different settings, with different people, and in different frames of mind, or set. A triangular relationship exists among the individual (set), the drug, and the environment (setting). During the experimentation stage, the user adjusts the three elements of this equation to determine the drug's effect.

Many systems that classify the stages of alcohol/drug use often call the experimental stage a *recreational* or *social use* stage. These terms tend to put alcohol/drugs in a more positive, emotion-laden frame of reference. The implication of the term *recreational* is that alcohol/drug use is no more than harmless recreational/social fun. This view overlooks the potential hazards and problems that may occur.

Parental guidelines during the experimental stage should include the following:

1. Talking with other parents and exchanging information about their children's behavior in the neighborhood, at neighboring homes, at school, or in the general community
2. Knowing where children are and who their friends are, as well as meeting the parents of their friends
3. Developing initiative, responsibility, and appropriate consequences for behavior
4. Evaluating the dynamics of the family and seeking professional help for early alcohol/drug educational advice and assessment
5. Being aware that a child is at-risk and seeking family counseling for alcohol/drug education, prevention, and treatment if there is a history of alcohol/drug problems in the family

Table 4.2 lists typical personality traits of adolescents who are frequent users or abstainers, compared to adolescents who are experimenters.

TABLE 4.2

Adolescent Personality Traits: Frequent Users and Abstainers Compared to Experimenters

Frequent Users (compared to experimenters)
- Not dependable or responsible
- Guileful and deceitful
- Opportunistic
- Unpredictable, unchangeable in attitudes and behavior
- Unable to delay gratification
- Rebellious and nonconforming
- Prone to push and stretch limits
- Self-indulgent
- Not ethically consistent
- Not having high aspirations
- Prone to express hostile feelings directly

Abstainers (compared to experimenters)
- Fastidious
- Conservative
- Proud of being "objective" and rational
- Overcontrolled and prone to delay gratification unnecessarily
- Not liked or accepted by people
- Moralistic
- Unexpressive
- Prone to avoid close interpersonal relationships
- Predictable in attitudes and behavior
- Not gregarious
- Not able to enjoy sensuous experiences
- Basically anxious
- Not straightforward and forthright with others
- Not physically attractive
- Not personally charming
- Not socially at ease

Source: Shedler and Block 1990.

Integrated Use

At the integrated stage of alcohol/drug use, the person spends more time, thought, and energy in the use of alcohol/drugs. It has become an integrated part of the individual's life. Whether adolescent or adult, the person begins to associate with others who use the same drug. At parties, the marijuana smokers congregate, the alcohol users belly up to the bar, and the polydrug users are the life of the party, drinking at the bar and smoking dope in the backyard.

The individual at the integrated stage buys the drug to make sure that the drug is available. For example, at this stage a person must have the alcohol/drug available when away from home for a vacation or a business trip. Obviously, alcohol/drugs are well integrated into the user's style of life.

Excessive Use

Even for experts, the excessive use stage is difficult to describe because there are different kinds of excessive use. Some people call this stage drug abuse; however, drug abuse is very arbitrary, emotion-laden, and difficult to define. The second Commission on Marijuana (1973) found that the term *drug abuse* had "no functional utility" and "had become no more than an arbitrary code word for that drug use which is presently considered wrong." The commission concluded that the facts of actual drug use are often not distinguished from feelings and opinions. The commission recommended that the term *drug abuse* be discontinued because of the emotion-laden, subjective interpretation of the term.

Excessive use is an increase in alcohol/drug use that results in significant problems or negative consequences. Users are putting increased time, thought, and energy into buying—perhaps selling—and using alcohol/drugs.

Some people use alcohol/drugs excessively in a periodic pattern, sometimes in the form of binges, which are excessive drug use within a period of 24 to 72 hours. Periodic excessive alcohol/drug use can occur just on weekends, every other week, once in a month, or even as infrequently as once every 3 months. When all the criteria for addiction are met, periodic excessive use is also defined as addiction.

Addiction

Addiction is the last stage. Based on our definition of addiction and the disease model, an addict cannot return to any of the previous stages of alcohol/drug use. The best recovery strategy is to abstain from alcohol/drug use and to participate in a 12-step recovery program. This usually involves an inpatient program; strong development in self-help support groups, such as Alcoholics Anonymous, Narcotics Anonymous, and Cocaine Anonymous; a relationship with a sponsor; and an aftercare treatment program on completion of the inpatient program. (See Chapter 11.)

Chronic alcoholics and drug addicts spend major portions of their lives addicted to alcohol/drugs. In this late stage of chronic addiction, they are extremely difficult to treat. (See Table 4.3.) Some new approaches are required for this population. Such programs provide basic needs for shelter, food, other health-related services, and educational and counseling services. These programs for chronic alcoholics have an emphasis on maintaining the individual's dignity while providing access to recovery services.

TABLE 4.3

Early and Late Stages of Alcohol/Drug Use

Early Stage	Late Stage
More freedom	Lack of freedom
Fewer risks and less damage	More damage
Possible abuse	Present abuse
No illness	State of illness
Linear operating factors	Vicious cycles

An alcoholic's arm sinking into a glass of booze.

AP/Wide World Photos.

✖ Jellinek's Types of Alcoholics

E. M. Jellinek (1960) believed that persons with certain types of alcoholism suffer through declining stages of functioning. He described five distinct types of alcoholism:

1. Alpha alcoholism: psychological dependence, in which alcoholics use drinking increasingly to help with their problems
2. Beta alcoholism
   a. Physical problems, such as cirrhosis of the liver or stomach problems, resulting from the consumption of alcohol
   b. No physical or psychological dependence
3. Gamma alcoholism
   a. Physical addiction, with withdrawal symptoms occurring whenever drinking is stopped
   b. Loss of control to regulate alcohol use
   c. Severe damage to health, financial, social, and interpersonal functioning
   d. Periods of abstinence (going on the wagon)

The alcoholic's life is limited, with significant negative consequences, as if he or she "is trapped in a shot glass."

AP/Wide World Photos.

4. Delta alcoholism
   a. Similar to gamma; however, the individual can control intake in given situations
   b. High degree of physical and psychological dependence, making abstinence, even for brief periods, impossible
5. Epsilon alcoholism: periodic, unpredictable drinking binges

TABLE 4.4

Stages of Recovery

Stage	Time Course*
Withdrawal	0–15 days
Honeymoon	15–45 days
The Wall	45–120 days
Adjustment	120–180 days
Resolution	180–360 days

From Richard Rawson et al., "Neurobehavioral treatment for cocaine dependency" in *Journal of Psychoactive Drugs* 22 (2): 159–71. Haight-Ashbury Publications, San Francisco, CA. Reprinted by permission.

*These generalized categories are rough estimates for periods of time when alcohol/drugs are not used. The actual time course for each stage of recovery may be quite different for each individual and alcohol or drug used.

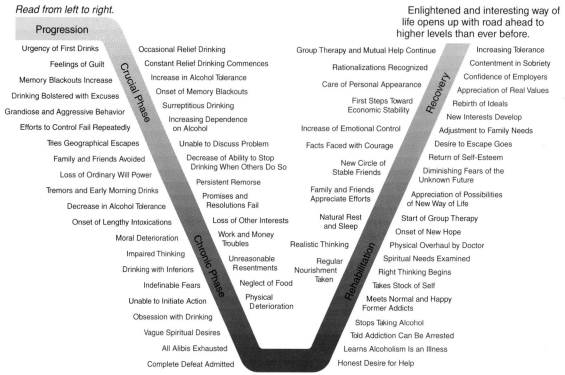

Read from left to right.

Progression

Urgency of First Drinks
Feelings of Guilt
Memory Blackouts Increase
Drinking Bolstered with Excuses
Grandiose and Aggressive Behavior
Efforts to Control Fail Repeatedly
Tries Geographical Escapes
Family and Friends Avoided
Loss of Ordinary Will Power
Tremors and Early Morning Drinks
Decrease in Alcohol Tolerance
Onset of Lengthy Intoxications
Moral Deterioration
Impaired Thinking
Drinking with Inferiors
Indefinable Fears
Unable to Initiate Action
Obsession with Drinking
Vague Spiritual Desires
All Alibis Exhausted
Complete Defeat Admitted

Crucial Phase

Occasional Relief Drinking
Constant Relief Drinking Commences
Increase in Alcohol Tolerance
Onset of Memory Blackouts
Surreptitious Drinking
Increasing Dependence on Alcohol
Unable to Discuss Problem
Decrease of Ability to Stop Drinking When Others Do So
Persistent Remorse
Promises and Resolutions Fail
Loss of Other Interests
Work and Money Troubles
Unreasonable Resentments
Neglect of Food
Physical Deterioration

Chronic Phase

Enlightened and interesting way of life opens up with road ahead to higher levels than ever before.

Group Therapy and Mutual Help Continue
Rationalizations Recognized
Care of Personal Appearance
First Steps Toward Economic Stability
Increase of Emotional Control
Facts Faced with Courage
New Circle of Stable Friends
Family and Friends Appreciate Efforts
Natural Rest and Sleep
Realistic Thinking
Regular Nourishment Taken

Recovery

Increasing Tolerance
Contentment in Sobriety
Confidence of Employers
Appreciation of Real Values
Rebirth of Ideals
New Interests Develop
Adjustment to Family Needs
Desire to Escape Goes
Return of Self-Esteem
Diminishing Fears of the Unknown Future
Appreciation of Possibilities of New Way of Life
Start of Group Therapy
Onset of New Hope
Physical Overhaul by Doctor
Spiritual Needs Examined
Right Thinking Begins
Takes Stock of Self
Meets Normal and Happy Former Addicts
Stops Taking Alcohol
Told Addiction Can Be Arrested
Learns Alcoholism Is an Illness
Honest Desire for Help

Rehabilitation

Obsessive drinking continues.

FIGURE 4.2   *Progression and Recovery of the Alcoholic in the Disease of Alcoholism*

From *Understanding Personality Problems and Addictions and Understanding Mood Disorders and Addictions,* 1993, Hazelden Foundation, Center City, MN.

Once an alcohol/drug problem is identified, the next step is recovery (Figures 4.2 and 4.3). Richard Rawson (1989) described a model for the stages of cocaine recovery, as seen in Table 4.4. This model also applies to alcohol or other drugs, although the time periods for each stage can be different and variable. Each stage of recovery is fully explained in Chapter 11.

✖ Diagnostic Categories

The *Diagnostic and Statistical Manual of Mental Disorders,* 4th edition, text revision (*DSM-IV-TR*) (American Psychiatric Association [APA] 2000) is a major reference used by mental health practitioners to diagnose both mental disorders and substance-related disorders.

The substance-related disorders are divided into two major categories:

1. *Substance use disorders.* These include substance dependence and substance abuse.
2. *Substance-induced disorders.* These include substance intoxication and substance withdrawal.

The *DSM-IV-TR* also describes substance-induced mental disorders (see Chapter 10 of this textbook).

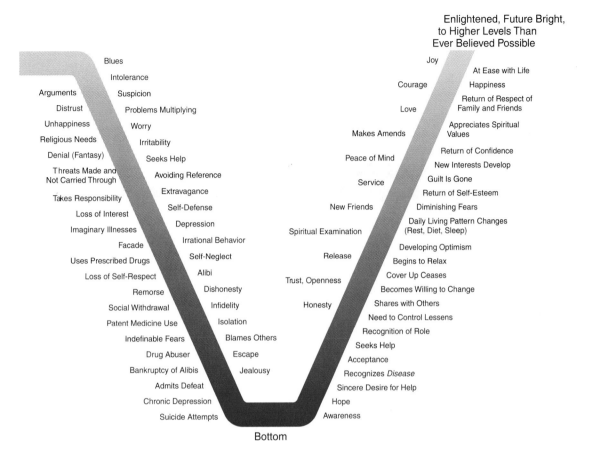

FIGURE 4.3   *Progression and Recovery of the Family Members in the Disease of Alcoholism*   The progression and recovery symptoms listed are based on the most repeated experiences of family members in the disease of alcoholism or other chemical dependencies. While not every symptom in the chart occurs in every member of every family, or in the same sequence, it does portray an average chain reaction. The entire process may take years, or it may occur in a very short time.

From *Understanding Personality and Addictions and Understanding Mood Disorders and Addictions,* 1993, Hazelden Foundation, Center City, MN.

Substance Abuse

Substance abuse is described by the following diagnostic criteria in the *DSM-IV-TR* (APA 2000):

A. A maladaptive pattern of substance use, leading to clinically significant impairment or distress, as manifested by one (or more) of the following, occurring within a 12-month period
   1. Recurrent substance use, resulting in a failure to fulfill major role obligations at work, school, or home (e.g., repeated absences or poor work performance related to substance use; substance-related absences, suspensions, or expulsions from school; neglect of children or household)
   2. Recurrent substance use in situations in which it is physically hazardous (e.g., driving an automobile or operating a machine when impaired by substance use)

3. Recurrent substance-related legal problems (e.g., arrests for substance-related disorderly conduct)
4. Continued substance use despite having persistent or recurrent social or interpersonal problems caused or exacerbated by the effects of the substance (e.g., arguments with spouse about consequences of intoxication, physical fights)

B. The symptoms have never met the criteria for substance dependence for this class of substances.

Substance Dependence

Substance dependence is described by the following diagnostic criteria in the *DSM-IV-TR* (APA 2000):

A maladaptive pattern of substance use, leading to clinically significant impairment or distress, as manifested by three (or more) of the following, occurring at any time in the same 12-month period:

1. Tolerance, as defined by either of the following:
   a. A need for markedly increased amounts of the substance to achieve intoxication or desired effect
   b. Markedly diminished effect with continued use of the same amount of the substance
2. Withdrawal, as manifested by either of the following:
   a. The characteristic withdrawal syndrome for the substance
   b. The same (or a closely related) substance is taken to relieve or avoid withdrawal symptoms.
3. The substance is often taken in larger amounts or over a longer period than was intended.
4. There is a persistent desire or unsuccessful efforts to cut down or control substance use.
5. A great deal of time is spent in activities necessary to obtain the substance (e.g., visiting multiple doctors or driving long distances), use the substance (e.g., chain-smoking), or recover from its effects.
6. Important social, occupational, or recreational activities are given up or reduced because of substance use.
7. The substance use is continued despite knowledge of having a persistent or recurrent physical or psychological problem that is likely to have been caused or exacerbated by the substance (e.g., current cocaine use despite recognition of cocaine-induced depression, or continued drinking despite recognition that an ulcer was made worse by alcohol consumption).

Substance Withdrawal

Substance withdrawal is described by the following diagnostic criteria (APA 2000):

A. The development of substance-specific syndrome due to the cessation of (or reduction in) substance use that has been heavy and prolonged.
B. The substance-specific syndrome causes clinically significant distress or impairment in social, occupational, or other important areas of functioning.

C.   The symptoms are not due to general medical condition and are not better accounted for by another mental disorder.

Substance Intoxication

Substance intoxication is described by the following diagnostic criteria (APA 2000):

A.   The development of a reversible substance-specific syndrome due to recent ingestion of (or exposure to) a substance. Note: Different substances may produce similar or identical syndromes.
B.   Clinically significant maladaptive behavioral or psychological changes that are due to the effect of the substance on the central nervous system (e.g., belligerence, mood lability, cognitive impairment, impaired judgment, impaired social or occupational functioning) and develop during or shortly after use of the substance.
C.   The symptoms are not due to a general medical condition and are not better accounted for by another mental disorder.

At each of the stages of recovery, individuals are vulnerable to relapse, or a return to alcohol/drug abuse or addiction. Therefore, all chemical dependency treatment programs must address relapse issues. Many experts agree that a longer-term inpatient or residential program is much needed (although financially difficult, due to limitations in insurance reimbursement and managed care). Experts agree that a 6- to 9-month inpatient program would be most effective, considering the high relapse rates. In addition, a one-year outpatient aftercare program would further enhance the probability of recovery without relapse. It is not surprising that the relapse statistics are high following the traditional 28-day inpatient stay, making it even more important to counsel patients in relapse prevention. (See Chapter 11.)

Many people find it extremely difficult to stop using alcohol/drugs. Danaher and Lichtenstein (1978) describe the natural cycle of smoking, which is similar to the cycle of alcohol/drug use (see Table 4.5).

⚔ **Vulnerability to Relapse**

Recovery from alcohol/drugs also involves the family of the alcoholic/addict. The family system is an integral part of the development of the disease. The most difficult work in recovery is dealing with family issues and relationships to help family members recover from dysfunctional patterns in the family system. (See Chapter 5.)

The most important task in assessing the potential for problems with alcohol/drugs is determining if there is a family history of alcohol or drug abuse and addiction. Family members may deny the extent of alcohol/drug use in their family. It might take additional questioning to clarify the true dimensions of family use of alcohol/drugs.

⚔ **The Family and Recovery**

Alcohol/Drug History

Some education for family members and the individual who may have a drug problem also might be necessary to establish a clear perception of the dimensions of

TABLE 4.5

Natural Cycle of Cigarette Smoking

Reasons for Starting

Availability	Social confidence
Curiosity	Modeling of peers, siblings, parents
Rebelliousness	Other reasons in the psychosocial domain
Anticipation of adulthood	

Reasons for Continuing

Nicotine addiction	Avoidance of negative effects (withdrawal)
Immediate positive consequences	Other reasons in the physiological
Signals (cues) in the environment	and psychosocial domains

Reasons for Stopping

Health	Aesthetics (feeling that it is bad, ugly,
Expense	and/or unbecoming)
Social pressure	Example to others
Self-mastery	Other reasons in the psychosocial domain

Reasons for Resuming

Stress	Alcohol consumption
Social pressure	Other reasons in the psychosocial domain
Abstinence violation effect	

From Brian G. Danaher and Edward Lichtenstein. *Becoming an Ex-Smoker,* copyright © 1978 Brian G. Danaher and Edward Lichtenstein. Reprinted by permission.

TABLE 4.6

Factors Enhancing the Reliability and Validity of Self-Reports Among Substance Abusers

The client is alcohol- and drug-free when interviewed.

Sufficient time has passed since last drink/drug use to allow clear responses.

Confidentiality is assured.

The setting is nonthreatening and nonjudgmental and encourages honest reporting.

The client does not feel pressure to respond in a particular way.

The client has no reason to distort reports (e.g., abstinence being a condition of parole).

The client is aware that corroborating information is available and will be collected (e.g., breath test, report of spouse) and that this information from other sources will be used to confirm what he or she reports.

Care is taken to ensure that questions are clearly worded and valid measurement approaches are used.

The assessment worker or therapist has a good rapport with the client.

The person administering the measures should be able to communicate clearly with the client.

Adapted from National Institute on Alcohol Abuse and Alcoholism (1990) and the Addiction Research Foundation (1994).

substance abuse and addiction (see Table 4.6). To assess an individual's alcohol/drug problem, counselors need the following information:

- Age of initial drug and alcohol use
- Frequency of use, amounts used, set and setting of use
- Patterns of use, binges, periods of nonuse
- Stage of current use—experimentation, integrated use, excessive use, addiction
- History of negative consequences—physical, psychological, financial, familial, and spiritual
- Medical history—conditions that might affect use of drugs/alcohol
- Use of coffee, cigarettes, and medication

Individual Vulnerability to Alcohol/Drugs

Counselors should determine the individual's vulnerability to alcohol/drug use:

What evidence is there of individual vulnerability?

- Primary alcoholism/drug addiction in the family system of origin
- Inherited or acquired mood disorder
- Psychosis
- Rejection or insensitivity to norms of behavior

What is the individual's attitude toward alcohol/drug use?

- Favorable, unfavorable, nonexistent

What are the environmental factors?

- Family, other

Are drugs available?

- Legally available, readily available illegally
- Individual has the necessary finances for drugs (Rankin 1978)

Counselors should also identify any other significant problems, especially other compulsive behaviors in the family—a family history of

- Alcohol/drug problems, gambling, workaholism
- Eating disorders—anorexia, bulimia, obesity
- Employment and financial problems
- Marital problems
- Psychiatric disorders—depression, anxiety, affective (feeling) disorders, and others

---

An extremely important area of assessment is the consequences of alcohol/drug use. Remember, the third criteria of addiction is "continued use despite adverse consequences."

    A client, who was referred for outpatient counseling after 120 days in a residential and extended care program, was now dealing with significant criminal, civil

❧
Consequences
of Alcohol/
Drug Use

and other legal problems, financial, marital, business, and relationship problems. He said, "You can do all the drinking and drugging you want as long as you are willing to pay the consequences."

Perhaps this is a straightforward way of looking at addiction, but it does point out the significant consequences that come with substance abuse and addiction. Pointing out the consequences may be a valuable tool in breaking through denial. A

TABLE 4.7

Consequences Related to Alcohol or Drug Use

Check below any PHYSICAL problems caused by or worsened by your use of alcohol or drugs:
- Convulsions with loss of consciousness
- Nasal sores, bleeding
- Chest congestion, wheezing
- Hepatitis or other liver problems
- Severe or frequent headaches
- Drug overdose requiring treatment in an emergency room or hospital
- Coughing up black phlegm
- Severe weight loss (without dieting)
- Sinus problems
- Ulcers or other stomach problems
- Heart palpitations
- Other (specify)

Check below any PSYCHOLOGICAL problems caused by or worsened by your use of alcohol or drugs:
- Irritability, short temper
- Panic attacks
- Violent thoughts
- Severe depression
- Memory problems
- Paranoia, suspiciousness
- Suicidal thoughts
- Other (specify)

Check below any SEXUAL problems caused by or worsened by your use of alcohol or drugs:
- Loss of sex drive
- Sex with strangers
- Sexuality out of control
- Sexual obsession or preoccupation
- Risking of AIDS through sexual behavior
- Other (specify)

Check below any RELATIONSHIP or SOCIAL problems caused by or worsened by your use of alcohol or drugs:
- Arguments with spouse or mate
- Thrown out of household
- Loss of friends
- Arguments with parents, brothers, or sisters
- Spouse or mate has threatened to leave or has already left
- Social isolation
- Other (specify)

Check below any JOB or FINANCIAL problems caused by or worsened by your use of alcohol or drugs:
- In jeopardy of losing my job
- Late to work
- Less productive at work
- In debt
- Already lost at least one job
- Missed days of work
- Missed opportunity for promotion or raise
- Behind in paying bills
- Other (specify)

Check below any LEGAL problems caused by or worsened by your use of alcohol or drugs:
- Arrested for possession of illicit substances
- Arrested for forging prescriptions
- Auto accident while driving under the influence
- Arrested for assaulting someone
- Arrested for embezzlement or check forgery
- Arrested for sale of illicit substances
- Arrested for DWI or DUI
- Arrested for violent or disorderly conduct
- Arrested for theft or robbery
- Other (specify)

From Washton 1995.

very common exercise used in most drunk driving programs is to have clients figure out how much their conviction has cost them. For some, the amount is staggering when they stop to consider the cost of legal fees, the diversion program, loss of work, and so on.

Arnold Washton (1995) asks several questions in the assessment stage about consequence covering—physical, psychological, sexual, relationship, job, financial, and legal consequences of alcohol/drug use (Table 4.7).

The denial of alcohol/drug problems is a major factor in the difficulty of assessment. There is widespread denial, not only by individuals who have drug problems but also by family and friends, as well as society at large. It is often difficult to break through denial and have the courage to admit a problem with alcohol/drugs. Family members often experience a sense of shame or embarrassment or feelings of responsibility for the alcohol/drug problem of a family member.

⚔ Denial— Problems in Accurate Assessment

The two major defense mechanisms used to deny problems with alcohol and drugs are minimization and rationalization. The following are common examples of minimizations and rationalizations of alcohol/drug problems:

"Now, if I drank and drugged like Shawn, then I would really have a problem."
"I use alcohol and drugs only on weekends; a person with a problem uses everyday."
"I never miss work, no matter how much [alcohol/drugs] I've used."
"The media are just trying to get you scared."
"I don't have a problem. Now, Tiffany has a problem. Why don't you get her into treatment?"

Additional consequences of minimization and rationalization include the following:

- Neglect; emotional, physical, or sexual abuse
- Loss—death, trauma, divorce, separation
- Numerous relocations and unstable home environment
- Parental dysfunction, creating feelings of parental unavailability and/or feelings of abandonment, rejection, or shame

---

The following 11 questions can help in identifying an adolescent alcohol/drug problem:

⚔ Identification of Adolescent Alcohol/Drug Problems

1. *Mood.* Has the child been extremely moody or more upset than usual? Adolescence is a time of fluctuations in mood. A child might be as happy as a lark one minute and quite despondent the next. Therefore, it is difficult to isolate change in mood as being related to alcohol/drug use. However, if a child's mood seems more intense than usual, it could be related to the irritability associated with withdrawal from marijuana, alcohol, or other drugs.
2. *Changes.* Are there some significant changes in the child's choice in friends, grades, dress, general hygiene, and responsibilities? Adolescence is a time of change, a time to explore different aspects of one's identity and personality.

However, when these changes are self-damaging and seem more than just the trying on of a different role, it could be a sign for concern.

3. *Responsibility.* Is the child more irresponsible about his or her commitments (e.g., chores, schoolwork, friends)? Is he or she not coming home on time or disregarding rules? It is common for young people to push limits and boundaries. However, doing this on a consistent basis or pushing boundaries beyond reasonable expectations may be a sign of alcohol/drug abuse.

4. *Motivation.* Is there a noticeable decrease in motivation, interest, or activity? Has the child shown disinterest in things he or she is normally interested in (e.g., friends, school, sports, extracurricular activities)? Loss of motivation is indicative of regular marijuana use. Alcohol and other drugs can also impair interest and/or performance in activities normally seen as pleasurable.

5. *School.* Are there signs of problems at school and difficulty in studying, completing assignments, and so on? Has the teacher complained that the youngster is sleeping or inattentive in class? Some common signs of problems are ditching school, having problems with teachers, acting out behavior, getting failing or lowered grades, and having fights and arguments with friends. School problems are usually the first sign of negative consequences that may be related to an alcohol/drug problem.

6. *Negative activities.* Is the child engaging in activities that are not healthy or productive and potentially damaging? Such activities include those that might provoke physical violence; emotional abuse of others; disregard for others' property; dangerous use of motor vehicles; weekend-long parties or excessive isolation and secrecy about activities; and no accountability or supervision of time. A youngster having problems with alcohol or other drugs will abandon old friends and seek out those with similar attitudes and behaviors.

7. *Lying, stealing, and cheating.* Is money, household objects, or personal property missing? Is alcohol, prescription medication, or perhaps a parent's own stash of drugs missing? Does the child make up stories and lie compulsively? The expense of alcohol/drugs can be overcome by taking things that can be used for cash or bartered for alchohol/drugs. It is probably not forgetfulness or memory loss that has caused things to be either "misplaced" or "missing."

8. *Community.* Has the child been in trouble with neighbors, storekeepers, or other community members? Have concerned friends, neighbors, relatives, or others talked about this child's behavior? Have former friends, teachers, or parents of the child's friends expressed concern or given information that indicates this child may have a problem with alcohol/drugs? You can't go on ignoring the problem when others in the community have seen the child's misbehavior or actual alcohol/drug abuse.

9. *Criminal justice problems.* Has the child been involved in an activity that has caused investigation or charges being made by the police? Examples of some of these behaviors include disorderly conduct, drunkenness, driving under the influence, stealing, bouncing checks, shoplifting, vandalism, fighting, and breaking and entering. As previously outlined, alcohol/drug use and antisocial behavior are highly correlated.

10. *Physical signs.* Are there physical signs of alcohol or drug use? Have some of the following been noticed?

- The smell of alcohol or marijuana on the breath or body
- Dilated pupils
- Increase in activity
- Grandiosity
- Talkativeness
- Extreme quietness
- Slurred or incoherent speech
- Bizarre behavior
- Moodiness
- Aggressiveness and show of temper
- Fatigue, lethargy

Has drug paraphernalia been found in the child's room (e.g., rolling paper, syringes, pipes [water pipes], mirrors, razors, baggies)?

11. *Parents.* Do you find yourself justifying your child's behavior? Are you saying things like the following?

- "He or she will grow out of it."
- "This is just a stage."
- "Kids will be kids."
- "I went through the same kind of behavior when I was a kid."

If so, you may be denying signs of alcohol/drug abuse. Remember: *Believe the behavior,* not necessarily what the person says.

What we learn from Case Study 4.1 is that it is not necessary to catch your children red-handed using alcohol/drugs. If there is enough evidence of possible alcohol/drug abuse, seek professional help early—don't wait until the problem gets out of hand.

✄ Alcohol/ Drugs and Suicide

Another key assessment issue with alcohol/drugs is the potential for suicide. Stanton and Landau-Stanton (1985) state that the "recognition of substance abuse as a suicidal endeavor stems from as far back as 1938 when Menninger likened addiction to chronic suicide." Others have since concluded that the high rate of deaths among addicts "is more than a result of living in dangerous environments and is to a great extent—if not primarily—" (Stanton and Coleman 1980). Table 4.8 highlights key facts about suicide.

Some common assessment questions for suicide are these:

1. Is there a family history of alcohol/drug problems, suicide, or depression?
2. Do you use alcohol/drugs to
   a. overcome bad/shameful feelings?
   b. deal with sleeping problems, depression, or stress?
   c. quiet suicidal or self-destructive thoughts?
3. Do you have suicidal thoughts?

Case Study 4.1

The Marijuana Search

Despite Mr. and Mrs. Green being aware of signs of drug use by their 13-year-old son, John, he kept denying he was using. John seemed to have an answer for everything. He would make them feel guilty for doubting his word and not trusting him. As time went on, the deceptions and lies got more and more complicated. John, despite being caught in these lies, insisted that he was not smoking marijuana. The parents were frustrated and felt the only way they could have their son acknowledge his problem was for them either to catch him using marijuana or to find his marijuana.

One day, while their son was out of the house, they searched his room. Despite looking everywhere in the room, they couldn't find any tangible evidence of marijuana use. Curiously, the room seemed cleaner and neater than usual—almost as if their son suspected a search was imminent. Perhaps he heard them talking on the phone to the neighbors when they suggested a search. By chance, the father decided to expand the search to other rooms in the house—the bathrooms, family room, bedrooms. They were searching the hall closet when they found what they were looking for. They unscrewed the rubberized handle of the vacuum cleaner and found a small stash of marijuana.

When their son came home, the parents calmly held a family meeting. They asked their son if he had any marijuana in the house. Again, he said he didn't. When they produced the marijuana and told him where they found it, the son didn't blink an eye while saying, "Oh, that stuff. I forgot all about it. I've been holding that for the kid down the block for months now—you know, the one who went into drug treatment. I forgot all about it."

Discussion Questions

Explain and describe "parental denial" in acknowledging their child's drug use.
Do you think parents have the right to search their kids' room, etc.?
What do you believe about drug testing of children,
By parents?
By schools? As a requirement for extracurricular activities . . .
Are drug tests reliable? Explain "false positives."
Class Project: Visit a drug testing lab and report on the procedure, tests available, and
    reliability of tests.

4.   How will you do it? Do you have a plan? (Assess the availability or means to commit suicide and the lethality of the means.)
5.   Have you previously had suicidal thoughts and have you attempted suicide before? How frequently do these thoughts occur?
6.   What role does alcohol/drug use have in relation to suicide? Does it make you more likely or less likely to follow through?
7.   On a scale of 1 to 10, how likely are you to kill yourself?
8.   How much do you want to die? to live?
9.   What would prevent you from committing suicide?
10. What might occur to make life worth living?

TABLE 4.8

The Facts About Suicide

1. Suicide is preventable. Most suicide victims do not want to die.
2. Suicide is the eighth leading cause of death and ranks ahead of homicide.
3. Talking about suicide does not cause someone to be suicidal.
4. Suicidal behavior is not inherited, but the risk is higher for family members who have lost a close relative to suicide.
5. The suicide rate is higher for the elderly than any other age group.
6. Suicide is the second leading cause of death among young people. Accidents are number one, but even some of these accidents could be suicides.
7. Suicide claims the lives of at least 30,000 people annually in the United States.
8. Five states have passed legislation providing for school suicide prevention programs. Federal legislation is still pending.
9. The incidence of suicide among young people has nearly tripled during the past three decades.
10. Three times as many men as women kill themselves, yet three times as many women as men attempt suicide.
11. More than 80 percent of people communicate their intent to kill themselves before they attempt to do so. They leave clues as to their distress and/or plans.

From the American Association of Suicidology, 4201 Connecticut Ave. NW, Suite 310, Washington DC 20008, (202) 237–2280.

Some questions to assess the intention of potential suicide are:

- Have you been thinking about suicide?
- Do you have a plan to take your life?
- Do you feel hopeless about the future?
- Do you think you are a burden to your loved ones?
- Are you feeling so bad you are considering ending your life?
- Do you ever wish you could go to sleep and never wake up?
- Have you ever wanted to stop living?

If a client is suicidal, an extremely important question to ask is "What would prevent you from committing suicide?" This will often lead to a dialogue and plan of action that will prevent suicide. Fortunately, the vast majority of suicidal people do not want to die so much as they want to find a way to live. Quinnett emphasizes the importance of the quality of the relationship between the counselor and the client as being pivotal to suicidal risk assessment. "Even clients in very high-risk groups will choose to live and will agree not to hurt themselves. However, if the counselor is perceived as frightened, angry or disinterested, the risk for suicide may be increased." A common practice involves a written contract with a client who may be suicidal. The client agrees to not take action or to call the therapist or a suicide hot line before making an attempt.

Silence is the enemy of recovery. (Alcoholics Anonymous)

Case Study 4.2

Alcohol, Depression, and Suicide

The names and details of this case study have been changed to maintain anonymity.

Cheryl, a 43-year-old manager of a telecommunications company, struggled with bouts of alcoholism and depression. She originally called, seeking help for marital problems. During the assessment session, Cheryl reported her struggles with alcohol and drugs. She admitted that she was probably addicted to cocaine. She was convinced that she could no longer use cocaine. She still struggled to control her drinking. Cheryl had been through one inpatient treatment program and sporadically attended AA but was able to sustain only short periods of abstinence. Her job was extremely stressful, demanding more of her time and energy. She frequently lost her temper with people she worked with. The counselor listened to her "gripes" about her husband and their marital problems but astutely brought the conversation back to Cheryl's alcohol abuse.

In the third session, Cheryl acknowledged the need to strengthen her efforts to seek recovery from alcohol. She began attending AA and was encouraged to obtain an AA sponsor and attend counseling sessions once a week, yet, as time went on, she got distracted from committing to AA and chose a sponsor whom she rarely interacted with. Despite the counselor's efforts to get her to develop a stronger recovery program, she resisted. In future sessions, Cheryl began to talk about overwhelming feelings of depression and suicidal thoughts. She was referred to a psychiatrist for evaluation and was put on antidepressant medication. At the same time, the counselor and Cheryl wrote a contract that she would not attempt suicide and, if she felt suicidal, she would call the counselor or the suicide helpline.

Several months into treatment, Cheryl's depression was stabilizing and she was attending AA meetings more regularly, but she still had not established an active relationship with a sponsor or others in the program. The counsel suggested a woman's recovery therapy group. Cheryl agreed and attended the therapy group each week. At this time, her marriage was headed for a divorce, and her job was getting worse. She eventually moved out of her house and rented an apartment. During this time, she lapsed back to using alcohol and was more depressed. The counselor and group encouraged her to get more active in AA and to continue with her medication. Unfortunately, Cheryl did the opposite. She stopped taking her medication, rarely went to AA, and immersed herself in her work. She spent excessive hours working overtime and eventually dropped out of group counseling, stating that her schedule and finances made it impossible to attend. Despite efforts by her counselor to have her continue in group at a reduced fee, Cheryl decided against it. She continued, only briefly, with her individual counseling. Despite the counselor's best efforts to point out the need for counseling and renewed recovery efforts, Cheryl did not follow through. She began to miss counseling appointments. The counselor pointed out her pattern of "isolating" and continued to try to reengage her into counseling and recovery. Despite the counselor's best efforts, Cheryl went to counseling less frequently and eventually stopped going.

Nine months later the counselor received news that Cheryl had killed herself. The combination of alcoholism, depression, marital problems, stress at work, and Cheryl's inability to seek connection with others had led to her suicide.

Discussion Questions

Describe the role "pride" and "shame" can play in not seeking help.

As a counselor, what boundaries would you set to deal with a client with suicidal ideation? Would you set up a contingency contract?

List some questions you might ask a client who you suspect may be suicidal.

What does "Silence is the enemy of recovery" mean?

What signs might make you aware of the potential for suicide?

Have you ever considered suicide? What is your view on suicide?

What conditions make one more vulnerable to suicide?

Case Study 4.3
Julia—Streetwise—Cocaine Freebase

The first time Julia walked into the cocaine recovery group, you knew her story was remarkable. She was 36, extremely streetwise, with strong common sense and a no-nonsense style, and would call "bullshit" on people. When she talked in the group, which was often, you listened. She had been there and had survived. She had done what it took to get her "freebase." She could con the best of them. She worked the inner-city streets as a prostitute but somehow retained her dignity. She could hold her liquor, snort the cocaine, but got lost when it came to freebase.

Just as she had worked so hard to get stoned, she worked on her recovery just as strongly. She was inspiration for other group members, and they admired her integrity.

Epilogue

Julia was another victim of cocaine freebase. There was no need for an assessment—she knew she was an addict. When the state took her children away from her, she hit bottom. She worked the program so strongly, and so thoroughly, that she not only got her children back, but she became an alcohol/drug counselor, and everyone wanted to get into her groups.

Discussion Questions

Julia is a unique individual, what qualities does she possess that might make her a good counselor in the future?

Do you think "losing her children" played a big part in her recovery? Is so, explain.

What are your personal feelings about Julia's story?

What do you think about Julia?

Considering Julia is a recovering freebase addict, who lives in the ghetto, and is still involved with a boyfriend (who is in jail), what do you think her chances are of staying sober? What does she need to do, to maintain sobriety?

The task of screening is to determine if an alcohol/drug problem exists. Screening inventories are often used by alcohol/drug counselors and mental health professionals, substance abuse treatment agencies, employee assistance programs, and other agencies to help identify a potential alcohol/drug problem.

❧ Alcohol/ Drug Screening Inventories

Michigan Alcohol Screening Test (MAST) and Drug Use Screening Inventory (DUSI)

The Michigan Alcohol Screening Test (see test on pages 128 and 129), better known as the MAST, is a brief, easily scored questionnaire. The MAST gives consistent and reliable (alpha of .95) results with a high validity ($r = .90$). The Drug Use Screening Inventory (DUSI) is a bit longer than the MAST. However, it not only helps identify adolescents and adults with alcohol/drug problems but also identifies areas of disturbance and their severity. These areas can then be addressed by referral to appropriate treatment. In addition to substance abuse, the major problem areas identified include behavior, health, psychiatric disorders, social competency, family system, school adjustment (for adolescents), work, peer relationships, and leisure/recreation (see the screening inventory on pages 130–141).

Marijuana and Cocaine Screening Questionnaires

The questionnaires are designed to sensitize individuals to symptoms that might indicate they have problems with either marijuana or cocaine. Individuals check those items that might apply to their use of either marijuana or cocaine. A yes answer to several questions may indicate problems requiring further assessment by a professional trained in alcohol/drug treatment.

Part of the problem in identifying drug dependence and addiction is the black-or-white perception many people have about drugs. People tend to put drugs into simplistic categories of good drugs versus bad drugs, licit drugs versus illicit drugs, and soft drugs versus hard drugs (Nowlis 1975). Public perceptions of drugs are based on limited information and personal, often emotional, viewpoints. (see Case Study 4.3)

Assessment

Once screening has established that a substance-abuse problem exists, the next step is to assess the nature, scope, and severity of the problem. A seasoned alcohol/drug treatment professional who specializes in alcohol/drug assessment and treatment services can conduct a basic assessment and establish a diagnosis. More time and energy are involved in further assessing the dimensions and depth of the substance-abuse problem (see Figures 4.4 and 4.5). The negative consequences—deficits in developmental skills, mood and personality disorders, family and marital impact of substance abuse, and other psychosocial factors—need to be assessed. This is essential in order to establish a clinical decision about treatment. A listing of assessment tools is found in Table 4.9.

MICHIGAN ALCOHOL SCREENING TEST (MAST)

Points			YES	NO
	0.	Do you enjoy a drink now and then?	___	___
(2)	*1.	Do you feel you are a normal drinker? (By normal we mean you drink less than or as much as most other people.)	___	___
(2)	2.	Have you ever awakened the morning after some drinking the night before and found that you could not remember a part of the evening?	___	___
(1)	3.	Does your wife, husband, a parent, or other near relative ever worry or complain about your drinking?	___	___
(2)	*4.	Can you stop drinking without a struggle after one or two drinks?	___	___
(1)	5.	Do you ever feel guilty about your drinking?	___	___
(2)	*6.	Do friends or relatives think you are a normal drinker?	___	___

* Alcoholic response in negative

MICHIGAN ALCOHOL SCREENING TEST (MAST) (*continued*)

Points			YES	NO
(2)	*7.	Are you able to stop drinking when you want to?	___	___
(5)	8.	Have you ever attended a meeting of Alcoholics Anonymous (AA)?	___	___
(1)	9.	Have you gotten into physical fights when drinking?	___	___
(2)	10.	Has your drinking ever created problems between you and your wife, husband, a parent, or other relative?	___	___
(2)	11.	Has your wife, husband (or other family members) ever gone to anyone for help about your drinking?	___	___
(2)	12.	Have you ever lost friends because of your drinking?	___	___
(2)	13.	Have you ever gotten into trouble at work or school because of drinking?	___	___
(2)	14.	Have you ever lost a job because of drinking?	___	___
(2)	15.	Have you ever neglected your obligations, your family, or your work for two or more days in a row because you were drinking?	___	___
(1)	16.	Do you drink before noon fairly often?	___	___
(2)	17.	Have you ever been told you have liver trouble? Cirrhosis?	___	___
(2)	**18.	After heavy drinking have you ever had Delirium Tremens (D.T.s) or severe shaking, or heard voices or seen things that really weren't there?	___	___
(5)	19.	Have you ever gone to anyone for help about your drinking?	___	___
(5)	20.	Have you ever been in a hospital because of drinking?	___	___
(2)	21.	Have you ever been a patient in a psychiatric hospital or on a psychiatric ward of a general hospital where drinking was part of the problem that resulted in hospitalization?	___	___
(2)	22.	Have you ever been seen at a psychiatric or mental health clinic or gone to any doctor, social worker, or clergyman for help with any emotional problem, where drinking was part of the problem?	___	___
(2)	***23.	Have you ever been arrested for drunk driving, driving while intoxicated, or driving under the influence of alcoholic beverages? (IF YES, How many times? _____)	___	___
(2)	***24.	Have you ever been arrested, or taken into custody, even for a few hours, because of other drunk behavior? (IF YES, How many times? _____)	___	___

* Alcoholic response in negative
** 5 points for delerium tremens
***2 points for *each* arrest

Scoring System: In general, five points or more would place the subject in an "alcoholic" category. Four points would be suggestive of alcoholism, three points or fewer would indicate the subject was not alcoholic.

Programs using the above scoring system find it very sensitive at the five point level and it tends to find more people alcoholic than anticipated. However, it is a screening test and should be sensitive at its lower levels.

References
Selzer, M. L. 1971. "The Michigan Alcoholism Screening Test (MAST): The Quest for a New Diagnostic Instrument." *American Journal of Psychiatry* 3: 176–81.

Selzer, M. L., A. Vinokur, and L. van Rooijen. 1975. "A Self-Administered Short Version of the Michigan Alcoholism Screening Test (SMAST)." *Journal of Studies on Alcohol* 36: 117–26.

DRUG USE SCREENING INVENTORY

DOMAIN I: SUBSTANCE USE

A. Drug Preference

1. How many times have you used each of the drugs listed below in the last month? Put an "X" in each box that applies to you.

	0 times	1–2 times	3–9 times	10–20 times	More than 20 times
Alcohol					
Cocaine/crack					
Marijuana/pot					
Stimulants/uppers					
LSD/mescaline					
Tranquilizers					
Pain killers					
Heroin/opiates					
PCP					
Sniff gases or fumes					
Other					

2. Circle the drugs that you think you may have a problem with.
3. Shade in the circle of the drug that you prefer the most.

Instructions: Answer *all* of the following questions. Even if a question does not apply exactly, answer according to whether it is mostly yes (true) or mostly no (false). Answer the questions as if they apply to you within the past year and leading up to the present time. Put a check mark (✓) in the box for each question.

B. Drug Involvement

	Yes	No
1. Have you ever had a craving or very strong desire for alcohol or drugs?	___	___
2. Have you ever had to use more and more alcohol or drugs to get the effect you want?	___	___
3. Have you ever felt that you could not control your alcohol or drug use?	___	___
4. Have you ever felt that you were "hooked" on alcohol or drugs?	___	___
5. Have you ever missed out on activities because you spent too much money on alcohol or drugs?	___	___
6. Did you ever break rules, miss curfew, or break the law because you were high on alcohol or drugs?	___	___
7. Do you change rapidly from very happy to very sad or from very sad to very happy because of drugs?	___	___
8. Have you ever had a car accident after using alcohol or drugs?	___	___

DRUG USE SCREENING INVENTORY (*continued*)

	Yes	No
9. Have you ever accidentally hurt yourself or someone else after using alcohol or drugs?	___	___
10. Have you ever had a serious argument or fight with a friend or family member after drinking or drug use?	___	___
11. Have you ever had trouble getting along with any of your friends because of alcohol or drug use?	___	___
12. Have you ever experienced any *withdrawal symptoms* following use of alcohol or drugs (e.g., headaches, nausea, vomiting, shaking)?	___	___
13. Have you ever had a problem remembering what you had done when you were under the effects of alcohol or drugs?	___	___
14. Do you like to play drinking games when you go to parties?	___	___
15. Do you have trouble resisting using alcohol or drugs?	___	___

DOMAIN II: BEHAVIOR PATTERNS

	Yes	No
1. Do you argue a lot?	___	___
2. Do you brag a lot?	___	___
3. Do you tease or do harmful things to animals?	___	___
4. Do you yell a lot?	___	___
5. Are you stubborn?	___	___
6. Are you suspicious of other people?	___	___
7. Do you swear or use dirty language a lot?	___	___
8. Do you tease others?	___	___
9. Do you have a bad temper?	___	___
10. Are you very shy?	___	___
11. Do you threaten to hurt people?	___	___
12. Do you talk louder than other kids?	___	___
13. Are you easily upset?	___	___
14. Do you do things a lot without first thinking about the consequences?	___	___
15. Do you do risky or dangerous things a lot?	___	___
16. Do you take advantage of people if you can?	___	___
17. Do you generally feel angry?	___	___
18. Do you spend most of your free time by yourself?	___	___
19. Are you a loner?	___	___
20. Are you very sensitive to criticism?	___	___

DOMAIN III: HEALTH STATUS

	Yes	No
1. Have you had a physical exam or been under a doctor's care in the last year?	___	___
2. Have you had any accidents or injuries that still bother you?	___	___
3. Do you sleep too much or too little?	___	___
4. Have you recently lost or gained more than 10 pounds?	___	___
5. Do you have less energy than you think you should have?	___	___
6. Do you have trouble with your breathing or with coughing?	___	___
7. Do you have any concerns about sex or trouble with your sex organs?	___	___
8. Have your ever had sex with someone who shot up drugs?	___	___

DRUG USE SCREENING INVENTORY (*continued*)

	Yes	No

9. Have you had trouble with abdominal pain or nausea in the past year? ____ ____
10. Have your eyewhites ever turned yellow? ____ ____

DOMAIN IV: PSYCHIATRIC DISORDER

1. Have you ever intentionally damaged someone else's property? ____ ____
2. Have you stolen things on several occasions? ____ ____
3. Have you gotten into more fights than most kids? ____ ____
4. Are you a fidgety person? ____ ____
5. Are you restless and can't sit still? ____ ____
6. Do you get frustrated easily? ____ ____
7. Do you have trouble concentrating? ____ ____
8. Do you feel sad a lot? ____ ____
9. Do you bite your fingernails? ____ ____
10. Do you have trouble sleeping? ____ ____
11. Are you nervous? ____ ____
12. Do you get easily frightened? ____ ____
13. Do you worry a lot? ____ ____
14. Do you have trouble getting your mind off things? ____ ____
15. Do people stare at you? ____ ____
16. Do you hear things that no one else around you hears? ____ ____
17. Do you have special powers nobody else has? ____ ____
18. Are you afraid to be around people? ____ ____
19. Do you often feel like you want to cry? ____ ____
20. Do you have so much energy that you don't know what to do with yourself? ____ ____

DOMAIN V: SOCIAL COMPETENCY

1. Do kids your own age dislike you? ____ ____
2. Are you usually unhappy with how well you do in activities with your friends? ____ ____
3. Is it difficult to make friends in a new group? ____ ____
4. Do people take advantage of you? ____ ____
5. Are you afraid to stand up for your rights? ____ ____
6. Is it very hard for you to ask for help from others? ____ ____
7. Are you easily influenced by other kids? ____ ____
8. Do you prefer doing things with kids much older than you? ____ ____
9. Do you worry about how your actions will affect others? ____ ____
10. Do you have difficulty standing up for your opinions? ____ ____
11. Do you have trouble saying "no" to people? ____ ____
12. Do you feel uncomfortable if someone gives you a compliment? ____ ____
13. Do people see you as not being a friendly person? ____ ____
14. Do you avoid eye contact when talking to people? ____ ____

DOMAIN VI: FAMILY SYSTEM

1. Has a member of your family (mother, father, brother, or sister) ever used marijuana or cocaine? ____ ____

DRUG USE SCREENING INVENTORY (*continued*)

	Yes	No

2. Has a member of your family used alcohol to the point of causing problems at home, at work, or with friends? ____ ____
3. Has a member of your family ever been arrested? ____ ____
4. Do you have frequent arguments with your parents or guardians which involve yelling and screaming? ____ ____
5. Does your family hardly ever do things together? ____ ____
6. Are your parents or guardians unaware of your likes and dislikes? ____ ____
7. Are there no clear rules about what you can and cannot do? ____ ____
8. Are your parents or guardians unaware of what you really think or feel about things that are important to you? ____ ____
9. Do your parents or guardians argue a lot with each other? ____ ____
10. Are your parents or guardians often unaware of where you are and what you are doing? ____ ____
11. Are your parents or guardians away from home most of the time? ____ ____
12. Do you feel that either of your parents or guardians don't care about you? ____ ____
13. Are you unhappy about your living arrangements? ____ ____
14. Do you feel in danger at home? ____ ____

DOMAIN VII: SCHOOL PERFORMANCE/ADJUSTMENT

1. Do you dislike school? ____ ____
2. Do you have trouble concentrating in school or when studying? ____ ____
3. Are your grades below average? ____ ____
4. Do you cut school more than two days a month? ____ ____
5. Are you absent from school a lot? ____ ____
6. Have you thought seriously about quitting school? ____ ____
7. Do you often not do your school assignments? ____ ____
8. Do you often feel sleepy in class? ____ ____
9. Are you often late for class? ____ ____
10. Do you have different friends at school than you did last year? ____ ____
11. Do you feel irritable and upset when in school? ____ ____
12. Are you bored in school? ____ ____
13. Are your grades in school worse than they used to be? ____ ____
14. Do you feel in danger at school? ____ ____
15. Have you ever failed a grade in school? ____ ____
16. Do you feel unwelcome in school clubs or extracurricular activities? ____ ____
17. Have you ever missed or been late to school because of alcohol or drugs? ____ ____
18. Have you ever been in trouble at school because of alcohol or drugs? ____ ____
19. Have alcohol or drugs ever interfered with your homework or school assignments? ____ ____
20. Have you ever been suspended? ____ ____

DOMAIN VIII: WORK ADJUSTMENT

1. Have you ever had a paying job that you were fired from? ____ ____
2. Have you ever stopped working at a job because you just didn't care? ____ ____
3. Do you need help from others to go about finding a job? ____ ____

Drug Use Screening Inventory (*continued*)

		Yes	No
4.	Have you been frequently absent or late for work?	___	___
5.	Do you find it difficult to complete work tasks?	___	___
6.	Have you ever made money doing something that is against the law?	___	___
7.	Have you ever used alcohol or drugs while working on a job?	___	___
8.	Have you ever been fired because of drugs?	___	___
9.	Do you have trouble getting along with bosses?	___	___
10.	Do you mostly work so that you can get money to buy drugs?	___	___

DOMAIN IX: PEER RELATIONSHIPS

		Yes	No
1.	Do any of your friends regularly use alcohol or drugs?	___	___
2.	Do any of your friends sell or give drugs to other kids?	___	___
3.	Do any of your friends cheat on school tests?	___	___
4.	Do your parents or guardians dislike your friends?	___	___
5.	Have any of your friends ever been in trouble with the law?	___	___
6.	Are most of your friends older than you?	___	___
7.	Do your friends cut school at lot?	___	___
8.	Do your friends get bored at parties when there is no alcohol served?	___	___
9.	Have your friends brought drugs or alcohol to parties in the past year?	___	___
10.	Have your friends stolen anything from a store or damaged school property on purpose during the past year?	___	___
11.	Do you belong to a gang?	___	___
12.	Are you bothered now by problems you are having with a friend?	___	___
13.	Is there no friend you can confide in?	___	___
14.	Compared to most kids, do you have few friends?	___	___

DOMAIN X: LEISURE/RECREATION

		Yes	No
1.	Compared to most kids, do you do fewer sports?	___	___
2.	Do you go out for fun on school nights without permission?	___	___
3.	On a typical day, do you watch more than two hours of TV?	___	___
4.	Are the parents absent at the parties you have gone to recently?	___	___
5.	Do you exercise less than most kids you know?	___	___
6.	Is your free time spent just hanging out with friends?	___	___
7.	Are you bored most of the time?	___	___
8.	Do you do most of your recreation or leisure activities alone?	___	___
9.	Do you use alcohol or drugs for recreational reasons?	___	___
10.	Compared to most kids, are you less involved in hobbies or outside interests?	___	___
11.	Are you dissatisfied with how you spend your free time?	___	___
12.	Do you get tired very quickly when you exert yourself?	___	___

Instructions: Go back over the answers and make sure that every question has either the yes or no box filled in with a check mark.

COCAINE SCREENING QUESTIONNAIRE

Check the box before any question to which you would answer yes.

❑   1. Are you using more cocaine than you plan to use and do you find that you are enjoying it less? That is, your tolerance is developing and despite not feeling very well, you continue to use.

❑   2. Are you experiencing three or more of the following physical signs?

❑ Excessive periods of fatigue   ❑ Itching, scratching, and/or skin lesions

❑ Sinus problems and nose bleeds   ❑ Trouble breathing and/or catching your
   breath   breath

❑ Chest pains and palpitations   ❑ Decreased appetite or weight loss

❑ Tremors and poor coordination   ❑ Headaches

❑ Light spots on the periphery of your vision   ❑ Hoarseness

❑ Sleep disturbances, sleepiness,
   or excessive sleeping

❑   3. Do you feel apathetic, disinterested, depressed; have you lost the ability to concentrate?

❑   4. Do you experience mood swings, irritability, short temperedness, emotional outbursts, rage or excessive sadness, paranoid and/or frantic bizarre behavior?

❑   5. As a result of cocaine use, have you been absent, late, or exhibited inappropriate behavior at work?

❑   6. Are family members and friends suggesting that you have a problem with cocaine and/or are you lying about your frequency of cocaine use?

❑   7. Are you reducing outside interests, withdrawing from, or in conflict with friends and family members?

❑   8. Are you experiencing financial and/or legal problems as a direct or indirect result of cocaine use?

❑   9. Are you injecting or freebasing cocaine?

❑   10. The morning after cocaine use are you feeling depressed, remorseful, guilty, and/or shameful about your behavior the night before?

If you checked the boxes before two or more of these questions you may have a potentially serious cocaine problem. Pursue further evaluation with a chemical dependency professional.

© Copyright, July 1988, Richard Fields.

MARIJUANA SCREENING QUESTIONNAIRE

Denial of marijuana dependence and addiction stems from misconceptions of the harmlessness of this drug. Current research clearly documents the physical, psychological, and emotional harm of marijuana in the 1990s.

This questionnaire is a tool to help those who might have a problem, or those individuals and family members concerned with others who might have a problem with marijuana. Check the box before any question to which you would answer yes.

❑   1. Are you smoking marijuana

    ❑ in the morning

    ❑ on a daily basis

    ❑ during work/school time

    (one or more checks is a yes answer)

❑   2. While under the influence of marijuana, do you experience any of the following symptoms?

    ❑ irritability

    ❑ anxiety

    ❑ tremors

    ❑ insomnia

    ❑ restlessness

    ❑ sweating

    ❑ feeling loss of control

    ❑ nausea, vomiting

❑   3. As a result of marijuana use, do you experience a loss of initiative and ambition and/or a withdrawal from customary interests and interpersonal relationships?

❑   4. After using marijuana have you experienced any of the following?

    ❑ a clouding of mental processes

    ❑ flashbacks

    ❑ delusions

    ❑ impaired thinking and confusion

    ❑ fear of brain damage

❑   5. Have others commented on your poor driving skills while under the influence of marijuana, and/or have you noticed impairment in perceptual motor skills, driving, decision making, and/or tracking and reaction time?

❑   6. As a result of using marijuana, have you experienced any adverse negative consequences (e.g., problems at work/school, accidents, difficulty in relationships, or mood swings)?

MARIJUANA SCREENING QUESTIONNAIRE (*continued*)

❏   7.   Do you think about using marijuana often (i.e., do events, time of day, or particular daily situations trigger the desire to use marijuana)?

❏   8.   Have you been unable to stop using marijuana for three months or longer without substituting other drugs, alcohol, or medication?

❏   9.   Do you use marijuana with cocaine, alcohol, and/or other drugs?

❏   10.   Do other members of your family have problems with marijuana, alcohol, and/or other drugs?

❏   11.   Do you use marijuana to alleviate stress, loneliness, depression, boredom, and/or problems in relationships?

❏   12.   Did you start using marijuana at a young age and/or have you been using marijuana regularly for several years?

If you checked three or more of these questions, consult a specialist in alcohol and drug assessment and treatment for further evaluation.

© Copyright, July 1988, Richard Fields.

Adult Substance Use Survey (ASUS)

The Adult Substance Use Survey (ASUS) is a screening instrument for adults, ages 19 and older.

The 60-item survey can identify potential problems of an emotional or mood adjustment, rebelliousness and antisocial attitudes and behaviors, defensiveness, and resistance to self-disclosure.

Please contact the Center for Addictive Research and Evaluation—CARE, 5460 Ward Road, Suite 140, Arvada, Colorado 80002 (303) 421-1261 for more information regarding use of the ASUS.

ASUS SCORING PROTOCOL

ITEM #	SCALE	VALUES
1–10	Involvement	a=0, b=1, c=2, d=3, e=4
11–31	Disruption	a=0, b=1, c=2, d=3, e=4
32–41	Social	a=0, b=1, c=2, d=3
42–50	Emotional	a=0, b=1, c=2, d=3
51–55	Defensive	a=3, b=2, c=1, d=0
56–60	Motivation	Not scored

Sum the total number of points for each scale.

ADULT SUBSTANCE USE SURVEY—ASUS

TO BE COMPLETED BY CLIENT

NAME   DATE OF BIRTH   DATE

AGE   GENDER: [ ] Male [ ] Female   YEARS OF SCHOOLING COMPLETED

ETHNICITY: [ ] Anglo [ ] Black [ ] Hispanic [ ] Native American [ ] Other

MARITAL STATUS: [ ] Single   [ ] Married   [ ] Separated   [ ] Divorced   [ ] Widowed

EMPLOYMENT: [ ] Employed   [ ] Unemployed 1–3 months   [ ] Unemployed more than 3 months

PRIOR ALCOHOL/OTHER DRUG OUTPATIENT TREATMENT: [ ] None [ ] 1–2 times [ ] more 2 times

PRIOR ALCOHOL/OTHER DRUG INPATIENT TREATMENT: [ ] None [ ] 1–2 times [ ] more 2 times

INFORMATION AND INSTRUCTIONS ON THE USE OF THIS SURVEY

This booklet contains questions about how you see yourself. Some questions have to do with your feelings and emotions and others have to do with the use of alcohol and drugs. The information you provide will be treated as strictly confidential and will only be used by your counselors. Be as honest as you can. This will help those who are working with you to understand your concerns and questions about yourself and about your use of alcohol and other drugs. For each question in this survey, circle the letter under the answer that best fits you. Please answer every question. NOW YOU MAY TURN THE PAGE AND BEGIN TO ANSWER THE QUESTIONS.

FOR EVALUATOR USE ONLY

EVALUATOR: _____   AGENCY: _____   CLIENT I.D. _____   DACOD: _____

1. AOD use involvement?	Minimal Low Moderate High
	0 1 2 3 4 5 6 7 8 9

4. Referral Source?

[ ] Vol: self.
[ ] Vol: agency
[ ] Court: DUI
[ ] Court: Adult
[ ] Other: _____

5. Referred:

[ ] None
[ ] Fur. Eval.
[ ] Reg. OP
[ ] Int. OP
[ ] Day OP
[ ] Resid. IP
[ ] SSC

2. AOD service readiness?	Minimal Low Moderate High
	0 1 2 3 4 5 6 7 8 9

2. AOD service need?	Minimal Low Moderate High
	0 1 2 3 4 5 6 7 8 9

ASUS Summary Profile

SCALE NAME	RAW SCORE	Low			Low-medium DECILE	RANK	High-medium			High		NUMBER IN NORM SAMPLE*
		1	2	3	4	5	6	7	8	9	10	
1. INVOLVEMENT1		0	1	2 3	4	5 6	7 8	9 10 11	12 13 14	15 17 20	21 26 40	645*
2. DISRUPTSYM1			0	1 2	3 4	5 6	7 8 9 10	11 15 18	19 26 32	33 39 46	47 58 77	609*
3. SOCIAL		0 1 3 4	5	6	7 8	9	10	11 12	13 14	15 17 18	19 22 31	613*
4. EMOTIONAL		0 1	2	3	4 5	6	7 8	9	10 11	12 13 14	15 18 30	643*
5. DEFENSIVE		0 1 2	3	4	5		6	7	8	9 10	11 12 15	602*
6. INVOLVEMENT2		1 2 3		4 5	6 7 8	9 10 11	12 14 15	16 17 19	20 22 24	25 26 29	30 34 40	229*
7. DISRUPTSYM2		0 1 3 11	12 18 21	22 27 29	30 34 36	37 40 43	44 46 48	49 52 54	55 56 57	60 63 64	65 68 75	229**

| | 1 | 10 | 20 | 30 | 40 | 50 | 60 | 70 | 80 | 90 | 99 |

PERCENTILE   *Adult Criminal Justice   **Public Hospital

Below is a list of several kinds of drugs that people use. Please choose the answer that best describes your use of these drugs by circling the letter under that choice on the test booklet. Circle "a" if you have never used the drug. For alcohol, it is the number of times in your lifetime that you have been intoxicated. For all other drugs, it is the number of times in your lifetime that you have used the drug. Then, indicate the number of times in the past 3 months you have been intoxicated on alcohol or you have used the other drugs by putting the letter under the choice that best fits you on the line on the right side of the page opposite the drug.

	Total Number of Times in Lifetime					
	Never used	1–10 times	11–25 times	26–50 times	More than 50 times	Times used drug in the past 3 months
1. Number of times intoxicated or drunk on alcohol (beer, wine, liquor, mixed drinks)	a	b	c	d	e	_____
2. Marijuana (pot, hashish, hash, THC)	a	b	c	d	e	_____
3. Cocaine (coke, snow, crack, rock, blow)	a	b	c	d	e	_____
4. Amphetamines/stimulants (speed, uppers, bennies, diet pills, crystal, black beauties, white crosses, pep pills)	a	b	c	d	e	_____
5. Hallucinogens (LSD, acid, peyote, mushrooms, mescaline, PCP, angel dust)	a	b	c	d	e	_____
6. Inhalants (rush, gasoline, paint, glue, lighter fluid, nitrous oxide)	a	b	c	d	e	_____
7. Heroin (horse, H, smack, junk)	a	b	c	d	e	_____
8. Other opiates or painkillers used for nonmedical reasons (codeine, opium, morphine, percodans, dilaudid, demerol, methadone)	a	b	c	d	e	_____
9. Barbiturates/sedatives used for nonmedical reasons (seconal, nembutal, amytal, doriden, quaaludes, dalmane, placidyl, sleeping medicines, blues, reds, yellows, ludes, etc.)	a	b	c	d	e	_____
10. Tranquilizers used for nonmedical reasons (Librium, Valium, Ativan, Xanax, Serax, Miltown, Equanil, meprobamates)	a	b	c	d	e	_____

	Never smoked	Do not smoke now	Up to half a pack a day	About a pack a day	More than a pack a day
11. Cigarettes (tobacco)	a	b	c	d	e

As a result of using or coming off any of the above drugs, including alcohol, indicate how often any of the following have happened to you.

		Never	1–3 times	4–6 times	7–10 times	More than 10 times
12.	Had a blackout (forgot what you did but was still awake).	a	b	c	d	e
13.	Became physically violent.	a	b	c	d	e
14.	Staggered and stumbled around.	a	b	c	d	e
15.	Passed out (became unconscious).	a	b	c	d	e
16.	Tried to take your own life.	a	b	c	d	e
17.	Saw or heard things not there.	a	b	c	d	e
18.	Became mentally confused.	a	b	c	d	e
19.	Thought people were out to get you or wanted to harm you.	a	b	c	d	e
20.	Had physical shakes or tremors.	a	b	c	d	e
21.	Became physically sick or nauseated.	a	b	c	d	e
22.	Had a seizure or a convulsion.	a	b	c	d	e
23.	Had rapid or fast heart beat.	a	b	c	d	e
24.	Became very anxious, nervous and tense.	a	b	c	d	e
25.	Was very feverish, hot, sweaty.	a	b	c	d	e
26.	Did not eat or sleep.	a	b	c	d	e
27.	Was weak, tired and fatigued.	a	b	c	d	e
28.	Unable to go to work or school.	a	b	c	d	e
29.	Neglected your family.	a	b	c	d	e
30.	Broke the law or committed a crime.	a	b	c	d	e
31.	Could not pay your bills.	a	b	c	d	e

Please choose the answer that best fits you for the following questions or statements.

		Never	1–2 times	3–4 times	More than 5 times
32.	When I was in my teen years, I got into trouble with the law.	a	b	c	d
33.	I was suspended or expelled from school when I was child or teenager.	a	b	c	d
34.	I have been in fights or brawls.	a	b	c	d
35.	I have been charged with driving under the influence of alcohol/drugs.	a	b	c	d
36.	As an adult, I have been in trouble with the law other than driving a motor vehicle.	a	b	c	d

		Always true	Not true	Somewhat true	Usually true
37.	I have had trouble because I don't follow the rules.	a	b	c	d
38.	I don't like police officers.	a	b	c	d
39.	There are too many laws in society.	a	b	c	d
40.	It is all right to break the law if it doesn't hurt anyone.	a	b	c	d
41.	Usually, no one tells me what to do.	a	b	c	d

		Yes, all the time	Hardly at all	Yes, sometimes	Yes, a lot
42.	Have you felt down and depressed?	a	b	c	d
43.	Have you been nervous and tense?	a	b	c	d
44.	Have you been irritated and angry?	a	b	c	d
45.	Have your moods been up and down—from very happy to very depressed?	a	b	c	d
46.	Do you tend to worry about things?	a	b	c	d
47.	Have you felt like not wanting to live or like taking your life?	a	b	c	d
48.	Have you had problems sleeping?	a	b	c	d
49.	Have you had disturbing thoughts?	a	b	c	d
50.	Are you discouraged about your future?	a	b	c	d

		Yes, a lot	No, never	Hardly at all	A few times
51.	Have you ever gotten angry at someone?	a	b	c	d
52.	Have you lied about something or not told the truth?	a	b	c	d
53.	Do you ever find yourself unhappy?	a	b	c	d
54.	Have you felt frustrated about your job?	a	b	c	d
55.	Do you hold things in and not tell others what you think or feel?	a	b	c	d

		For sure yes	For sure no	Maybe no	Maybe yes
56.	Do you want help with an alcohol problem?	a	b	c	d
57.	Are you willing to not use or to give up the use of alcohol?	a	b	c	d
58.	Are you willing to not use or to give up the use of drugs other than alcohol?	a	b	c	d
59.	Do you feel you are being forced into getting help?	a	b	c	d
60.	Have you been honest with the answers you have given to these questions?	a	b	c	d

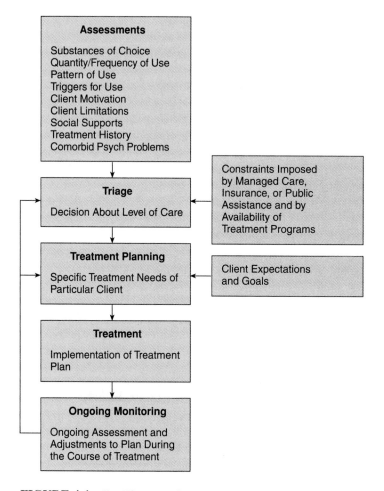

FIGURE 4.4   *Key Elements of Treatment Decision Making*

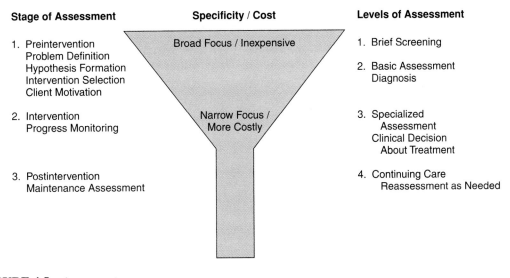

| Stage of Assessment | Specificity / Cost | Levels of Assessment |

1. Preintervention
   Problem Definition
   Hypothesis Formation
   Intervention Selection
   Client Motivation

2. Intervention
   Progress Monitoring

3. Postintervention
   Maintenance Assessment

Broad Focus / Inexpensive

Narrow Focus /
More Costly

1. Brief Screening

2. Basic Assessment
   Diagnosis

3. Specialized
   Assessment
   Clinical Decision
   About Treatment

4. Continuing Care
   Reassessment as Needed

FIGURE 4.5   *Assessment*

TABLE 4.9

Examples of Instruments and Interviews Appropriate for Use in Multidimensional Assessments of Substance Use Disorders Across Different Stages of the Assessment Process

Stage of Assessment	Assessment Domain	Examples of Instruments	References
Screening	Alcohol use	CAGE Questions Two Item Alcohol Screening Questions NET T-ACE TWEAK Alcohol Use Disorders Identification Test (AUDIT) Michigan Alcohol Screening Test (MAST) Brief Michigan Alcohol Screening Test (bMAST) Short Michigan Alcohol Screening Test (sMAST)	Mayfield et al. 1974 Cyr and Wartman 1988 Russell 1994 Sokol et al. 1989 Russell et al. 1991 Saunders et al. 1993 Selzer 1971 Pokorny et al. 1972 Zung 1984
	Drug use	Two Item Alcohol and Drug Screening Questions Drug Abuse Screening Test (DAST)	Brown et al. 1997 Skinner 1982
Problem assessment	Alcohol use patterns	Time-Line Follow Back Form-90 Comprehensive Drinker Profile (CDP) Alcohol Use Inventory (AUI)	Sobell and Sobell 1992 Miller 1996 Miller and Marlatt 1984 Wanberg et al. 1977
	Drug use patterns	Addiction Severity Index (ASI) Drug History Questionnaire (DHQ) Individual Assessment Profile (IAP)	McLellan et al. 1992 Sobell et al. 1995 Flynn et al. 1995

TABLE 4.9 (*continued*)

Examples of Instruments and Interviews Appropriate for Use in Multidimensional Assessments of Substance Use Disorders Across Different Stages of the Assessment Process

Stage of Assessment	Assessment Domain	Examples of Instruments	References
	Diagnoses	Psychiatric Research Interview for Substance and Mental Disorders (PRISM)[a]	Hasin et al. 1996
		Diagnostic Interview Schedule (DIS)	Robins et al. 1981
		Schedules for Clinical Assessment in Neuropsychiatry (SCAN)	Wing et al. 1990
		Composite International Diagnostic Interview (CIDI)	Robins et al. 1988
		Alcohol Use Disorders and Associated Disabilities Interview Schedule (AUDADIS)	Grant and Hasin 1990
	Outcome expectancies— alcohol	Negative Alcohol Expectancy Questionnaire (NAEQ)	Jones and McMahon 1993
		Alcohol Expectancy Questionnaire (AEQ)	Brown et al. 1987
		Drinking Expectancy Questionnaire (DEQ)	Young and Knight 1989
		Alcohol Beliefs Scale (ABS)	Connors and Maisto 1988
		Effects of Drinking Alcohol (EDA)	Leigh 1987
		Comprehensive Effects of Alcohol Scale (CEAS)	Fromme et al. 1993
	Outcome expectancies—drugs	Cocaine Expectancy Questionnaire (CEQ)	Jaffe and Kilbey 1994
		Cocaine Effect Expectancy Questionnaire—Likert (CEEQ-L)	Schafer and Fals-Stewart 1993
		Cocaine Effect Expectancy Questionnaire (CEEQ)	Schafer and Brown 1991
		Marijuana Effects Expectancy Questionnaire (MEEQ)	Schafer and Brown 1991
	Relapse risk	Substance Abuse Relapse Assessment (SARA)	Schonfeld et al. 1993
		Cocaine Relapse Interview (CRI)	McKay et al. 1996
		Cocaine High-Risk Situations Questionnaire (CHRSQ)	Michalec et al. 1992
		Situational Competency Test (SCT)	Chaney et al. 1978
		Reasons for Drinking Questionnaire (RFDQ)	Zywiak et al. 1996
		Reasons for Heroin Use Questionnaire (RFHUQ)	Heather et al. 1991
		Relapse Situation Appraisal Questionnaire (RSAQ)	Myers et al. 1996
	Coping: substance-related	Coping Behaviors Inventory (CBI)	Litman et al. 1983
		Problem Skills Inventory (PSI)	Hawkins et al. 1986
		Alcohol Specific Role Play Test (ASRPT)	Monti et al. 1993
	Coping: general	Ways of Coping Checklist (WOC)	Folkman and Lazarus 1980
		COPE	Carver et al. 1989
		Coping Responses Inventory (CRI)	Moos 1995
	Self-efficacy—alcohol	Alcohol Abstinence Self-Efficacy Scale (AASE)	DiClemente et al. 1994
		Drinking Refusal Self-Efficacy Questionnaire (DRSEQ)	Young et al. 1991
			Miller et al. 1994
		Individualized Self-Efficacy Survey (ISS)	Annis et al. 1987
		Inventory of Drinking Situations (IDS)	Annis and Graham 1988
		Situational Confidence Questionnaire (SCQ)	

T A B L E   4 . 9   (*c o n t i n u e d*)

Examples of Instruments and Interviews Appropriate for Use in Multidimensional Assessments of Substance Use Disorders Across Different Stages of the Assessment Process

Stage of Assessment	Assessment Domain	Examples of Instruments	References
	Self-efficacy—drugs	Inventory of Drug-Taking Situations (IDTS)	Annis and Graham 1991
		Drug Abuse Self-Efficacy Scale (DASES)	Martin et al. 1995
		Situational Confidence Questionnaire—Heroin (SCQ-Heroin)	Barber et al. 1991
Personal assessment	Personality	California Psychological Inventory (CPI)	Gough 1975
		NEO Personality Inventory	Costa and McCrae 1992
		Personality Research Form (PRF)	Jackson 1994
	Psychopathology	Minnesota Multiphasic Personality Inventory (MMPI-2)	Hathaway et al. 1989
		Millon Clinical Multiaxial Inventory (MCMI-II)	Millon 1992
		Psychological Screening Inventory (PSI)	Lanyon 1970
	Emotional state	Symptom Checklist-90 (SCL-90)	Derogatis 1977
	Anger	State-Trait Anger Inventory	Spielberger et al. 1983
		Multidimensional Anger Inventory	Siegel 1986
	Anxiety	State-Trait Anxiety Inventory	Spielberger et al. 1970
		Beck Anxiety Inventory	Beck et al. 1988
	Depression	Beck Depression Inventory (BDI)	Beck et al. 1961
		Center for Epidemiologic Studies Depression Scale (CES-D)	Radloff 1977
		Inventory to Diagnose Depression (IDD)	Zimmerman and Coryell 1987
	General life/social function	Addiction Severity Index (ASI)	McLellan et al. 1992
		Psychosocial Functioning Inventory (PFI)	Feragne et al. 1983
Treatment-related factors	Readiness to change	Stages of Change Readiness and Treatment Eagerness Scale (SOCRATES)	Miller and Tonigan 1996
		Readiness to Change Questionnaire (RTCQ)	Rollnick et al. 1992
		University of Rhode Island Readiness to Change Assessment (URICA)	McConnaughy et al. 1983
		Desire for Help Scale (DHS)	Simpson and Joe 1993
		Intrinsic/Extrinsic Motivation to Quit Questionnaire (IEMQ)	Curry et al. 1990 McBride et al. 1994
	Barriers to treatment	Barriers to Treatment Instrument (BTI)	Allen 1994
		Reasons for Delaying Seeking Treatment (RDST)	Cunningham et al. 1993
		Fears About Treatment Questionnaire (FTQ)	Oppenheimer et al. 1988

TABLE 4.9 (concluded)

Examples of Instruments and Interviews Appropriate for Use in Multidimensional Assessments of Substance Use Disorders Across Different Stages of the Assessment Process

Stage of Assessment	Assessment Domain	Examples of Instruments	References
	Reasons for seeking treatment	Treatment Seeking Scale (TSS)	Cunningham et al. 1994
		Treatment Motivation Questionnaire (TMQ)	Ryan et al. 1995
		Readiness for Treatment Scale (RTS)	Simpson and Joe 1993
		Reasons for Giving Up Drugs and Alcohol	Murphy and Bentall 1992
		Reasons for Coming to Treatment Questionnaire (RCTQ)	Oppenheimer et al. 1988
		Circumstances, Motivation, Readiness, and Suitability Scales (CMRS)	DeLeon et al. 1994
	Treatment goals	Treatment Goals Inventory (TGI)	Glaser and Skinner 1981
	Treatment services utilization	Treatment Services Review (TSR)	McLellan et al. 1992
Collateral information	Collateral reports	Form-90	Miller 1996
		Comprehensive Drinker Profile (CDP)	Miller and Marlatt 1984, 1987

[a]PRISM was formerly known as the SCID-A

Source: McCrady, Barbara S., and Elizabeth E. Epstein. *Addictions: A Comprehensive Guide Book.* Cary, NC: Oxford University Press, 1999.

References

American Psychiatric Association. 2000. *Diagnostic and statistical manual of mental disorders.* 4th ed., text rev. Washington, D.C.: Author.

Danaher, B. G., and E. Lichtenstein. 1978. *Becoming an ex-smoker.* Englewood Cliffs, N.J.: Prentice Hall.

Jellinek, E. M. 1960. *The disease concept of alcoholism.* New Haven, Conn.: Hillhouse Press.

Nowlis, Helen. 1975. *Drugs demystified.* Paris: UNESCO Press.

Rankin, James G. 1978. *Core knowledge of the drug field: A basic manual for trainers.* Toronto: Addiction Research Foundation.

Rawson, Richard. 1989. *Cocaine recovery issues: The neurobehavioral model.* Beverly Hills, Calif.: Matrix Institute on Addictions.

Shedler, Jonathan, and Jack Block. 1990. Adolescent drug use and psychological health: A longitudinal inquiry. *American Psychologist* 612.

Smith, David, and Donald Wesson. 1988. *Treating cocaine dependence.* Center City, Minn.: Hazeldon Foundation.

Stanton, M. D., and S. B. Coleman. 1980. The participatory aspects of indirect self-destructive behavior. In *The many faces of suicide,* edited by N. L. Farberow. New York: McGraw-Hill.

Stanton, M. D., and Judith Landau-Stanton. 1985. Treating suicidal adolescents and their families. In *Handbook of adolescent and family therapy,* edited by M. P. Mirkin and S. L. Koman. New York: Gardner Press.

Washton, Arnold M. 1995. *Psychotherapy and substance abuse: A practitioner's handbook.* New York: Guilford Press.

Family

5

Substance Abuse and Family Systems

❖ **Chapter in Review**

The alcoholic/drug addict family system is a system in disequilibrium, often trying to counterbalance the extent of the problem with denial. Therefore, instead of *dysfunctional family system,* we can use the term *imbalanced family system.* This term is recommended because it is a more accurate description and avoids the shame connotations of the term *dysfunctional.*

Families have specific rules, alliances, and patterns of communication. The alcoholic/addict family system has survival roles—chief enabler, family hero, family scapegoat, lost child, and family mascot. Enabling behaviors include avoiding and shielding, attempting to control, taking over responsibilities, and rationalizing and accepting.

During family recovery, the family goes through the stages of grieving—denial, anger, bargaining, depression/feeling, acceptance.

⚔ Families as Systems

Initially, one must look at the family as a system. Some key elements of family systems are that they all have rules, values, verbal and nonverbal methods of communicating, boundaries, roles, and patterns of interaction. Systems always seek some level of homeostasis, or balance. Alcoholism and drug dependency are dysfunctional elements in family life. The result is a disequilibrium, or imbalance, forcing family members to compensate and give up aspects of their own sense of self in an attempt to keep the family in balance. One could describe the alcoholic/addict family system as having a top-heavy top that tries to spin in a functional pattern but instead swerves to one side and skids in a diagonal direction until it stops. The individuals in this system are all compensating in different yet similar ways. It's as if they are walking around with a heavy weight on one shoulder; they have to either lean to one side to walk properly or use all their energy to try to compensate and look as if they are walking upright. Both positions require a great deal of energy. Family therapist Carl Whitaker (Whitaker and Napier 1978) has described the family as the source of all kinds of electrical energy, with positive and negative voltages.

Virginia Satir (1967), a famous family therapist, was the first to describe the family using the metaphor of a mobile: if the wires on one of the pieces of the mobile are twisted, the mobile spins improperly. Instead of a delicately balanced mobile, each piece gets entangled and out of balance at the slightest breeze. A well-balanced mobile, or family system, sways and flexes with the strong gusts and heavy winds of life. The family with alcohol/drug problems is described as an imbalanced, or dysfunctional, family system. In a healthy family, the system is flexible and fluid, open (not rigid), predictable (not inconsistent), and balanced in meeting both the individual's and the family's needs.

Looking at the family as a system is imperative in addressing the problem of alcohol/drug de-

---

The names and circumstances of case studies in this chapter have been changed to maintain anonymity.

pendence and addiction. If the family system does not change and the family members do not do their recovery work, the same dysfunctional styles of communication and interaction make the alcoholic/addict at risk for alcohol/drug relapse or the development of another dysfunctional behavior.

To effectively treat the alcoholic/addict, the rest of the family system also needs treatment. The dysfunctional aspect of the disease has affected all family members. The high alcohol/drug relapse rate is often attributable to the lack of recovery by the family members. Too frequently, the alcoholic/addict is the focus of help, and the family members deny their own enabling and codependent behavior. The messages from the family are "Just fix the alcoholic/addict" and "Just get him or her to stop using alcohol/drugs and then everything will be O.K."

Functional and dysfunctional systems.

Annie Bauger.

Family members avoid being active in treatment because they resist looking at their own behavior; they fear getting in touch with painful feelings, which may be overwhelming.

Another fear is whether the family system can survive reexperiencing these feelings. They wonder, "Has the family been hurt beyond repair?" and "Will the family be able to work through the violations of the past?" These questions and others need to be addressed for the effective recovery of the alcoholic/addict and the family members.

The expression *dry drunk* refers to the alcoholic/addict who is abstaining from alcohol/drug use but either is unaware of other behavioral, personality, and relationship problems or is choosing not to address these maladaptive behaviors. The overall behavior and personality styles of dry drunks are very similar to when they were using alcohol/drugs. Essentially, they have chosen not to deal with the underlying issues that contributed to the negative aspects of their personalities. For some, it is certainly enough that they are sober. Others who are still experiencing feelings of depression, fear, rage, and anxiety may decide to get help and address the problem.

After 1 to 5 years of being sober, many recovering alcoholics/addicts realize that they are still having problems, especially in interpersonal relationships. This is often described as the addict's "second bottom." The first bottom is the realization that they can no longer continue to use alcohol/drugs. The second bottom is the realization that they are still not having fun, due to unresolved personality issues. They ask themselves the question "Now that I am years sober, am I having fun yet?" The answer frequently is "No, my life is more manageable but I'm still not feeling better."

The family of the alcoholic/addict also goes through a kind of dry drunk. The family may glow in the joy of the alcoholic/addict's initial sobriety and may now feel validated that he or she is, indeed, okay. From the viewpoint of friends, neighbors, and community, he or she "did the right thing." There is no discounting that the family members were courageous in struggling to get the alcoholic/addict into treatment. However, they must continue the struggle to develop a healthier family system. In many cases, the family returns to old dysfunctional patterns. It is fair to say that recovery from the diseases of alcoholism and drug addiction is an ongoing process for the individual and the family.

✖ Family Rules

Each family makes decisions and choices based on the rules, boundaries, and alliances of family members. Families have rules about who, when, and how feelings are expressed.

Family rules often involve rules of communication—who is allowed to express feelings, how they are expressed, and how they are received.

Rules in the alcoholic/addict family system often focus on ways to communicate and believe in order to deal with the substance-abusing person. This often involves secret keeping, or what Claudia Block (1981) referred to as the three rules that children of alcoholics often learn to live by: "Don't talk. Don't trust. Don't feel."

> Talking, especially about the substance abuse, might cause even more problems. Trusting usually leads to disappointment when parents do not come through with their promises. Feeling is too painful, and expression of feelings is not allowed because it might cause more trouble. (Lawson and Lawson 1998)

✖ Imbalanced vs. Dysfunctional

Nathan Ackerman first coined the term *dysfunctional family* in 1958, when referring to alcoholic family systems. Throughout the literature of the alcohol/drug and mental health fields—and even in this textbook—we frequently use the term *dysfunctional* in describing families, systems, relationships, parenting, behavior, and individuals. The term *dysfunctional* is frequently a shame-based, negative label, with a negative emotional tone. Labeling them as dysfunctional discourages families and individuals who are struggling with the problems of alcohol/drug dependence. Many people have been annoyed and discouraged at being told they are dysfunctional. It sounds hopeless. For example, what good does it do to tell a patient, relative, or friend, "You come from a shame-based, dysfunctional family system" or "You have a codependent, enabling, dysfunctional relationship with your spouse and children"? This doesn't really help the person and shames him or her, making the person feel helpless and hopeless. Most people feel a sense of betrayal in even thinking about their families in such a derogatory manner.

Instead of using *dysfunctional,* replace it with the term *imbalanced,* for this is truly what we are looking at—an imbalance in the individual and in the family members' lives. Remember Satir's image of an out-of-balance mobile. It is so much more hopeful to seek treatment if one has the expectation of becoming balanced. It is also a far more positive approach.

There is truly an emotional imbalance in the alcoholic/addict family system. The term *imbalance* gives hope that there is a way to get help and better manage the system. The goal is to establish balance and order by addressing the problems in the family.

There are different kinds of imbalance in family systems. Alcohol/drugs serve a different function in each of these imbalanced systems. Next we will examine rigid, ambiguous, overextended, and distorted family systems to better understand imbalanced family systems. In each family system, the drug of choice and its function are for illustration, not an empirically proven fact.

Rigid Family Systems

Rules—Strict interpretation of the rules with no exceptions; inflexibility with no extenuating circumstances. The rules keeper (usually a critical/judgmental father or mother) is exempt from the rules.

Values—"There is only one way to do things and that is the right way—my way." Things are always black or white, right or wrong.

Motto—"Do it right, or else."

Communication—Linear, hierarchical. The father is usually dominant, powerful, and unapproachable. The mother softens the impact of the father's harshness. Or the mother is critical-judgmental, often moralistic and controlling, and the father goes along with the mother, deceptively avoiding conflict and the rage of the mother.

Drugs of choice—Alcohol and/or heroin, other sedative hypnotics, and narcotic analgesics.

Functions of drug—Suppress feelings, especially anger, and stay numb to the trauma in this family system.

Ambiguous Family Systems

Rules—We have rules but we don't enforce them, and we change them if someone is annoyed or inconvenienced.

Values—Forever changing, based on the situation.

Motto—"Keep peace at all costs; avoid conflict."

Communication—Mixed messages that are confusing. "Do what you know we want, without us letting you know what it is we want."

Drugs of choice—Alcohol and/or heroin, marijuana, and hallucinogens.

Functions of drug—Suppress feelings of discomfort, kill pain, shut out reality, and/or distort reality.

Overextended Family Systems

Rules—Be productive, get busy, stay on the move.

Values—Look good, achieve, do it with willpower, feelings are for wimps.

Motto—"We can achieve anything we set our minds to." "The right stuff."

Communication—Feelings are not expressed or integrated; decisions are based on results and what will please the parents.

Drugs of choice—Cocaine, methamphetamine, and other stimulants, alcohol.

Functions of drug—Keep on working/doing, even though feelings are not congruent with work or intimate relationships.

Distorted Family Systems

Rules—Don't let outsiders know we are crazy. Act as if we were a normal family, just a bit eccentric.

Values—Maintain an illusion of normalcy, despite significant physical, emotional, and interpersonal problems of the family. Keep outsiders guessing about us. Motto—"Aren't most families like ours?"

Communication—Mixed messages; parents and children are unavailable and have limited common perceptions of situations.

Drugs of choice—Alcohol, hallucinogens, marijuana, and inhalants.

Functions of drug—Distort reality, which is already distorted, to try and make sense, or no sense, of it.

✖ Satir's Family Patterns of Communication

Virginia Satir, author of *Conjoint Family Therapy* (1967) and *Peoplemaking* (1972) and co-author of *Helping Families to Change* (1976), emphasizes the feeling component of family patterns of communication. She describes a dysfunctional family as one that maintains rules that do not fit the reality of what is felt and believed.

Satir's work is monumental and popular. According to Satir, individuals with poor self-concepts see pots that are half-empty. Individuals with the ability to differentiate (i.e., those with good self-concepts) see their pots as half-full. The former group feels hopeless and negative; the latter group is positive and hopeful.

Satir identified the following dysfunctional styles as well as a functional style of communicating:

1. Placaters discount themselves. Their goal is frequently to avoid conflict and to avoid others' anger. Their communication patterns feature the following:
   a. Words that agree and avoid conflict: "Whatever you want is O.K." The placaters' worth is based on others accepting, not rejecting, what they say.
   b. Bodies that placate: "I am helpless." The placaters' worth is based on being physically available, even when that may not be consistent with what they feel.
   c. Feelings: "I am worthless." Placaters believe they have no choices but to be dependent in dysfunctional relationships because there is no way out, and they are not strong enough or worth the struggle.
2. Blamers elevate themselves by discounting others. Their goal is to avoid looking at themselves, their own issues, and their own responsibility. Others' feelings are often discounted. If others would only do it the right way—which is their way—then things would work out. Their communication patterns feature the following:
   a. Words that are critical, judgmental, shaming put-downs: "You never do anything right." "It's all your fault."
   b. Bodies that blame: "I am more powerful, more dominant."
   c. Feelings: "It is your fault that I am unhappy."
3. Intellectualizers discount their own feelings. Their goal is to place rigid emphasis on the cognitive to figure out problems, to deny the role feelings play in relationships and decisions, and to avoid the emotional impact of

feelings. Intellectualizers are the brains, the computers, the cognitive persons who think, "If I can only understand this, I'll be OK." They often feel that, if they can only find that missing piece of the puzzle, they will find the cause of their problems. They fail to integrate the key elements of the puzzle—their feelings—and fail to realize that the puzzle may not be solvable, especially with their linear approach. Their communication patterns feature the following:

a. Words that are extremely logical: "That makes sense and is reasonable."
b. Bodies in control or shut down
c. Feelings: "I am vulnerable and feel threatened when I get in touch with my feelings, especially feelings of vulnerability."

4. Distracters discount context. Their goal is to keep others and themselves away from painful feelings, to distract and avoid conflict. Distracters are the elusive, sometimes charming, magicians. They are difficult to hold accountable or responsible because they keep the focus elsewhere, not on themselves. Many alcoholics and addicts are masters of this style of communication and avoid or deny their problems with alcohol and drugs. Their communication patterns feature the following:

a. Words that are confusing and irrelevant. They are unable to establish clarity or to set specific goals.
b. Bodies that act as if they are somewhere else when the content gets too specific and focused. They want to frustrate, discount, and escape from others.
c. Feelings: "Nobody cares. I am not happy."

According to Satir, **leveling** is the healthy state of communication. Words, body, and feelings are consistent with the message. The individual is congruent and acts in a congruent fashion.

Wegscheider-Cruse's Alcoholic/Addict Family System Survival Roles

⚹ Family
System Roles

Sharon Wegscheider-Cruse was trained by and has worked closely with Virginia Satir. Wegscheider-Cruse is best known for her books *The Family Trap* (1976) and *Family Reconstruction Therapy—the Living Model* (1994). She is a leader in the field of adult children of alcoholics and family reconstruction and has popularized the concept of survival roles in the alcoholic/addict family system. These roles are labeled in terms of the coping mechanisms members use to survive in a dysfunctional alcoholic/addict family. They include the chief enabler, family hero, family scapegoat, lost child, and family mascot.

The *chief enabler* assumes primary responsibility for the chemically dependent family member. The chief enabler shelters and protects, even denies, the dysfunctional aspects of a family member's alcohol/drug use. The major enabling approaches are the following:

1. Avoiding and shielding
2. Attempting to control

3. Taking over responsibilities
4. Rationalizing and accepting
5. Cooperating and collaborating (Nelson 1988)

The *family hero* is the achiever, the responsible child, the good child, the model child. The family hero is often the firstborn, who escapes the dysfunctional aspects of the alcohol/drug family through personal achievement. The family's sense of self-worth is often the conscious or unconscious responsibility of this family member. Unfortunately, the family hero achieves for the family and ignores personal feelings, values, and goals. The family hero in adulthood often experiences a depression or sense of loss due to the incongruency of internal feelings with external behaviors. The hero may be outwardly successful but feel like a charlatan, or empty inside. When this conflict is not dealt with, the family hero is vulnerable to alcohol/drug problems and/or problems in interpersonal relationships.

The primary function of the *family scapegoat* is to divert the family members away from the real issues in the family (e.g., marital discord, marital infidelity, or parental alcohol/drug problems) and the painful emotionality of these family issues. The family members can then blame the scapegoat for all of the family problems. The family scapegoat often exhibits acting-out behavior in school and at home, antisocial behavior, and substance abuse due to underlying feelings of anger and resentment.

The *lost child's* role (see Case Study 5.1) is often the most tragic. This is the child whose primary function is to allow the dysfunctional family—especially the parents—to expend less energy. This child often identifies with the pain of his or her parents and other siblings and wants to decrease the family members' level of pain by not contributing to the problem, perhaps even taking on the family's pain. The family inadvertently reinforces this child for not having needs. The child denies feelings and needs, frequently disconnecting emotionally and even physically from the family. At some point, the child can no longer deny personal feelings and pain. Thus, lost children frequently get overwhelmed with emotions and are at risk for suicide.

The primary function of the *family mascot* is to divert attention away from the family issues and family pain. The mascot uses humor, silliness, and even self-disparaging ineptness (making fun of oneself) as a way of diverting the family from its pain. Frequently, the mascot discounts a sense of self as the price to pay for calm in the family. As a result, the mascot may feel unworthy of love, unless able to alleviate someone's pain.

These are just a few family roles. The roles are stereotypic classifications for purposes of identifying some common role features in dysfunctional, or imbalanced, family systems. Please note that the roles are illustrations of dysfunctional patterns of family interaction and should not be used to pigeonhole someone into a static classification. Usually, people maintain a variety of traits from each of the roles. Family roles may also change based on different family situations and adjustments in the family process.

Other important family therapists—Salvador Minuchin, Theodore Lidz, Lieman Wynne, James Framo, Ron Jackson, and Jay Haley—emphasize a systems approach in their work with families and changing dysfunctional patterns of family communication and interaction. These family therapists have different styles, theo-

Case Study 5.1

The Lost Child

Michelle

Michelle was beginning her senior year in high school when her family began therapy. At that time, her stepbrother, Jack, was heavily into drugs (marijuana, hallucinogens, speed, and cocaine) and alcohol. Her other sisters were extremely angry with Jack's attitude and behavior. Michelle was an A student and student body president. She was on the cross-country team and very popular. She had a quiet, affable presence and acted older than her 17 years. She was the only one in the family to whom Jack related. During the course of treatment, it was very difficult for Michelle to express any feelings. Even in individual sessions, she would deny feeling any pain or negative emotions.

Later that year, Michelle was accepted to a college a few hours' drive from home. During her first semester away at school, despite good study habits, she ended up dropping a course and receiving C grades. Also, she didn't make any friends at school. Michelle was running on the college track team but was unmotivated and not running to her true potential. This was quite traumatic for Michelle because she had been so popular and such a good student and athlete in high school. Michelle set up an individual counseling appointment during her college break. For the first time, she was in touch with her pain and grief. If she had not reached out for help, Michelle would have been another college student unable to cope with the pressures or to deal effectively with backlogged feelings, which eventually might have caused her to take her own life.

Discussion

This case illustrates the family role of the lost child. The lost child role takes many forms, but the essential theme is a child who appears on the surface to be doing extremely well but who in truth is foundering. The goal of the lost child is to be self-sufficient and not take any energy away from the family—a family that is struggling with other problems (e.g., alcohol/drug abuse and addiction). Unfortunately, the lost child is not dealing with her or his own feelings and can eventually be overwhelmed by them. The lost child is the family member who is at risk for suicide.

As adults, lost children are often high achievers. They affirm the family through their drive to success, but often are unable to identify or give voice to their own feelings. This is often exhibited in problems with intimacy, empathy, and connection with others.

---

ries, and methods of working with families. Some see the entire family together in a counseling session. Others may see family members separately or sometimes see the father and son, mother and daughter, or just the children. Family therapists even use a multigenerational approach that includes grandparents, or an expanded family approach of including other relatives. The key element of all of these approaches is looking at the family as a system, a system that is affected and changed by the actions and events in the lives of each of the family members.

Family Roles Played Out at the Dinner Table

The Green family, like many families, had the ritual of having dinner together. When the children were younger, the minor irritations of "spilled milk" (literally and metaphorically) gave rise to Dad's rage. Mr. Green was usually exhausted at dinnertime, stressed out by his job. Mr. Green's father was a mean-tempered, negative, emotionally disconnected, and nasty alcoholic, who didn't model any form of connection or caring toward his children. Mr. Green, like his father, had little patience with his children and would lose his temper easily. As the children got older, the dinner table became a battle zone. The youngest child was the "lost child," the middle child the "scapegoat," and the oldest child the "hero."

The middle child (the scapegoat) would spark the battle by antagonizing his father, challenging him. This son would argue politics, religion, current events, and so on, taking a position that would irritate his father. This son was the brightest child, aware and well read, and would use these skills to mock his father's ignorance on issues.

Mr. Green would soon escalate and explode. The youngest child (lost child) would plead for a truce, which was ignored. She would burst into tears and retreat to her room. The oldest child (the hero) would make jokes and tell the family they were too serious about all this. Sometimes this approach worked, but many times it didn't. Mr. Green would usually explode, grab his dinner plate, and retreat to the den. The oldest child was aligned and enmeshed with his mother. Mom would then sit down by this son and blame the middle child (scapegoat) for causing the conflict.

This is just one scenario of family roles and alliances. The family imbalance is played out night after night at the dinner table.

Five Styles of Managing Anxiety

Harriet Lerner (1997) describes five styles or roles of managing anxiety—underachievers, overfunctioners, blamers, pursuers, and distancers (see Table 5.1). Anxiety about substance abuse in the family often leads to these coping roles.

Enabling Behavior

In an attempt to avoid recognizing problems, the family enables the continued use of alcohol/drugs and other dysfunctional behaviors. Enabling is described as an unhealthy doing-for, or killing with kindness (Table 5.2). Parents may have good intentions in enabling their children. Their lack of insight into the dynamics of the enabling process, however, causes problems to continue and to get progressively worse. (See Case Study 5.2)

> Protecting one's child is normal and appropriate, but overprotection can cause problems. Enablers overprotect and find it difficult to separate what their child needs from what their child wants. The price of overprotection is prolonging the dependency of immaturity and thereby aiding the progression of chemical dependency. (MacDonald 1984)

Enabling behavior has been defined as taking responsibility for someone else's lack of responsibility, or softening the consequences for someone's irresponsibility. Enablers are under the delusion that no one knows about the problems and they can

TABLE 5.1

Five Styles of Managing Anxiety

Underfunctioners

- tend to have several areas where they just can't get organized.
- become less competent under stress, thus inviting others to take over.
- tend to develop physical or emotional symptoms when stress is high in either the family or the work situation.
- earn such labels as the "patient," the "frail one," the "sick one," the "problem," the "irresponsible one."
- have difficulty showing their strong, competent side to intimate others.

Overfunctioners

- know what's best not only for themselves but for others as well.
- move in quickly to advise, rescue, and take over when stress hits.
- have difficulty staying out and allowing others to struggle with their own problems.
- avoid worrying about their own personal goals and problems by focusing on others.
- have difficulty sharing their own vulnerable, underfunctioning side, especially with those people who are viewed as having problems.
- may be labeled the person who is "always reliable" or "always together."

Blamers

- respond to anxiety with emotional intensity and fighting.
- have a short fuse.
- expend high levels of energy trying to change someone who does not want to change.
- engage in repetitive cycles of fighting that relieve tension but perpetuate the old pattern.

- hold another person responsible for one's own feelings and actions.
- see others as the sole obstacle to making changes.

Pursuers

- react to anxiety by seeking greater togetherness in a relationship.
- place a high value on talking things out and expressing feelings, and believe others should do the same.
- feel rejected and take it personally when someone close to them wants more time and space alone or away from the relationship.
- tend to pursue harder and then coldly withdraw when an important person seeks distance.
- may negatively label themselves as "too dependent" or "too demanding" in a relationship.
- tend to criticize their partner as someone who can't handle feelings or tolerate closeness.

Distancers

- seek emotional distance or physical space when stress is high.
- consider themselves to be self-reliant and private persons—more "do-it-yourselfers" than help-seekers.
- have difficulty showing their needy, vulnerable, and dependent sides.
- receive such labels as "emotionally unavailable," "withholding," "unable to deal with feelings," from significant others.
- manage anxiety in personal relationships by intensifying work-related projects.
- may cut off a relationship entirely when things get intense, rather than hanging in and working it out.
- open up most freely when they are not pushed or pursued.

Source: *The Dance of Anger* by Harriet Lerner, Ph.D., 1997, HarperCollins.

continue to cover them up. The reality is that others are aware of the problems and are directly and indirectly letting the family know they need help. Only the family maintains this denial to the real dimensions of the problem.

T A B L E   5 . 2

Enabling Behavior

Charles Nelson (1988) identified the following four styles of enabling behavior.

Avoiding and Shielding

Avoiding and shielding constitute any behavior by a family member that covers up or prevents the user or the family member from experiencing the full impact of the harmful consequences of the drug use. Enabling behavior includes

- Making up excuses to avoid social contact during drinking and drugging periods
- Side-stepping or avoiding participation in discussions about drugs
- Taking alcohol, sedatives, and/or other drugs to try to lower one's own anxiety or stress about a family member's problems with drugs
- Not standing up for one's rights in fear of the family member going into a binge cycle of drug use
- Cleaning up the family member's vomit after an alcohol/drug episode
- Staying away from home as much as possible to get away from the situation
- Shielding the addict from a crisis that could send her/him into therapy
- Telling the alcoholic to leave until he/she quits drinking but then immediately going out and looking for that family member
- Helping the addict keep up appearances or cover up around relatives, friends, neighbors, or her/his employer

Attempting to Control

Attempting to control is any behavior by a family member that is performed with the intent of taking personal control over the alcoholic/addict's use of the drug. Enabling behavior includes

- Trying to buy things that might divert the addict from drug use (sports equipment, tools, car, house, etc.)
- Spending the night at a hotel or motel to get the user to quit

- Spending the night at a friend's house to get the user to quit
- Screaming, yelling, swearing, or crying in an attempt to get a family member to stop drinking or drugging
- Threatening to hurt oneself in an attempt to get a family member to quit
- Threatening physical violence to get the user to quit
- Checking or measuring the addict's drug stash to determine how much he has been using
- Encouraging the addict to do the drug at home to avoid more problems away from home
- Using or withholding sex as a way to control a partner's alcohol/drug use
- Throwing away, hiding, or destroying the family member's stash or paraphernalia

Taking Over Responsibilities

Taking over responsibilities is any behavior by the family member designed to take over the user's personal responsibilities (e.g., finances, household chores, or employment). Enabling behavior includes

- Cleaning the family member's drug paraphernalia when left out
- Waking the alcoholic in time for work
- Reminding the user to eat at times
- Staying home from work to take care of the family member's problems resulting from drug use
- Preaching to the addict about her failures as a warning about the personal effects of the drug use
- Doing the family member's chores
- Waiting hand and foot on the family member
- Paying all the bills
- Taking a second job to cover the bills piling up after money has been diverted to drugs
- Covering the alcoholic/addict's bad checks

Rationalizing and Accepting

Rationalizing and accepting are any behavior by the family member that conveys a rationalization or

TABLE 5.2 (*continued*)

Enabling Behavior

acceptance of the alcoholic/addict's use of the drug. Enabling behavior includes

- Believing and/or communicating that the family member's episodes of drug use were only isolated instances and not patterns of use

- Believing and/or communicating that the use of the drugs was safe
- Believing and/or communicating that the family member's use of drugs increased that person's self-confidence

Case Study 5.2

Enabling Behavior

Jerome

Jerome's marijuana use and related behaviors were driving his family crazy. Mom tried persuasion and pleading to Jerome's sense of "doing the right thing." She picked up after Jerome, believed his stories, denied his abuse of marijuana, and buffered him from his dad's anger.

Dad vacillated from trying to control the situation, to buying and doing things for Jerome. He would "throw money" at the problem and then get angry when Jerome was irresponsible. This cycle continued for quite some time. The family entered family counseling, but most sessions were just "rag on Jerome sessions." Mom and Dad decided to do their own individual counseling, which eventually led to marital counseling. Eventually they stopped blaming each other for Jerome's problems, diminished their enabling behavior, and held Jerome responsible for his behavior. Progress was slow but eventually led to all three of them feeling like they were a more functional and balanced family.

Discussion

Enabling behavior is not the domain of just one family member. Usually both parents, and even siblings, enable in an imbalanced family system. Until all family members can take responsibility for their own enabling behavior, rather than blaming each other, the family will continue to have problems.

Family counseling can be effective if family members work with a therapist who is trained in both family systems and alcohol/drug treatment. Often individual therapy, or some form of individual work (e.g., Alanon), is necessary before the family can work together.

✗ Stages in Family Recovery from Substance-Abuse Problems

Families have a wide range and variety of reactions to alcohol/drug problems, yet there are some common, generalizable patterns to a family's response.

One model describes the following stages in the family's adjustment to the substance-abuse problem:

1. Denial and minimizing
2. Tension and isolation
3. Frustration and disorganization
4. Attempts to reorganize, shifts in family member alliances
5. Separation in roles, escape
6. Reorganization without the addict/alcoholic
7. Recovery and reorganization with the addict/alcoholic

The application of the stages of grieving can also be used as a model to describe the stages in recovery for the alcoholic/addict and their family members.

1. Denial
2. Anger
3. Bargaining
4. Feeling (or depression)
5. Acceptance

Often the stages are positioned differently or combined. Remember, such models are meant to highlight different aspects of the recovery process, not to describe a rigid linear process.

Denial

At the denial stage (see Table 5.3), family members rarely acknowledge that something is wrong, although they sense something might be different about their family. The spouse or family members may seek help in an indirect, nonspecific manner, such as talking to friends and/or relatives. Unfortunately, those friends and relatives often reinforce the denial. One such example is the following:

Denial Transaction Between Mary and Her Sister-in-Law, Maureen

Mary: The other night at the party, do you think Harry drank too much?
Maureen: Oh, that happens to everyone once in a while.

TABLE 5.3

Denial Stage in Imbalanced Family Systems

Feelings—embarrassed, humiliated, shamed
Defenses—minimization, rationalization
Linkage to society—friends and relatives "maintain the denial"
Motto—"Normal family illusion"

Mary: You don't think he has a problem with alcohol, do you?

Maureen: No, of course not. He drinks like most of us in the family, and we certainly don't have a problem. You're overreacting.

In reality, Harry and Maureen grew up in alcoholic family systems and they both have drinking problems.

Anger

Anger is an effective defense to keep family members from talking about issues and feelings that might indicate an alcohol/drug problem in the family. Anger can be expressed as verbal, physical, emotional, and/or sexual threats, abuse, and/or violation. Anger can be actual or threatened rejection and abandonment. Alcoholics/addicts use anger to blame and shame other family members as inadequate and responsible for their predicament. In reality, the anger is a way for the alcoholic/addict to avoid feelings of shame, to control others in the family, and to deny responsibility for problems in the family system.

Once in recovery, many adolescent and adult patients/clients admit that causing a conflict or big fight was a way to get out of the house and use alcohol/drugs. Many clients rationalized that they were already in trouble with the family, so what was the difference if they got into more trouble?

An adolescent patient/client once described her alcoholic/addictive family system as "raging and ragging" (nagging): "Dad is the one who rages around the home, and Mom attempts to control him by ragging at Dad and everyone else. It is no wonder that I don't spend much time at home."

The combined effect is an unsafe, unpredictable family system with underlying feelings of confusion, fear, anxiety, and shame and sometimes immobilizing trauma.

This conflict among family members creates a climate of confusion and a lack of clarity as to what is an appropriate approach to the problem of alcohol/ drugs. The result is often a trial-and-error approach. At first, family members try extreme control or rigid threats: "The next time you use alcohol/drugs, I will . . ." (not let you in the house, confine you to your room for one month, get a divorce or separation). When this doesn't work, the next approach might be to let go, or to try to ignore the addictive

The Garden of Eden: Enabling behavior.

Callahan, distributed by Levin Represents.

TABLE 5.4

Anger Stage in Imbalanced Family Systems

Feelings—confusion, fear, anxiety
Defenses—"raging and ragging"
            control to chaos
            trial and error
Linkage to society—search for magical solutions
Goal—cover-up real issues and feelings

behavior completely, as if the addict didn't exist. The resulting pattern of control-release is chaotic. This trial-and-error approach creates further anger, confusion, and feelings of hopelessness.

At this stage, the family might go beyond relatives and friends and talk to a minister, priest, rabbi, family physician, or school counselor. The family members may be vague in disclosing the degree to which alcohol/drugs are used. At this stage, family members are still not quite sure they need help and are embarrassed in seeking help. They may start to get help, get frightened, or be resistant to experiencing the pain associated with acknowledging the problem and then back off from getting help. See Table 5.4.

Bargaining

The bargaining stage (see Case Study 5.3) is usually preceded by a major crisis. The family can no longer deny or ignore the problem and cannot cover up the feelings of frustration and anger. The family is essentially saying, "We have had enough of this; it's too chaotic." The family is still not ready to effect change in the system; instead, the goal is to strike some arrangement or bargain. Being held hostage by the addict, the family is willing to pay a ransom to have the addict stop bothering them with outrageous behavior. Unfortunately, the ransom often goes beyond what is reasonable or tolerable, and the family initially agrees to do almost anything to survive in this chaos. Many of the bargains are financial or object-related: "If you stop abusing alcohol/drugs, I'll buy you. . . ."

The underlying and false assumption of most bargains is that the addict can stop using. The assumption is that the addict can override the drive and allure of the alcohol/drugs for a reward. Unfortunately, the drive to use alcohol/drugs is stronger than the reward of the bargain, and willpower alone is not strong enough to overcome the drive to use alcohol/drugs.

Some of the bargains are far more subtle. Couples, families, and friends develop lives based on the bargain of maintaining addiction. See Table 5.5. Following are some common bargains related to alcoholism and drug addiction, and their weaknesses:

TABLE 5.5

Bargaining, Feeling, and Acceptance Stage in Imbalanced Family Systems

Goal—"maintain the chaos of addiction"
Bargains—compromise values
        love/hate—let go/hold on
        avoid making a decision
        confused—doesn't know what is appropriate
Depression/feelings—feelings are experienced
Acceptance
  there is a problem
  on road to recovery

Case Study 5.3

A Bargain that Doesn't Work

Marilyn

Marilyn is a very bright, attractive, outgoing 17-year-old. She puts forth minimal effort at school and barely passes her classes, despite her superior intelligence.

She smokes marijuana regularly, drinks alcohol, uses cocaine, and has begun freebasing cocaine. She has been staying out late, and sleeping in every day during the summer. This is the second marriage for her mother, and Marilyn's mother and father are always trying to bribe Marilyn to get her to straighten out. Bribes have included a new car, clothes shopping excursions, and vacations. There have been so many conflicts at home between Marilyn, her mother, and her stepfather, that her real father has agreed to let Marilyn live in the condo on the waterfront for the rest of the summer. It only took a few weeks for the place to be trashed, and the police became regular visitors to Marilyn's parties. Her parents also became aware of Marilyn's freebase cocaine use and took her in for an alcohol/drug evaluation.

Discussion

Bargaining doesn't work and is a temporary solution. Marilyn was not held accountable for her behavior, school grades, and drug use. The parents were avoiding these issues and related conflicts by blindly hoping that Marilyn would somehow mature and grow out of this stage. They kept on giving her things and buying (no pun intended) her stories.

In the "bargaining" stage, they avoided the reality of feeling what was really going on, and accepted that Marilyn had significant problems. But they avoided the first and biggest problem—her drug abuse.

- *Let's ignore the addict's behavior and it might just stop.* The more you ignore the destructive behavior, the more intense and dramatic the situation becomes.
- *Let's separate or withdraw from the addict temporarily.* Unless there is strong therapeutic and personal support, the addict feeds on the partner's or family members' weaknesses. The individual usually does not have the support to break the codependent dance of addiction. (See Chapter 7.)
- *Avoid making a decision; maybe it will get better with time.* It's very rare that a spontaneous recovery occurs from alcohol/drugs. In Chapter 9 we discuss alcohol/drug intervention and "raising the addict's bottom" in an attempt to salvage and avoid further damage. Rarely do addicts decide on their own to get help. Sometimes it is so late that scary consequences are involved, such as the threat of physical harm, criminal justice and legal problems, job and financial problems, or death.

At the bargaining stage, family members might seek help from experts in the field because their bargains are not working and they need advice and direction. Even when family members are fortunate in finding a counselor who knows about alcohol/drug intervention and treatment, the family members may still not follow through. The attitude at this stage is still a form of bargaining. The therapeutic bargain is to fix the identified patient (the addict) so the bargainer can avoid feeling pain. In some situations, family members may even sabotage counseling to avoid the pain of looking at their roles in the dysfunction. In a distorted sense, the failure of the trained professional validates the failure of the family member: "If the counselor can't help, then I guess we didn't do such a bad job." Many families seeking counseling soon find out that addiction is a family disease and effective treatment involves the entire family.

Feeling

At the feeling stage, family members can no longer deny, cover up with anger, or bargain their feelings away. Many feelings come to the surface and are easily accessed. Family members are crying at the slightest provocation, anxious to the point of being hypervigilant (checking things out obsessively), and in some cases feeling immobilized. These feelings are undeniable and force the family to seek help.

Acceptance

At the acceptance stage, the family has recognized that they have a problem. They are ready to do the work necessary to heal and develop healthier ways of relating. Recognizing that all the family members are suffering, they have the courage to get help. At this stage, the alcoholic/addict and the family members have begun to work on the problem. This is when treatment and recovery begin.

References

Lawson, Ann, and Gary Lawson. 1998. *Alcoholism and the family: A guide to treatment and prevention.* 2d ed. Gaithersburg, Md.: Aspen.

Lerner, Harriet. 1997. *The dance of anger.* New York: HarperCollins.

MacDonald, Donald Ian. 1984. *Drugs, drinking and adolescents.* Chicago: Year Book Medical.

Nelson, Charles. 1988. The style of enabling behavior. In *Treating cocaine dependency,* edited by D. E. Smith and D. Wesson. Center City, Minn.: Hazeldon Foundation.

Satir, Virginia. 1967. *Conjoint family therapy.* Palo Alto, Calif.: Science and Behavior Books.

Satir, Virginia. 1972. *Peoplemaking.* Palo Alto, Calif.: Science and Behavior Books.

Satir, Virginia, and Michele Baldwin. 1983. *Satir: Step by step—A guide to creating change in families.* Northvale, N.J.: Aronson, Jason.

Wegscheider-Cruse, Sharon. 1976. *The family trap.* Palo Alto, Calif.: Nurturing Network.

Wegscheider-Cruse, Sharon, et al. 1994. *Family reconstruction therapy: The living model.* Palo Alto, Calif.: Science and Behavior Books.

Whitaker, Carl, and Augustus Y. Napier. 1978. *The family crucible.* New York: Harper & Row.

Parenting

Impact on Alcohol/Drug Use and Abuse

❖ **Chapter in Review**

Parental imbalance is defined as parents who lack knowledge and skills in parenting. These parents have unrealistic expectations of their children and are insensitive to the needs of their children.

Imbalanced families often have difficulty in setting appropriate boundaries. Boundary inadequacy is defined as the inability to set consistent and appropriate boundaries in relationships, as evidenced by ambiguous, overly rigid, and invasive boundaries. Triangulation is another form of boundary inadequacy, in which the parent-child affiliation is established at the expense of the peripheral parent. Frequently, these problems in boundary setting lead to physical and sexual violations and emotional and psychological abuse. This is especially true in alcohol/addict family system.

Parents who use/abuse alcohol or drugs model the same behavior in their offspring. Conversely, family cohesion, flexibility, and communication clarity can positively influence a child against using/abusing alcohol or drugs.

This chapter focuses on six factors that influence a child's use/abuse of alcohol or drugs later in life:

1. Parent-child bonding
2. Temperament of the child
3. Parenting styles and the quality of the parent-child relationship
4. Parental imbalance and boundary setting
5. Parents' use/abuse of alcohol and drugs
6. Other family system variables

Poor bonding is described in the context of separation stress, leading to feelings of abandonment and rejection. The six key elements of abandonment depression in adults are feelings of homicidal rage, suicidal depression, panic, hopelessness and helplessness, emptiness and void, and guilt.

The child's temperament is described as a behavioral characteristic present at birth, or within the first few months. Certain temperaments put the individual more at risk for substance abuse. A so-called difficult temperament puts the individual at risk for problem behaviors, including substance abuse. A difficult temperament includes high activity level, low flexibility, task orientation, mood instability, and social withdrawal.

Shame plays a major role in devastating the parent-child relationship. Shame is a deep-rooted feeling that results from traumatic childhood experiences. Shame is defined as the self looking in on itself and finding itself lacking. When shame attaches to feelings, those feelings are usually escalated (e.g., anger + shame = rage).

This chapter concludes with a description of the imbalanced life cycles of families and the difficulty in getting fathers of

The names and circumstances of case studies in this chapter have been changed to maintain anonymity.

alcoholics/addicts to be involved in family counseling. Noble ascriptions are described as a way to engage fathers to get involved in family treatment.

Some of the parenting variables that influence a child's use and abuse of alcohol/drugs later in life are

- Parent-child bonding
- Temperament of the child
- Parenting styles and the quality of the parent-child relationship
- Parental imbalance and boundary setting
- Parents' use/abuse of alcohol or drugs
- Other family system variables

These factors are the major focus of this chapter.

The parent-child bond is an extremely potent, primary relationship that greatly influences behavior. Maccoby and Martin (1983) describe the parent-child bond as unique among human relationships. Nothing is as powerful as the bonding between parent and child. Extraordinary feats of strength and sacrifice have come to be identified with this strong bond. Examples of the parent-child bond include the incredible adrenaline-induced strength of a father saving a child who is pinned under an automobile and the dedication and perseverance of a mother who protects her child from the drug- and crime-infested streets of the inner city.

✄ Parent-Child Bonding

The child's development is often impaired as a result of a poor bond between parent and child. Self-concept, social and interpersonal relationships, achievement, and identity are negatively affected by inadequate parent-child bonding.

A positive, caring relationship is essential for healthy development. The effective parent establishes bonding experiences that develop a positive regard for the child and reinforces a positive sense of self. When a parent loses this positive bonding with a child, the child's sense of loss and anger may never be assuaged. This loss is often found in alcoholic/addict family systems.

Often, because of certain circumstances, parents are not available. A variety of conditions may take the parents from the child—death of a parent, a parent away at war, divorce, illness, mental breakdown, criminal-justice problems, financial problems, job relocation (e.g., military), and so on. All of these circumstances prevent bonding between child and parent and are extremely disruptive to the child's life. (See Case Study 6.1.) The child may even suffer depression as a result of times when he or she felt abandoned or rejected.

Certainly, the parent's alcoholism/drug addiction also makes the parent either unavailable or inconsistent in the quality of the parent-child relationship.

Patrick Carnes, author of numerous books on sexual trauma and addiction, describes the importance of developing healthy bonds with caring adults outside of the family system for children who have been sexually violated/traumatized by a family member. In an interview in *Professional Counselor Magazine*, Carnes states, "One of the things that emerges in trauma literature is why some kids, who have the same identical history of trauma, rebound from that and have resiliency. As near as I can tell from the literature and what I have seen clinically, the primary factor is the

Case Study 6.1

Early Bonding—Being Available in the "Now"

Karen

Karen was very young—18 years old—when she had her first of two children. Over the next few years, she was extremely depressed. Perhaps it was the responsibility of two young children and being tied to the house or the constant conflicts with her husband that caused Karen to decide to leave. It was an extremely difficult decision to leave two toddlers. However, at the time, her own survival seemed more important.

Twelve years later, Karen was in counseling. She was 34 years old and struggling with the fact that her 14-year-old son, Gary, was addicted to alcohol/drugs. Over the past 2 years Gary had been in and out of outpatient counseling programs and was now in his second inpatient alcohol/drug program. Karen was needing some support in setting boundaries with Gary. She first needed to talk about her guilt at abandoning him when he was 2 years old. She had left the home, had filed for divorce, and had given custody of both children to Gary's father.

As the counseling proceeded, it became clear that her own alcohol use had contributed dramatically to her problems in those early years in the marriage. It was a few years after leaving the marriage that she acknowledged her own alcoholism. Even though she had been in recovery from alcohol and drugs for several years now and extremely active in Alcoholics Anonymous (AA), she was still experiencing dramatic problems in relationships. Over several sessions, she was able to talk about her own childhood and revealed that her father had sexually violated her. Although she had talked about this several times in previous counseling sessions and during her inpatient alcohol/drug program, she was now able to see that this contributed to her own fears of abusing her own children. She slowly began to accept how her alcoholic behavior prevented her from bonding with her own children. After some time, she was able to accept that she could not recapture those lost years with her children. She could not compensate for the lack of bonding during those formative years, no matter how available she was for Gary and his younger sister today. She began to recognize that her own attempts to compensate for those early years had resulted in her enabling Gary's alcohol and drug use. It took Karen some time to grieve and accept that she missed those early developmental years. She realized that there was a permanent loss in bonding, a loss that could never be recaptured.

Discussion

At age 18, Karen was not really capable of providing adequate nurturing and nourishment to her infant children. Her own depression, alcoholism, and history of sexual violation, along with the developmental reality that she was 18 years old, contributed to her inability to be present with her children. The constant conflicts with her husband made an impossible situation even more difficult.

The guilt of her having "abandoned" her toddlers caused her to indulge her so when they did get reunited. It is important that her therapist not judge Karen but help her work through her own issues—the first of which is that she cannot recapture all those lost years—and help her grieve, and accept what she can do to develop relationship with her son. It is also important to acknowledge the reality that their relationship might not develop, but that she can persevere and maintain her availability to her son "in the now."

ability of children to have healthy bonds around them that are not traumatic. As an antidote to trauma bonding, you need healthy bonds" (Carnes 1995).

Two prevailing hypotheses regarding parental bonding in adolescent substance abusers are the *overinvolvement hypothesis* and the *functional hypothesis* (Volk et al. 1988). The overinvolvement hypothesis is that one parent (frequently the mother) is overly involved in the adolescent's life to compensate for the lack of availability by the other parent. The functional hypothesis is that the adolescent's substance abuse distracts the family from focusing on other familial problems, such as marital discord, infidelity, and parental abuse of alcohol/drugs.

Abandonment Depression

A young child needs nurturing and connection with a caring parent. James Masterson (1976), in his work with borderline-personality-disordered individuals, identifies an affective (feeling) disorder that he labeled "abandonment depression." Masterson believes that a significant separation stress precipitates abandonment depression (see Table 6.1). It is also likely that this separation occurs early in life, at 18 to 24 months of age. The individual suffering from abandonment depression is metaphorically described as "a hollow eggshell with the insides removed." All the good stuff—the nutrients, the seed, the juices of life—has been removed, has rotted, or has been destroyed by a lack of nurturing.

The six key elements of abandonment depression are

1. Homicidal rage
2. Suicidal depression
3. Panic

TABLE 6.1

Childhood Experiences of Abandonment and Rejection

- Lack of physical and emotional availability of parents
- Negative blaming; verbal and nonverbal behavior or attacks
- Mixed messages (double binds), saying one thing and meaning something else
- Unreasonably high expectations or standards; ambiguous expectations of behavior, performance, and affect
- Lack of warmth, sensitivity, security, safety, or high regard for feelings, situations, and conflicts
- Discounting of the child's sense of self or physical and psychological boundaries
- Disparaging, blaming, and generally rejecting attitude about the child's difficulty with developmental tasks
- Disregard, ridicule, blaming, teasing, or other verbal and nonverbal behavior that is either rejecting or shaming
- Threats to abandon or leave a child in a joking or real manner
- Negative and rejecting statements, actions, and comments about something that is of minor or major importance to the child

4. Feelings of hopelessness and helplessness
5. Emptiness and void
6. Guilt

Perhaps the parent is ill, suffering from depression, or withdrawn due to a personality and/or psychiatric disorder and finds it hard to nurture his or her child. Maybe the parent didn't grow up in a family system that modeled nurturing, caring, and empathetic connection with the children. Masterson (1976) describes three elements that may produce separation stress in children:

1. *Nature:* Possible genetic or constitutional deficiencies such as inability to tolerate separation anxiety or to synthesize positive and negative effects as well as such conditions as attention deficit disorders and developmental disharmonies.
2. *Nurture:* "Maternal libidinal unavailability for the child's move toward separation-individuation or self-activation (i.e., the mother is unable or has difficulty in identifying, acknowledging, and supporting the child's emerging self-activation, experimentation, and exploration). The reasons for maternal libidinal unavailability may be many—death, divorce, physical or emotional illness, etc."
3. *Fate:* "Any accident of fate that impairs the child's ability to separate and/or individuate. On the separation side, events such as death or divorce can prevent the mother from being emotionally available. On the individuation side, events can impair or prevent the child from practicing his emerging individuation. For example, the child may be sickly or in a restricted environment."

Impact of Early Abandonment on Adult Interpersonal Relationships

Individuals suffering from abandonment depression express complaints having to do with intimacy. They have difficulty emotionally entering into healthy relationships and are unable to differentiate their needs from others' needs. They experience difficulty in identifying and communicating feelings or in accepting feelings and communication from others. There is either a fusing of others into self or a fission, causing them to break away emotionally from others.

Masterson (1976) described persons suffering from abandonment depression as experiencing difficulty in establishing intimacy in relationships due to a limited capacity for spontaneity, empathy, and sensitivity. These persons have difficulty in making an emotional commitment to a relationship. Such individuals experience twin fears—the fear of losing (abandonment), which leads to clinging behavior, and the fear of being engulfed (smothered), which leads to feelings of depersonalization, shutting down, distortion of reality, and desensitization (numbing, disconnecting from the body).

At first, using alcohol and drugs to facilitate feeling in interpersonal relationships may seem effective; however, as time goes on, this becomes dysfunctional and destructive. Persons feeling pain also use alcohol/drugs to alleviate the core feeling of abandonment.

Another option those suffering feelings of abandonment may choose is to enter into dysfunctional and/or alcoholic/addict relationships, or relationships with individuals emotionally and physically unavailable.

The *Diagnostic and Statistical Manual of Mental Disorders* (American Psychiatric Association, 1994) lists diagnostic criteria for borderline personality disorder, which include the following. These often result from early childhood experiences of abandonment.

1. Impulsivity or unpredictability in at least two areas that are potentially self-damaging
2. A pattern of unstable and intense interpersonal relationships
3. Inappropriate, intense anger or lack of control of anger
4. Identity disturbances manifested by uncertainty about several issues relating to identity, such as self-image, gender identity, long-term goals or career choice, friendship patterns, values, and loyalties
5. Affective instability

✖ Child's Temperament

Each child has his or her own temperament. Temperament is described as a behavioral characteristic that researchers believe is present at birth, within the first few months of life, and during infancy (Garrison and Earls 1987; Kohnstamm, Bates, and Rothbart 1989).

There is emerging evidence that extremes in certain temperament traits, such as high activity level, emotionality, attention span, and sociability, are associated with children of alcoholics. These temperaments also put the child at risk for alcoholism/drug addiction and other problem behaviors. The parents of these children are faced with challenges beyond the average parenting techniques. Early evaluation and early intervention are essential to address the issues of children with these temperaments. Children who exhibit these genetically determined temperaments may benefit from prevention efforts, that include special educational and counseling programs. Parents also benefit from parenting skills and education in helping these children to cope better.

Aspects of temperament may predict the behavior problems and substance abuse problems that frequently arise during adolescence. There also appear to be gender differences in temperament that put children at risk for behavior problems and substance abuse. A study by Block, Block, and Keyes (1988) found that nursery school girls who were low in ego resiliency and ego control were using marijuana at age 14, and boys' marijuana use was predicted by low ego control but not by early ego resilience. Masse and Tremblay (1997), in a study of kindergarten boys, found that high novelty seeking and low harm avoidance measured at age 6 predicted early onset of cigarette smoking, drunkenness, and other drug use in adolescence. Dobkin, Tremblay, Masse, and Vitaro (1995), in a study of 755 six-year-old boys, found that disruptive behaviors (fighting, hyperactivity, oppositional behaviors) measured at 6 years of age predicted having been drunk or using other drugs—or both—prior to age 14.

Some clusters of temperament related to substance use/abuse are labeled as a "difficult temperament"—high activity level, low flexibility and task orientation, mood instability, and social withdrawal (Lerner and Vicary 1984, Ohannessian and

Hesselbrook 1995). Tubman and Windle (1999) described a difficult temperament as higher activity level, lower task orientation, inflexibility, a withdrawal orientation, biological arrhythmicity, and low positive mood, as a predictor of higher levels of alcohol problems among adolescents. In a study by Martin, Kaczynski, Maisto, and Tarter (1996) a cluster of temperament traits was a predictor of the number of drugs used by adolescents. That cluster included dispositional traits characterized by heightened negative affect (depressed mood and anxiety) and behavioral undercontrol, reflecting impulsivity, aggressivity, acting out, and sensation seeking.

The research on temperament has primarily been on the traits that predict substance use and abuse and problem behaviors. There are temperament traits that may function as a protective factor, especially for high-risk groups. One such study measured the influence of cuddly, affectionate temperament style in infancy and early childhood. This longitudinal Kauai study of low socioeconomic children of alcohol-abusing parents found decreased risk for alcohol-related and other adverse outcomes in adolescence and adulthood. The explanation was that these children had resiliency as a result of more frequent and stronger social and emotional support (Werner and Smith 1999).

✖ Parenting Styles and the Quality of the Parent-Child Relationship

A *supportive* parent with a healthy relationship with her or his child is less likely to have a child who gets involved with alcohol/drugs.

Rollins and Thomas (1979) explained the differences between a supportive and controlling parent. They defined a supportive parent as possessing "parental behaviors toward the child such as praising, encouraging, and giving physical affection, which indicate to the child that she or he is accepted, approved of, and loved." In contrast, the controlling parent is defined as having "parental behavior toward the child which is intended to direct the child's behavior in a manner acceptable to the parent."

The goal of parenting is to develop a high level of parental support and a moderate level of parental control. Parents who are highly rigid, authoritarian, and controlling tend to have children who are resentful, frustrated, and angry. These children are then prone to problem behaviors, causing them to rebel or passive-aggressively get back at the rigid parent. "Children whose relationships with their parents lacked love, warmth, and closeness and exhibited signs of hostility, have children who exhibit increased levels of substance abuse, delinquency, and dysfunctional coping strategies" (Johnson and Pandina 1991).

The children of parents who are unable to establish moderate control and effective disciplining techniques often experience problem behaviors and associate with other children who have problem behaviors.

The availability of the parent(s) is extremely important in the child's development, as is the quality of the parent-child relationship. Frequently, parents will spend a quantity of time with their children and mislead themselves into thinking they are effectively developing the relationship. The quality of the parent-child relationship is the essential ingredient. The parent needs to be fully present, listening reflectively, and exchanging ideas, while giving full attention to the child. Quality time also involves understanding, touching (hugging), playing, and sharing. Making a genuine, heart-to-heart connection is at the core of a good parent-child relationship.

TABLE 6.2

Characteristics of Shameful Experiences

1. Unexpected exposure; being judged on a vulnerable aspect of oneself
2. Feeling as if there is a loss of choice
3. Feeling out of place, flawed, defective, or inadequate
4. A threat to the core of one's identity
5. Mistrust in ability to perceive things properly; unsure of self in making decisions or relating to people
6. Trust of self and others is jeopardized; boundaries are distorted; and physical, emotional, and/or sexual violations may occur.
7. Difficulty in assessing what is reality
8. Feeling helpless, powerless, and trapped, with no way out (Fossum and Mason 1986).

Parenting Styles That Shame Children

Shame is a deep-rooted feeling, often a result of traumatic childhood experiences that are excessively shaming (e.g., sexual, physical, and emotional abuse). (See Table 6.2.) Parental imbalance and parenting dysfunction are at the core of these feelings of shame. Merle Fossum and Marilyn Mason (1986) defined shame as "the self looking in on itself and finding the self lacking or flawed." Individuals may feel exposed, vulnerable, and fearful that others know they are feeling inherently bad and inadequate. Shame is more powerful than simple embarrassment, which is a temporary situation with little long-term impact. In shame, people feel that they will never recover from the negative way others see them.

Shame is a feeling that has an integral role in the individual's development. "Shame is a basic, natural human emotion, which in moderation is adaptive, healthy, and absolutely essential for development. We could not eliminate shame even if we wanted to. It's inbred in the species" (Kaufman 1989).

Sigmund Freud used the word *guilt* to describe feelings of shame. Erik Erikson, in his description of the human life cycle, outlined two developmental stages that focused on guilt and shame: (1) autonomy versus doubt and shame and (2) initiative versus guilt.

Growing up in an alcohol/addict family system or an imbalanced family system creates a foundation of shame. Additional feelings of shame are perpetrated by peers, the school system, other institutions, and other authority figures in the child's life. These shame-based messages are internalized by children. The result is a vicious pattern of feelings and behavior, which perpetuates the feelings of shame.

Individuals from shame-based family systems often feel that (1) there is no hope for change; (2) shame is inescapable and inevitable; (3) shame is exterior-based, not an internal process; and (4) they are bad, no good, flawed, or worthless as individuals (Fossum and Mason 1986). For these individuals, feelings of shame can include thoughts like these:

No matter what I do, it's never going to be good enough, so why try?

Each time I try, I fail, anyway. The result is always negative.

I must try so much harder than others. It's so much easier for others, so I must be
    inferior and inadequate.

You have to be perfect to be O.K.

Look at _____. Now, if I could only be like them.

It's never going to get any better, no matter how hard I try.

If only others would feel good. Then I would be happy.

    Shame is a fascinating topic because it affects us all in some way (see Table 6.3). Most individuals can overcome feelings of shame and grow as a result of it, getting on with their lives. However, some individuals have been shamed dramatically and frequently, especially during early developmental years, and are unable to overcome it. These individuals are at risk for alcoholism and drug dependence or developing relationships with alcoholics/addicts. Too much trauma creates shame which leads to feelings of hopelessness and helplessness.

    There is almost a resignation that life is painfully unfulfilling—not worth trying to change. Expectations and aspirations are only indirectly acknowledged, for fear of reexperiencing rejection and shame. Shame-based individuals perceive themselves as trapped, inescapably destined to again experience the shame message of self-inadequacy and powerlessness. The shame-based orientation is external. The individual's sense of self is formed by others' evaluations and judgments of his or her performance and behavior. The orientation is outside (external world) in versus inside (internal self) out. Three characteristics—no hope, inescapable shame, and an exterior base—are found in shame-based systems and shame-based individuals.

    In contrast, in a balanced family system, the individual has a much healthier way of approaching life and others. The individual receives feedback from the world and evaluates the feedback. The individual then chooses to make changes or adjustments in decision making, goal setting, and interpersonal communication, based on his or her evaluation of the validity of the feedback. The major focus is on *hope* and *choice*.

    In a balanced-system, individuals can recognize their mistakes and not feel that they are the mistake. They can make amends to those who might have been hurt

---

TABLE 6.3

Shame

Definition: self looking in on self, finding the self lacking or feeling exposed—"seen"—in a public way and wanting to cover—feeling hunted

Shame-Based System	Balanced System
1. No hope—hopelessness	1. Hope—choice
2. Inescapable	2. Can make amends
3. Exterior-based	3. Internally based

Source: Fossum and Mason 1986.

by their mistakes and can learn from their errors. The experience is valued, and there is an opportunity for self-growth. Individuals from a balanced family system have an orientation that is inside out (internal). These individuals relate well to and have empathy for others, balancing their own sense of self with the judgments and reactions of others.

The following are ways to avoid shame in early childhood:

1. Parents should provide unconditional love. They should let their child know that they really like him or her. Talking; touching with affection; hugging; and, most important, paying attention to the child are some of the ways in which parents express unconditional love.
2. Parents should provide safety, nurturance, security, and care.
3. Parents should communicate clearly with and support their spouse or partner.
4. Parents should resolve conflicts with their spouse or partner (invoking the Alcoholics Anonymous motto "Would you rather be right or happy?").
5. Parents should play with their infants and children.
6. Parents should be available and enjoy the growth and development of their children.
7. Parents should recognize that at times parenting is overwhelming—they need to take a break and get support.
8. Parents should protect their children from others who may hurt, violate, or shame them.
9. At times, when parents "don't like their child's behavior" or are frustrated and annoyed, parents need to minimize the impact.
10. Parents should use appropriate discipline and good judgment in parenting and learn about parenting by taking classes on parenting and child development.
11. Parents should seek help from teachers, family members, counselors, doctors, clergy, and so on when "shame-based" family issues arise. They should not isolate or deny (minimize or rationalize) these issues but take early, proactive action, which can prevent a more significant problem later on.
12. Parents should encourage children to express themselves (what they feel and think) in play, verbal and nonverbal communication, and other activities.

Parents' Shame

Parents who have not done a good job of parenting may experience feelings of shame. Gomberg (1988) describes this parental shame as falling short of expectations in being a good parent. Jessup (1983) also describes a sense of failure for mothers that is shameful. Eliason and Skinstad (1995) describe the deep sense of identity and self-esteem that many women gain from their children.

> When they perceive failure at meeting the needs of their children, the sense of hopelessness that follows can be devastating. The sense of shame . . . about mothering in substance using women has been heightened by the media's attention to Fetal Alcohol Effects and 'cocaine babies' in recent years. This press is often sensationalized and contains blatant mother-blaming implications (Eliason and Skinstad 1995).

Shame and Feelings

Shame-based messages that are internalized have a major impact on feelings. When shame is attached to normal, everyday feelings, it tends to escalate those feelings. For example, when an internalized shame-based message is attached to normal, everyday feelings of frustration or anger, it tends to escalate those feelings to rage (anger + shame = rage). The person feeling shame then directs this rage toward others, blaming and holding them responsible for feelings of anger and frustration. The rage violates others, pushes them away, and creates more of a feeling of isolation, loneliness, and hopelessness with no way out. This out-of-control emotional freight train picks up speed from all the memories of shame experienced in the family of origin. Some may think that the way to slow down this runaway emotional pain is to self-medicate with alcohol/drugs. Unfortunately, this temporary solution may even speed up the emotional turmoil or cause it to be repeated. When people do not deal with feelings of shame, this pattern continues. The next time, even less anger and shame are needed for the escalation to rage. (See Table 6.4.)

One of the largest domains of shame is human sexuality, as evidenced by our society's problems in establishing intimate and caring relationships. We will look at three areas in particular: adolescent sexual identity, sexual violation, and drugs and sex.

Adolescent Sexual Identity and Shame

The developmental task of exploring and defining one's sexual identity is probably the most difficult task of adolescence. Shame-based messages by parents, schools, institutions, and peers may be devastating to adolescents and delay the development of a secure sense of sexual identity. Shame-based messages include the following:

T A B L E   6 . 4

Affect-Shame Binds

anger + shame = rage

anxiety + shame = panic

fear + shame = terror

sadness + shame = depression

depression + shame = despair

despair + shame = suicidal thoughts

suicidal thoughts + shame = suicide attempt

hurt + shame = pain

pain + shame = trauma (deep or chronic pain)

trauma + shame = phobia

phobia + shame = loss of reality

unavailability + shame = lack of trust of others

lack of trust of others + shame = paranoia

paranoia + shame = loss of reality

You are bad if you _____. (masturbate, are feeling sexual, are aroused, etc.)

Having sexual feelings before marriage is unnatural.

Sex is dirty.

That's all that men want. Men are bad and evil.

Women use sex to manipulate you to get what they want.

Don't watch television; it promotes sexual arousal.

In our family, we don't talk with others about sex.

Sexual Violation and Shame

Sexual violations are common in alcoholic/addict and imbalanced family systems. Children often feel responsible for sexual violation, as if they caused the violation (e.g., I must be responsible for this sexual feeling in others because I am so cute, attractive, shy, or outgoing). Usually, the violation is not talked about or is enabled by the mother or, in some cases, the father. When told of the violation, the parent often denies that it happened or that it is possible and rationalizes the action: "Your uncle is that way with everyone. Try to stay away from him." Such parents fail to adequately protect children from future violations. When the behavior is acknowledged by children, usually no one in the family seeks therapeutic help for the victim and/or the perpetrator. Families deny sexual violations for fear of exposing the inappropriate and violating behavior and to avoid familial shame. Instead of families getting help, they maintain denial and scapegoat the victims by not acknowledging the violations or their pain. They take no or limited action to prevent future violations to the victim or to someone else.

Drugs, Sex, and Shame

Cocaine, marijuana, alcohol, methaqualone, and other drugs are often described as sex drugs, or aphrodisiacs. At early stages, alcohol/drugs do reduce inhibitions. This confuses people who define them as aphrodisiacs. In reality, all drugs impair performance, especially at middle and later stages of use.

Under the influence of alcohol/drugs, individuals also experience impaired judgment and may take part in sexual activities in which they would not normally engage if they were sober. The shame of these sexual experiences can be devastating, so they use alcohol/drugs to blot out these feelings of shame. This can become a vicious, negative, addictive cycle. This cycle involves alcohol/drug use, followed by sexual activity, followed by feelings of shame. More alcohol/drug use follows (to numb the feelings of shame), succeeded by sexual activity and more shame and feelings of loss of control.

Additional Characteristics of Shame and Abandonment
Rejection Sensitivity

Feelings of shame and abandonment can make individuals extremely sensitive to rejection, so much so that they choose not to try to grow and develop. Persons suffering from rejection sensitivity avoid situations that may be potentially shaming for fear of the situation triggering feelings of abandonment or rejection. Healthy individuals can tolerate shame, rejection, or abandonment and respond adaptively to these feelings by making the necessary adjustments and healthy choices in their lives.

Fear and Difficulty Making Decisions

Feelings of rejection, abandonment, and shame result in a variety of fears. Some of these fears are so traumatic that individuals cannot choose to change extremely uncomfortable situations. The fears of failure that may activate or trigger feelings of rejection, abandonment, and shame are so great that individuals choose to maintain self-effacing, even violating situations, instead of choosing healthy, growth-oriented paths.

The fear of success can also bring fears that, once some level of success is attained, it will fall apart and return the individual to previous feelings of failure and rejection. People then sabotage the gains in anticipation of deeper feelings of shame, rejection, and abandonment. What is missing is belief in themselves, their own self-worth, and their emerging talents, skills, and capabilities.

Poor Frustration Tolerance

When goals are blocked, even temporarily, persons who feel abandoned and rejected cannot tolerate this frustration. Such individuals believe there are no alternative choices or solutions to their blocked goals. Poor impulse control and self-destructive thinking may cause people to self-sabotage the progress they have made.

Other Reactions and Defenses

Common reactions and defenses to avoid feelings of abandonment and rejection include being overly defensive, extremely critical, or judgmental; showing rage or distorted thinking; and masking true feelings and emotions. People in pain deny the real issues and feelings by being overly defensive and critical of others. These persons view the world as being similar to the depriving, rejecting, and abandoning mothers and fathers they knew while growing up. Their distorted thinking tells them that the world will respond to them in the same way.

❧ Parental Imbalance and Boundary Setting

In her review of the literature, Carol L. Kempher (1987) identified various factors that contribute to parental imbalance. Often parents are imbalanced as caregivers; sometimes they are overwhelmed by problems of their own. (See Table 6.5.) This prevents them from providing the kind of care, support, structure, and healthy encouragement that children require to effectively develop and grow. Kempher summarized these characteristics of parental imbalance:

1. Increased alcoholism, drug use, and nicotine dependence
2. Increased antisocial or sexually deviant behavior in parents
3. Increased mental and emotional problems, such as depression, personality disorders, or narcissism
4. Increased marital conflict
5. Increased parental absenteeism due to separation, divorce, or death

Parents who are not aware of their own emotional and psychological issues may deny the impact their anger, rage, and physical and emotional unavailability have on their children. Parents play an integral role in the development of their children.

TABLE 6.5

Parental Imbalance

Chemically dependent and/or imbalanced parents often

- Lack knowledge and skill in parenting
- Have unrealistic expectations and lack information on what is developmentally appropriate behavior at various ages
- Are insensitive to the special needs of their children
- Have decreased family-management skills
- Have inappropriate disciplining techniques and maintain inconsistent, rigid, or ambiguous boundaries
- Have decreased positive responses to and reinforcement of their children
- Have decreased parental involvement and poor bonding or parent/child attachment

It is natural and essential for parents to set appropriate boundaries with their children. Boundaries act as guideposts for children to bump into as they test their own independence and developmental skills. Good boundaries are a sign of good communication, respectful negotiation, and connection between parents and children. Poor boundaries escalate conflict and frustration, leading to disrespect and poor communication.

It is natural for children to test the limits of parental authority as they explore their own capacity for taking on more responsibility as they grow up. Poor boundary setting causes children to be exposed to situations before they have the developmental skills to handle the situations.

Boundaries are not rules for behavior of children; nor are they processes of limit setting. Boundaries exist between each member of the family, between subsystems, and between the family and society. These are the rules of interaction and the methods of functioning (Lawson and Lawson 1998).

Minuchin (1974) defined three types of boundaries: Clear boundaries are essential to balanced families. Enmeshed and disengaged boundaries are characteristic of imbalanced families.

Clear boundaries allow mutual respect and concern by allowing separateness for each member yet maintaining closeness. Freedom and flexibility in these healthy relationships are developed by clear, direct, and understanding communication. Clear boundaries allow children to develop, grow, and differentiate from the family. Individuation can be accomplished only when clear boundaries are functioning within the family system.

Enmeshed boundaries are inflexible, are unyielding, and leave no room for differences. Differentness or separateness is not tolerated; individuation is not a goal of enmeshed relationships. Families with enmeshed boundaries view differentness as disloyalty and as a threat to the rules of the system. The needs of the individual are subjugated to the needs of the parents or system. Satisfying the parents' definition of unity and sameness is stressed. Individual boundaries are blurred, and the individual is often swallowed up by the system. Individuals discount their own feelings, needs, and desires; they feel smothered and numb. They often use alcohol/drugs to counteract these feelings and the underlying resentment and anger.

Disengaged boundaries are overly rigid, with little or no opportunity for communication. Individuals in families that maintain disengaged boundaries have little sense of belonging, often feeling isolated from one another. The family also isolates from community and society. The parents are emotionally unavailable to each other, to the children, and, for that matter, to anyone else.

Boundary Inadequacy

Boundary inadequacy has been defined as the inability to set consistent and appropriate boundaries in relationships. The three major forms of boundary inadequacy identified by Eli Coleman and Phillip Colgan (1986) are ambiguous, overly rigid, and invasive.

Ambiguous boundary inadequacy involves a pattern of double messages exchanged within the relationship. The double messages create an atmosphere of tension wherein the recipient of the communication can never be sure what can be believed. The inability of the communicator to send clear messages lays the groundwork for the cycle of ambiguity to begin.

Overly rigid boundary inadequacy is characterized by patterns of behavior wherein smooth and efficient functioning is a priority over being responsive and adaptable. Adherence to a preset code of behavior is maintained, regardless of intervening situational variables, wherein roles are played and rules are strictly enforced.

Invasive boundary inadequacy involves patterns of behavior wherein an imbalance of power is used to objectify people. Other people become objects for the person to use in satisfying all needs (e.g., sexual and physical abuse).

Boundary Ambiguity

Boss and Greenberg (1984) use the term *boundary ambiguity* for confusion in family members' perceptions of who is in and out of the family and who is performing various family roles and tasks. The alcoholic family system organizes around the alcoholic or the family member(s) who exhibit dysfunctional behavior. In recovery, the family is challenged to reorganize as a viable system or become dysfunctional with continued boundary ambiguity (i.e., the dry-drunk family).

Ziter (1988) describes the alcoholic/imbalanced family as going through four recovery stages to overcome boundary ambiguity. These stages are very similar to the grieving stages of denial, anger, bargaining, depression, and acceptance described earlier in this chapter.

- *Stage 1—Clustering.* This is described as an early denial stage, when the family members sacrifice in order to maintain family harmony. The family task at this stage is to assure themselves that a family exists and to try to keep the alcoholic in the family system.
- *Stage 2—Conflict.* The reality of the situation is beginning to be understood at this stage. Individual differences are penetrating the denial system, and the family members are experiencing the stress and uncertainty of these ambiguous differences. It is at this stage that anger replaces denial to control family differences.

FIGURE 6.1 *Triangulation*

- *Stage 3—Individuation.* At this stage of family recovery, the family members are able to recognize the individuality of each person. The family's task is to support each other in exploring "self" while negotiating living together. Boundaries are becoming clearer.
- *Stage 4—Connection.* Family members are making connections with each other. There is a new way of relating that perhaps was not experienced before—an intimate linking. Mutuality emerges, and family members maintain boundaries through their own assertiveness and the respect of other members.

One can see how family members move from a system with imbalance and boundary ambiguity to a balanced system with connection and clarity in boundaries.

Eli Coleman (1987) underscored the importance of setting appropriate boundaries for members of imbalanced families:

> Developing skills at boundary setting is an essential ingredient in the recovery from chemical dependency or codependency. For many it is learning to say "no" to someone's request for physical, sexual, or emotional intimacy. Through saying "no," the individual learns that he or she can have a personal boundary and have it respected. This leads to a clear sense of self-wants and self-desires and it develops a sense of power and control in interpersonal relationships. After learning to say "no," the individual can learn to say "yes," and not lose a sense of individuality.

Triangulation—Another Boundary Issue

Jay Haley, a noted family therapist, defined triangulation (Figure 6.1) as at least two adults involved in an offspring's problem, where the parent-child dyad is pitted against a more peripheral parent, stepparent, or grandparent. The triangle may involve a parent's lover, an estranged parent, or another relative (Haley 1971).

The destructive nature of the triangle is that the parent-child dyad, or alliance, is established at the expense of the peripheral parent. (See Case Study 6.2.) Often the parent-child dyad creates a marital conflict. The parent is overly enmeshed in this alliance, seeking the child's favor despite the reality of the situation.

Kandel and Andrews (1987) postulated that parents can influence their offspring's behavior by modeling actions and defining norms, by controlling the child's susceptibility to the influence of others, and by providing positive attachments.

The modeling of drug use and alcohol use by parents, inadequate supervision of children, and lack of physical and emotional availability are factors that may put children at risk for substance abuse.

�ખ Parents' Use/Abuse of Alcohol and Drugs

Case Study 6.2

Triangulation—It Takes 3 or More to Tango

John and Mary and Michelle

John and Mary have significant marital problems. John is the head of the fire department for the county in which they reside and escapes the conflicts at home by spending much of his time with the men at the various fire stations. The couple actively attend community events and act as if their marriage were perfect. Their adopted 16-year-old daughter Michelle knows the truth. Michelle frequently argues with her mom to the point of hysteria. Mary often gives Michelle reason to be angry by giving her ambiguous, mixed messages (e.g., I want to be close to you, yet I don't trust you because you are stealing my husband, whom I can no longer hold in the marriage). Mary buys Michelle clothes and jewelry but is emotionally cold and unavailable. Mary has no insight into the way she antagonizes Michelle. Michelle is very bright but acts out her frustration with her mom by ditching classes, stealing things from her dresser, and being extremely flirtatious with boys. John and Michelle maintain an enmeshed dyadic alliance. John is frustrated with his wife's coldness, emotional and sexual unavailability, and constant arguments with Michelle and nagging of him. Michelle makes sexual overtures to young men while with her father and makes other sexually inappropriate remarks. In effect, she is flirtatious with her father; they are acting out their unconscious desires to be intimate with each other. These unconscious conflicts put more pressure on Michelle and she has begun to use alcohol/drugs excessively and to have sex with numerous young men. At this point, the family has sought counseling, a process that involves unraveling this triangulation and establishing clearer boundaries and lines of communication.

Discussion

All parties in this case are involved quite dramatically in this triangulation. It will take a skilled therapist to unravel the lines of triangulation and prevent any of the family members from permanently sabotaging the process. The therapist must establish a climate of trust, integrity, and competency to help this family. The three family members will not succeed at setting appropriate boundaries unless all of them agree to persevere in the process.

   The counselor will need support in this case and might involve other "consultant counselors" who will communicate clearly and directly with the primary counselor. This demonstrates (recapitulates) to the family that members of a system can work together effectively. The counselor must also expect that when issues become uncomfortable, each family member is capable of sabotaging progress and the process. Observing and commenting on that as a natural element of the process of counseling is recommended as a way to reengage family members.

✷ Other Family System Variables

Grace M. Barnes (1990) describes the three major family system variables necessary to prevent problem behaviors by children: **family cohesion, flexibility,** and **communication clarity.**

   Cohesion is defined as the emotional bonding of family members toward each other. Family members respect one another, support each other, and have appropriate boundaries. Cohesion is not possible if family members are enmeshed or disengaged from each other. Instead, there is a balance in roles, tasks, and ability to resolve conflicts.

Flexibility is the family members' ability to alter family roles and rituals in response to situational stress.

Communication clarity is the ability of family members to develop coalitions and to understand each other.

Parental competence is described by Burton White, director of the Harvard Preschool Projects, as the ability and willingness of parents to

- Sensibly design the world of the child
- Serve as a child's personal consultant
- Set limits effectively, for the sake of the child (not the parent) (White, Kaban, and Attanucci 1979)

Interestingly, adolescents in single-parent and stepparent families report more alcohol use than do adolescents in traditional families (Burnside et al. 1986). A study of high school students (Barnes and Nindle 1987) reported a tendency for adolescents living with both natural parents to have fewer alcohol-related problems.

Older siblings can exert a tremendous influence of alcohol/drug use on younger children in the family. Often it is an older sibling who initiates younger brothers and sisters into the rite of alcohol and drug use. The older sibling frequently has better access to alcohol/drugs and is often a more experienced user. Sometimes it is older cousins, stepbrothers/sisters, or friends of the family who initiate alcohol/drug use. Adolescents who have close, quality relationships and good communication with their parents are less likely to be influenced negatively by older siblings or peers.

The adolescent's positive sense of self, attainment of developmental skills, and ability to individuate also minimize negative peer influence. Studies have indicated that the level of closeness and trust in the parent-child relationship determines the choice of positive peer relationships.

Children who grow up in an abstinent family system may also develop alcohol/drug dependence and addiction. People who become alienated from their abstinence backgrounds may use excessive drinking to express their frustration with early rigid familial, religious, and community teachings. Problem drinking or excessive drug use is symbolic of a rebellion or revolt against early family values that became overly rigid. Sometimes alcohol/drug problems skip a generation as well. The child growing up in an alcoholic/addict system decides to "never be like his or her alcoholic/addict dad or mom" and chooses to abstain from any alcohol/drug use as an adult. The genetic predisposition for alcoholism/drug addiction is still passed on to his or her children, who may develop problems with alcohol/drugs, even though they grew up in a household where there was no parental use of alcohol/drugs.

The size of the family may also influence alcohol and drug use by children. As the number of siblings increases, the family becomes more complex in role relationships and tasks. Some children may experience increasing levels of frustration (blocked goals). In very large families, parents may be more controlling/coercive, less available, and less supportive, resulting in problem behaviors by some of the children and perhaps overly responsible (codependent) behaviors by siblings. This is illustrated in Case Study 6.3.

Case Study 6.3

Family System Variables

Jane

Jane grew up with four sisters. Dad's alcoholism was denied for most of their childhood. It was Jane's responsibility to take care of Mom emotionally. When Mom experienced chronic fatigue, Jane took care of the other, younger sisters, giving them dinner, getting them to bed, and trying to keep them quiet. Despite her efforts, Mom's physical symptoms increased in frequency. The other sisters didn't seem to be as affected by Mom's pain and Dad's alcohol use. It took Mom's "nervous breakdown" and her being hospitalized for a month in a psychiatric hospital for the other children to recognize the problem. Jane and her next younger sister were now responsible for the house. The middle sister began drinking during this time, and the youngest seemed to spend more time playing quietly by herself.

A few months after Mom returned home, Dad started attending AA meetings. Mom still experienced fatigue and physical pain, but less frequently. Jane went away to college, rarely visiting, immersing herself in studies, and marrying right out of college. The middle sister declared she was gay and went off to school 3,000 miles from home. The youngest and next to oldest stayed close to home, alternating the emotional caretaking of both Mom and Dad.

It was only in later years that the sisters started to share their memories of their painful childhood. Each had sought counseling for various relationship problems. Each had learned about being an adult child of an alcoholic. They were now beginning to heal by talking about their recovery. Mom was now actively pursuing interests outside of the home and spending time on her own. Dad was several years sober now and beginning to communicate more effectively with his daughters.

Discussion

Here is a case where many family system variables affect all family members—the father's alcoholism, the mother's major depression and chronic headaches, a psychiatric hospitalization of the mother that left the children as caretakers and housekeepers, and many other variables implied in growing up in this family system.

A number of good outcomes have occurred over the years, despite these problems. Dad is attending Alcoholics Anonymous; Mom is getting out and her headaches and pain are more manageable; and, probably the most important development, the adult children are talking to each other about their experiences growing up in this family system. There are signs of remarkable resilience in the parents and the children. (For more on the resilient self, see Chapter 7.)

Imbalanced Life Cycles of Families

Jay Haley (1971) described the following major stages in the family life cycle:

1. Relationships between families through unattached young adults
2. Joining of families through marriage
3. Family and the young child
4. Family and the adolescent
5. Launching of children
6. Later life

Case Study 6.4

Adopting a Surrogate Family

Steve

At the age of 8, Steve was always with his friend Joe's family. He would have breakfast and dinner with them and spend most of his free hours playing with Joe and talking with Joe's parents. When Steve had problems, concerns, or conflicts, he would talk to Joe's parents and not discuss the issues with his own family.

Discussion

One could make a calculated guess that Steve adopted his friend's family because there were problems/imbalances in his own family. Often children will go elsewhere to find the support, nurturance, and comfort they do not have in their own immediate family. Sometimes an aunt, a grandmother, a teacher, a counselor, a clergyman, or some other significant person becomes a mentor or surrogate parent.

As a result of the imbalance in alcoholic/addict family systems, developmental and interpersonal tasks are impaired at each stage of the family life cycle.

Relationships Between Families and the Joining of Families

During the first two stages, the relationships between families are often filled with conflict and tension. Cooperation between families is difficult because the alcoholic/addict family system is trying to deny, minimize, and cover up the family secret of alcoholism/addiction. This results in the families' inability to develop trust and closeness.

Family and the Young Child

At the third stage, the family is either isolated or involved with other families that have similar problems with alcohol/drugs. The child is the innocent victim at this stage. The young child is often embarrassed by his or her parents' unpredictable behavior. As a result, the child frequently prefers playing at other children's homes and rarely invites other children to his or her home. Often, children from alcoholic/addict homes literally adopt their friends' parents. Becoming stepchildren, they spend a great deal of time with their friends' families.

Family and the Adolescent

The fourth stage is the time of most turmoil. Tumultuous even in the balanced family system, adolescence becomes even more dramatic in an imbalanced family system. The adolescent's exploration of a healthy personal identity is incongruent with the imbalanced, unhealthy alcoholic/addict system. The conflict of holding allegiance to the family, imbalanced as it is, and exploring self through individuation and differentiation creates tremendous guilt and anxiety for adolescents. If this conflict is unresolved, adolescents can either internalize their own frustration and anger and develop an imbalanced sense of self or act out their anger in a demonstrative and destructive manner. The acting-out behavior often includes problems with alcohol/drugs, sexual promiscuity, problems in school and with authority figures, and criminal-justice problems. The internalized anger is sometimes more subtly manifested in the need for constant approval from peers, a poor self-concept, insecurity, or fears of abandonment and rejection.

Launching of Children

During the fifth stage, when the children are launched, the parents' alcohol and drug use usually intensifies. The empty-nest syndrome forces the parents to look at the dissatisfaction in their own marital system. The usual way to avoid the issues of marital imbalance is to increase the use of alcohol/drugs.

Of course, adult children of alcoholics/addicts are at risk for creating imbalanced relationships with their partners and for recapitulating the family of origin by developing imbalanced family systems as well. If there is no help, the result is the repetition of the same imbalanced system from generation to generation.

Later Life

In the sixth stage, the issues intensify in an alcoholic/addict family system. Consciously or unconsciously, the adult recognizes the imbalanced patterns of relating during childhood. Adult children of alcoholics/addicts enter treatment as they notice the imbalances in their own lives. Contacts with their parents in these later years may bring highly emotionally charged conflict to the forefront, making it difficult to have caring or effective relationships with their parents. If the parents are still using alcohol/drugs, this even further intensifies the difficulty in maintaining or developing better relationships. Working through the stages of grief and accepting the painful limitations of these imbalanced relationships are other developmental tasks for adult children. Healing may occur before the parents die. Perhaps the legacy of alcoholism/addiction will not be passed on to the next generation.

How does a counselor get resistant family members to participate in counseling? Alcoholic/addict families are among the most difficult families to get into treatment, whether the setting is inpatient, residential, or outpatient treatment. Families often abdicate responsibility for the alcoholic/addict's problems. It is too difficult for them to admit their feelings of embarrassment, shame, and personal feelings of inadequacy in trying to control family members' abuse of alcohol/drugs. Mason (1958) reported that, of 1,000 eligible parents of alcoholics/addicts, only 30 to 40 would appear at monthly parent-staff meetings and almost none of these attended more than three times.

Not only are family members resistant to attending sessions but also the alcoholics/addicts themselves often sabotage family involvement. Alcoholics/addicts are often self-protective of their families, not wanting them to experience more pain. Alcoholics/addicts may even feel a sense of betrayal in assisting counselors to get the rest of the family involved. This would be disloyal to the rules of the imbalanced, enmeshed family system.

For many alcoholics/addicts, having their spouses or other family members involved in treatment might blow their cover. Alcoholics/addicts may have lied or deceived counselors in giving inaccurate or distorted information about their alcohol/drug use, family interactions, or other information. There is also fear that counselors would blame, criticize, or shame other family members; then these family members would get back at the alcoholics/addicts.

The fathers of alcoholics/addicts are by far the most difficult family members to get into family sessions. A large percentage of these fathers have alcohol/drug problems themselves and don't want this brought to the attention of the counselor (the same may hold true for mothers). The father is difficult to engage in the process of family therapy because he has generally been unavailable to the drug user and other family members. The father is often angry and defensive.

I have heard many a father say, "Since nobody ever listened to me or allowed me to follow through in what I thought would work in the first place, I am angry and don't want to get involved." The truth of the matter is that most fathers are frightened by the emotional content of counseling and profess not to believe in counseling. They see therapists as invading the family systems the fathers have tried to control. Fathers are also trying to avoid their own emotional pain and issues.

In an attempt to engage fathers in treatment, Labate (1975) recommends a kind of romancing of the father by acknowledging the positive intentions that the father possesses, emphasizing that the father's participation in treatment is needed to make treatment successful. Labate suggests the following:

1. Reassuring the father that he is important
2. Pointing out that changes depend on his participation
3. Making the father aware that he has the power to sabotage treatment
4. Noting that the father has choices, such as transferring to another counselor, who might work with him individually
5. Placing responsibility for change squarely on the father's shoulders
6. Getting the father to consider realigning his priorities (e.g., choosing his family's happiness over acquisition of more material goods)

Labate's strategies can be used on any family member of the alcoholic/addict—the spouse, brothers, sisters, or other family members—who may have the same resistance to family treatment.

⚔ Fathers of Alcoholics/ Addicts— Dealing with Resistance

"Anyone working with addicts' families for the first time is impressed with the tremendous defensiveness that most of them show. It sometimes seems as if they are just waiting for the therapist to cast even a minor aspersion so they can protest or perhaps abort therapy prematurely" (Stanton et al. 1982). In approaching alcoholics/addicts and family members in treatment, it is essential that the counselor's style be nonpejorative, nonjudgmental, sensitive to the patient's issues of shame, and

⚔ Noble Ascriptions to Counteract Defensiveness

in no way blaming. Duncan Stanton suggested that the treatment be put in the context that each family member's intentions were and are noble and that there is a good reason or adaptive function for even the most destructive behavior. For example, anger, frustration, and generally attacking behavior can be relabeled as "a concern that is painful to tolerate," rather than "You are really angry for no reason" or "There he goes again, using anger to hurt and control us." Destructive enabling behavior can be nobly ascribed as "It is difficult to see your child in pain, pain that you would prefer that the child not go through."

"Simply defining problems as interactional or familial stumbling blocks serves to have them viewed as shared, rather than loading the blame entirely on one or two members—'we're all in this together'" (Stanton et al. 1982). This approach does not abandon the therapist's role in challenging the thoughts, beliefs, and behaviors that might hinder the family from becoming more functional. Instead, the counselor expresses perspectives and viewpoints in a human, caring, and nonshaming manner, facilitating trust in the therapeutic alliance. The ascribing of noble intentions or characteristics takes the shame out of the therapeutic work—shame that would inevitably cause one or more family members to sabotage treatment.

References

American Psychiatric Association. 1994. *Diagnostic and statistical manual of mental disorders.* 4th ed. Washington, D.C.: Author.

Barnes, Grace M. 1990. Impact of the family on adolescent drinking patterns. In *Alcohol and the family,* edited by R. Collins et al. New York: Guilford Press.

Barnes, Grace M., and M. Nindle. 1987. Family factors in adolescent alcohol and drug abuse. *Pediatrician* 14:13–18.

Boss, P., and J. Greenberg. 1984. Family boundary ambiguity: A new variable in family stress theory. *Family Process* 23:535–46.

Burnside, M. A., et al. 1986. Alcohol use by adolescents in disrupted families. *Alcoholism: Clinical and Experimental Research* 10:274–78.

Carnes, Patrick. 1995. Patrick J. Carnes: Riding the tides, navigating counseling's turbulent waters [Interview]. *Professional Counselor Magazine,* December, pp. 47–52.

Coleman, Eli. 1987. *Chemical dependency and intimacy dysfunction.* New York: Haworth Press.

Coleman, Eli, and Phillip Colgan. 1986. Boundary inadequacy in drug dependent families. *Journal of Psychoactive Drugs* 18:21–30.

Dobkin, P. L., R. E. Tremblay, L. Masse, and F. Vitaro. 1999. In *Alcohol use among adolescents,* edited by M. Windle. Thousand Oaks, Calif.: Sage.

Eliason, M. J., and A. H. Skinstad. 1995. Drug/alcohol addictions and mothering. *Alcoholism Treatment Quarterly* 12(1): 83–95.

Fossum, M., and M. Mason. 1986. *Facing shame: Families in recovery.* New York: W. W. Norton.

Garrison, W. T., and F. J. Earls. 1987. Temperament and child psychopathology. *Developmental Clinical Psychology and Psychiatry* 12.

Gomberg, E. S. L. 1988. Shame and guilt issues among women alcoholics. *Alcoholism Treatment Quarterly* 5:139–55.

Haley, Jay. 1971. *Changing families: A family therapy reader.* New York: Grune & Stratton.

Jessup, M. 1983. *Chemically dependent women in San Francisco: A status report.* San

Francisco: California Department of Public Health, San Francisco Community Substance Abuse Services.

Johnson, Valerie, and Robert J. Pandina. 1991. Effects of the family environment on adolescent substance use, delinquency, and coping skills. *American Journal of Drug and Alcohol Abuse* 1(17): 71–88.

Kandel, D. B., and K. A. Andrews. 1987. Processes of adolescent socialization by parents and peers. *International Journal of Addiction* 22:319–42.

Kempher, Carol. 1987. Special populations: Etiology and prevention of vulnerability to chemical dependency in children of substance abusers. In *Youth at high risk for substance abuse,* edited by B. S. Brown and A. R. Mills. NIDA monograph. Washington, D.C.: U.S. Department of Health and Human Services.

Kohnstamm, G., J. Bates, and M. K. Rothbart. 1999. In *Alcohol use among adolescents,* edited by M. Windle. Thousand Oaks, Calif.: Sage.

Labate, K. 1975. Pathogenic role rigidity in fathers: Some observations. *Journal of Marriage and Family Counseling* 1:69–79.

Maccoby, E., and J. A. Martin. 1983. Socialization in the context of the family: Parent-child interaction. In *Handbook of Child Psychology,* vol. 4, edited by E. M. Hetherington. New York: Wiley.

Mason, P. 1958. Mother of the addict. *Psychiatric Quarterly Supplement* 32:189–99.

Minuchin, Salvador. 1974. *Families and family therapy.* Cambridge, Mass.: Harvard University Press.

Rollins, B. C., and D. L. Thomas. 1979. Parental support, power, and control techniques in the socialization of the child. In *Contemporary theories of the family,* vol. 1, edited by W. R. Burr et al. New York: Free Press.

Stanton, Duncan M., et al. 1982. *Family therapy of drug abuse.* New York: Guilford Press.

Tubman, J., and M. Windle. 1999. In *Alcohol use among adolescents,* edited by M. Windle. Thousand Oaks, Calif.: Sage.

Volk, R. J., et al. 1988. Family systems of adolescent substance abusers. *Family Relations* 38:266–72.

Werner, R. J., and C. A. Smith. 1999. In *Alcohol use among adolescents,* edited by M. Windle. Thousand Oaks, Calif.: Sage.

White, B., B. Kaban, and J. Attanucci. 1979. *The origins of human competence: The final report on the Harvard Preschool Project.* Lexington, Mass.: Lexington Books/D. C. Heath.

Ziter, MaryLou Politi. 1988. Treating alcoholic families: The resolution of boundary ambiguity. *Alcoholism Treatment Quarterly* 5:221–33.

Growing Up in an Alcoholic Family System

❖ **Chapter in Review**

Alcoholism affects the children of alcoholics, not just the alcoholic and spouse. Adults who were children in alcoholic family systems (adult children of alcoholics) are vulnerable to having feelings and behaviors that are characteristic of post-traumatic stress disorder.

Children of alcoholics tend to distrust their own feelings and to deny reality.

Codependency is defined in this chapter as continual investment of self-esteem in the ability to influence or control feelings and behaviors in the self and others in the face of obvious adverse consequences.

Alcoholism is a family disease, where the family is centrally organized around the alcoholic's behavior and/or drinking. Codependency and enabling behavior, plus denial, end up perpetuating both the alcoholism and the alcohol-related problems. The marriage is also at risk, with sexual and intimacy problems.

One of the results of growing up in an alcoholic system is that interpersonal relationships are often imbalanced in the form of overattachment, overseparation, and codependent dances.

Grief is a feature of recovery from growing up in an alcoholic system. Second-order change is one technique to change family interaction. The 11 curative factors of group therapy are outlined as a way for adult children of alcoholics to pursue recovery.

This chapter focuses on children of alcoholics. In the 1980s this was an emerging issue that shifted the focus away from the alcoholic/addict to the children in the alcoholic/addict family system.

Alcoholism is a family disease that includes codependency, enabling behavior, and marital discord. The children in an alcoholic system, much like the nonalcoholic spouse, compensate to keep the system in homeostasis. The family is organized around the alcoholic's behavior and drinking. The alcoholism is the central organizing principle around which the family focuses.

Children growing up in an alcoholic/addict family system experience traumas, which result in specific adult behavioral characteristics and developmental disabilities. Adult children of alcoholics (ACAs) have trouble establishing effective boundaries in relationships and are often either overseparated or overattached in partner relationships. Recovery for adult children involves dealing with unresolved feelings of childhood grief and working through feelings of shame, abandonment, and rejection.

By understanding the healing and recovery process for adult children, perhaps this pattern of imbalance can be broken for the next generation.

✖ The Adult Children of Alcoholics Movement

In the 1980s, one of the most significant alcohol/drug issues brought to the attention of the general

---

The names and circumstances of case studies in this chapter have been changed to maintain anonymity.

public was the awareness of the characteristics of adult children of alcoholics. Children who grew up in alcoholic families are now adults, hence the term *adult children of alcoholics*. These adults report difficulties in establishing effective, intimate, interpersonal relationships.

The talent and dedication of people such as Timmen Cermak, Claudia Black, Stephanie Brown, Janet Woititz, Sharon Wegscheider-Cruse, Robert Ackerman, and Lori Dwinell created an awareness of the trauma of growing up in an alcoholic family system. Because of this awareness, our society not only has recognized but today is dealing with how the imbalanced aspects of alcoholism affect all family members.

In 1979, a *Newsweek* article about adult children of alcoholics reported the early work of Claudia Black (1982) and Stephanie Brown, who both described and labeled the characteristics of ACA. Brown (1988) described the reaction after the *Newsweek* article as "a prairie fire of interest." The proliferation of articles, materials, books, general information, workshops, and speakers on ACA issues was dramatic from 1979 to the late 1980s. Adult children of alcoholics were finally recognized as a treatment population that had generally been ignored for years. This explosion of interest was in direct proportion to the neglect and oversight that occurred as professionals focused myopically on the alcoholics, while ignoring the children who grew up in alcoholic families. Bosma appropriately described children of alcoholics in 1972 as *victims in a hidden tragedy*. In 1983, the National Association for Children of Alcoholics (NACOA) was formed. Timmen Cermak, one of the founders, was its first president. Numerous planning meetings established the NACOA as a central organizing force in disseminating information, providing direction, and developing resources for adult children of alcoholics. The NACOA organized national conferences to provide a forum for the dissemination of ACA treatment information for both professionals and the lay public.

In 1983, the NACOA developed some basic facts about children of alcoholics in its charter statement:

- An estimated 28 million Americans have at least one alcoholic parent.
- More than half of all alcoholics have an alcoholic parent.
- Children of alcoholics are at the highest risk of developing alcoholism themselves or marrying someone who is alcoholic.
- In up to 90 percent of child abuse cases, alcohol is a significant factor.
- Children of alcoholics are frequently victims of incest, child neglect, and other forms of violence and exploitation.

The popularity of the ACA movement also brought with it some concerns for overgeneralization and a lack of clinical foundation. Appropriately, this point is made by one of the pioneers of the movement.

> Like many social movements, the sudden recognition, widespread interest, and emotional intensity have been powerful and helpful for many children and adults. However, there continues to be a lack of a solid clinical research and theoretical foundation on which to base important decisions for intervention, education, prevention, and treatment. (Brown 1988)

Characteristics of Adult Children of Alcoholics

Following are some of the behavioral characteristics of ACAs:

1. Fear of losing control
2. All-or-none, black-or-white thinking
3. Fear of experiencing feelings
4. Overdeveloped sense of responsibility or irresponsibility
5. Difficulty with intimacy and with asking for what is wanted or needed
6. Flashbacks of childhood but many memory gaps
7. Feelings of being little, or like a child, when under stress
8. Unreasonable loyalty
9. Addiction to excitement
10. Difficulty relaxing
11. Feelings of guilt, abandonment, and/or depression
12. Tendency to confuse love with self-pity
13. Backlog of shock and grief
14. Compulsive behaviors
15. Living in a world of denial
16. Guessing at what is normal
17. Tendency toward physical symptoms (e.g., headaches, gastrointestinal problems)

Growing Up in an Alcoholic Home as Post-Traumatic Stress Disorder

Timmen Cermak (1984) stated that the effect of growing up in an alcoholic family system is analogous to the post-traumatic stress disorder (PTSD) (see Case Study 7.1) of war veterans or survivors of the Holocaust because the same coping mechanisms are used. The soldier who helplessly watches as a buddy is shot and killed shuts down his own emotions to survive the trauma, which can later be reexperienced in a safe environment. This same reaction of shutting down emotionally occurs in the children of alcoholics. After these children become adults, they reexperience feelings of childhood traumas and suffer chronic symptoms of acute anxiety, depression, sleep disturbances, and nightmares, as well as an inability to work or function effectively at daily activities.

The following major symptoms of PTSD are similar to symptoms experienced by the ACA:

1. Reexperiencing the trauma, as evidenced by
    a. Nightmares
    b. Recurrent obsessive thoughts
    c. Sudden reemergence of survival behavior in the face of events that resemble the original trauma
    d. Emotional overload
2. Psychic numbing, as evidenced by
    a. A sense of depersonalization
    b. A sense of not fitting into one's surroundings
    c. A feeling of emotional anesthesia
    d. Constriction of emotions, especially in situations demanding intimacy, tenderness, or sexuality

Case Study 7.1

The ACA and Post-Traumatic Stress Disorder

Joe

Joe was a client who had experienced both the trauma of growing up in an alcoholic family system and post-traumatic stress as a result of military service in Vietnam. Joe was referred to me by a colleague, who was counseling Joe's 12-year-old daughter.

Joe came home drunk one evening, went to his daughter's bedroom to kiss her good night, and began crying and talking about how unhappy he was. Although there was no sexual violation, the daughter was extremely upset by her father's behavior. She was frightened and concerned about his drinking and his deep emotional sadness.

Joe was one of those patients for whom I initially had very little hope; he turned out to be a case that reinforced my belief in the inherent goodness in people. Joe was 25 minutes late for his first counseling session. Joe insisted that his lateness was due to a business appointment and wondered why I was so concerned with time. He believed that his only problem was his business. He said, "If I could only get out from under the financial pressure, everything would be back to normal." Joe agreed to come back for counseling to help with stress management although he felt that his daughter needed assistance, not him.

Gradually, I was able to establish a therapeutic bond with Joe. Once I got to know him, I soon realized that he had the heart of a puppy dog and he had suffered significant disappointments and trauma in his life.

Joe's alcoholic father, who was well-read and extremely bright, owned his own business. His dad spent most of his time drinking at the office and the local bar while discussing many topics with his customers and friends; he was well versed in politics, philosophy, religion, physics, even psychology. Although he was a friendly and entertaining drunk with his friends, he was emotionally unpredictable at home. At times, Joe's dad was maudlin about his childhood and his father's death when he was eight. At other times, he raged around the house, screaming resentments for his need to work so hard to support his wife and children. Once Joe was so angry with his father that he took a baseball bat and was going to smash him in the face.

Sometimes Joe felt sorry for his father and put him to bed after a drinking binge; when things got to be overwhelming, Joe just ran out of the house. On those evenings, Joe frequently went down to the school and threw rocks at the classroom windows. This and similar aggressive behavior kept him in trouble throughout his childhood. Joe was extremely bright and, despite his aggressive behavior, pulled good grades in high school. Because he spent more time drinking than studying in college, in 1968 his military deferment was revoked.

In the service, Joe was put through training for military intelligence and could have avoided Vietnam if his alcoholism and aggressive anger hadn't gotten him into trouble with his top sergeant. In Vietnam, Joe's major job was to fly to battle zones after conflicts and get a body count for Vietnamese and American soldiers.

Joe felt sadness for the Vietnamese children; he described them stealing, cheating, and manipulating the GIs to survive. It reminded him of his own childhood anger and aggressive behavior. In counseling sessions, Joe initially denied the emotional trauma of his experiences in Vietnam. He insisted that he had had it good, compared with others. Joe suffered from this traumatic exposure as well as from survivor's guilt. He experienced all the traditional signs of post-traumatic stress: sleep disorders and nightmares, night sweats, inability to concentrate,

(continued on next page)

Case Study 7.1 (*continued*)

The ACA and Post-Traumatic Stress Disorder

Joe

hypertension, disorientation, and explosive temper. All of these symptoms were complicated by his alcoholism.

After a year and a half of individual counseling, followed by group counseling with other ACAs, Joe was able to maintain sobriety, grieve the loss of his father, and grieve his experiences in Vietnam. After some time in counseling, Joe and some other group members visited the Vietnam War Memorial in Washington, DC. This was an important event in his painful journey to recovery.

Discussion

This case illustrates the many layers of pain that are often covered up by denial, alcohol/drugs, anger, and withdrawal. Joe was very unhappy and depressed, and he felt shame and guilt about his own behavior. Although he initially couldn't admit or ask for help, he did continue to come back. For many clients like Joe, it is important to recognize that it is hard for them to ask for help, admit their vulnerability or pain to themselves and others, and see that recovery is possible.

Joe is one of those rewarding and remarkable stories that validate the need for the counselor to hang in there, not abandon him, not get angry with him, but hold him responsible for his behavior and recognize that progress is slow.

---

  e. Lack of feelings during times of stress
  f. Sudden experience of a wall between the self and the feelings
  g. Confusion instead of having feelings
  h. A lump in the throat instead of allowing feelings to emerge or pressure and tightness in the jaw, shoulders, or other parts of the body
  i. Feelings that emotions will be overwhelming if one gets in touch with them

3. Hypervigilance, as evidenced by
  a. Inability to relax
  b. Frequent startle responses
  c. Chronic anxiety
  d. Panic attacks

4. Survivor guilt, as evidenced by
  a. Chronic depression
  b. A sourceless sense of guilt

5. Intensification of symptoms by exposure to events that resemble the original trauma

In order to constitute post-traumatic stress disorder, the trauma must be significant. Severe emotional or physical abuse and/or sexual violation can be so traumatizing to the child that symptoms of PTSD might occur. Unfortunately, the diagnosis of PTSD has frequently been used too loosely, without evidence of significant trauma. Just growing up in an alcoholic family does not mean one suffers from PTSD. Cermak is using PTSD as a model to understand the symptoms of ACA, not as a generalized label.

Children in alcoholic families learn to distrust their own observations (what they see and hear) and feelings (what they sense), and they feel powerless to change the family system. They cannot speak out and cannot trust their feelings because the rules in an alcoholic family system are don't talk, don't feel, and don't trust. Because these children distrust their own observations and feelings, they must wonder or guess at what is normal. At a time when most functional families are providing structure, discipline, and natural consequences for their children's behavior, alcoholic families provide control; rigidity; fear; irresponsibility; immaturity; and, most important, *unpredictability*. Children in alcoholic families try to control the behavior of the alcoholic parent and the codependent spouse by becoming super-responsible and trying to do everything correctly to obtain the parent's approval. They soon find out that, despite their best efforts to be perfect, the parent always finds fault with something. While desperately trying to predict or control the behavior of their parents, children do not realize that alcoholism and drug addiction is a disease that results in unpredictable behavior.

❈ Childhood in an Alcoholic Home

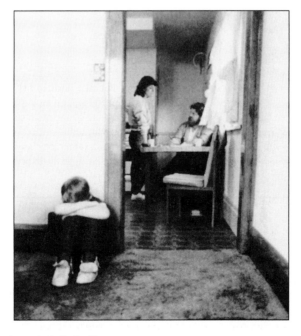

Child growing up in an alcoholic family.

Case Study 7.2

Rejection Sensitivity

Frank

A colleague, old friend, and workshop training partner of mine tells a story of his fear of rejection. Growing up in an imbalanced, alcoholic family system, Frank learned how to defend against shame by being likable and by avoiding conflict. He figured that, if everyone liked him and he avoided conflict, he would not be subject to rejection, attack, or shame. Unfortunately, his likable quality put him in a real dilemma back in the third grade.

As Frank tells the story, his classmates really liked him and nominated him for third-grade class president. Normally, he would be just likable enough, but not too popular, because that would bring the unwanted attention he feared. That year, there were no outstanding choices for class president, and his likable, nonaggressive style became the qualities that the class wanted in its president. His classmates reacted to the nomination with genuine acceptance and encouragement. Frank felt this put him in a lose-lose position. Frank thought that, if he ran and lost, he would experience tremendous feelings of rejection and shame. If he ran and won, he would disappoint his classmates by being an inadequate class president, unable to meet the responsibilities of the office. Ultimately, this would lead to the same feelings of rejection and shame. Either way, Frank felt he would be rejected and shamed. His only choice was to reject the nomination for office. He did this rather adroitly by taking the nomination as an opportunity to lend his support to another, more popular classmate. "Thanks for the nomination," he said, "but my support goes to Larry. He would make a far more capable class president than me, and he was the one I had intended to nominate." Unfortunately, Frank missed out on the opportunity to grow from experiencing what it is like to run for office and perhaps the opportunity to be class president.

Discussion

This case illustrates how growing up in an alcoholic family can cause the ACA to choose to avoid the attention of others (public domain) and to not take positive risk that can produce growth. For Frank, the fear of losing the election was much bigger than if it were "just an election." A loss would rekindle in Frank waves of rejection and strong feelings of personal inadequacy and shame. So Frank played it safe by deflecting the attention and supporting another person. This was a life pattern that would later cause him to regret the decisions he had made. A healthier response would have been to run in the election, gain the experience, sort out the results, and move on.

Identification of Children of Alcoholic Families

Robert Ackerman (1978) described various behavioral characteristics of children of alcoholics, including the following:

- Being superachievers or perfectionists or exhibiting efforts that go far beyond the reasonable criteria of every task
- Exhibiting an inordinate need to control their environment and therefore becoming anxious with the slightest threat to their security (e.g., a teacher's

comment on homework or an unusually low grade may provoke emotional upset)
- Displaying social disengagement from or excessive attention to the peer group (as an isolated loner or a class clown)
- Exhibiting signs of physical neglect (untidiness, soiled clothing, poor hygiene) and/or physical abuse (bruises, cuts, etc.)
- Being unable to concentrate and sometimes showing marked variations in academic performance, especially when parents are in a binge pattern of alcohol use or in codependent conflict

---

The alcoholic family swears an allegiance to the family secret of alcoholism. Family members dedicate themselves to denying that Dad and/or Mom is out of control. The children hope that perhaps their family secret will change and continually explore ways to make it change.

Sometimes this becomes an almost magical quest by the children to find that special way of being or ritualistic behavior that can make Dad and/or Mom change. Children give up their own sense of self in their search for the key that will change their parents' dysfunctional behavior.

A friend tells this story illustrating how children's feelings are discounted: When the alcoholic dad falls down, drunk, and spends the night on the front lawn, still in his work clothes, does the child really believe Mom's explanation? "You know your dad loves astronomy; he came home late last night, lay down to gaze at the stars, and, since he was tired from working late, just fell asleep, gazing at the constellations."

Children must maintain the *illusion of normalcy,* the illusion that their families are normal. The child defensively maintains the belief that this is what other families go through.

Howard Clinebell (1985) reported that the following factors produce damage in the lives of children of alcoholics:

1. *Role reversal:* Children may undertake parental duties because the parent is unable to be responsible or because the parent forces responsibilities on the children. The alcoholic may be treated as a child and, in return, act helpless. In incestuous families, the daughter and mother often switch roles.
2. *Unpredictability:* An inconsistent and unpredictable relationship with the alcoholic emotionally deprives the children.
3. *Unavailability:* The nonalcoholic, inadequate parent is struggling with major problems; because this parent's own needs are unmet, he or she is unable to attend to the needs of the children.
4. *Social isolation:* The damaging factor is the social isolation of the family, as protection from further pain and suffering, due to embarrassment.

Even periods of parental sobriety have negative effects on the children in alcoholic families. This is due primarily to the inconsistency and shattered hope that this time it will be different. The alcoholic father "inspires the natural love of his offspring, who build there from an ideal father image of omnipotence and loving

✴ Denial of Feelings in an Alcoholic Family

kindness. This disillusionment of the drunken episode is shattering to the frail super-ego structure of the child who is subjected to alternating experiences of exalted hopes and blighting disappointments" (Newell 1950).

❦ Perspective of the Child in an Alcoholic Family

M. Cork (1969) interviewed 115 children living in alcoholic families in an attempt to understand the child's perspective. Cork found that the children react to the alcoholic family system in a number of common ways. The interviewed children in alcoholic families

1. would not go to a friend's house because they would not dare reciprocate and invite friends to their homes due to the unpredictability and embarrassing behaviors of their parents.
2. were angry at everybody.
3. were preoccupied at school with worry about what would happen when they returned home.
4. envied their friends who seemed to have fun with their families.
5. felt alone when they were only children.
6. felt neglected when both parents were drinking.
7. felt they had to be parentlike, especially if the mother was drinking.
8. worried about each parent's loneliness if the parents were separated; wished for their parents to reunite, even if their home was calmer during the separation; seemed to feel an even deeper loss if the alcoholic parent moved out of the house.
9. were unable to separate and individuate from their parents as adolescents; it was difficult to break away from somebody with whom they had no ties; one child poignantly said, "I want to be somebody, but I feel like nobody."

TABLE 7.1

Problems of Children in Alcoholic Families

Physical Neglect or Abuse	Acting-Out Behaviors	Emotional Reaction to Alcoholism and Chaotic Family Life	Social and Interpersonal Difficulties
Serious illness	Involvement with	Suicidal tendencies	Family relationship problems
Accidents	police and courts	Depression	Peer problems
	Aggression	Repressed emotions	Adjustment problems
	Alcohol and other	Lack of self-confidence	Feeling different from norm
	drug abuse	Lack of life direction	Embarrassment
		Fear of abandonment	Overresponsible
		Fear of future	Feeling unloved and unable to trust

From G. Lawson, James S. Peterson, and Ann Lawson, *Alcoholism and the Family: A Guide to Treatment and Prevention,* Aspen Publications, 1983. Reprinted by permission of G. Lawson.

TABLE 7.2		

Problems of Alcoholic Families Affecting More Than One Person

Marital	**Parental**	**Cross-Boundaries—** **Parent and Child Relationships**
Marital instability	Inadequate parenting	Physical and sexual abuse of children
Prolonged separation	Lack of structure	Parentification of children (child becomes the parent)
Divorce	Inconsistencies	
Death of a spouse	Emotional neglect of children	Role reversal
Physical abuse of a spouse	Inability or unwillingness to perform parental duties	Family conflict
		Isolation of family from society
		Isolation of individual family member within the family
		Incongruent communication (mixed messages)
		Lack of trust between family members
		Family secrets

From G. Lawson, James S. Peterson, and Ann Lawson, *Alcoholism and the Family: A Guide to Treatment and Prevention,* Aspen Publications, 1983. Reprinted by permission of G. Lawson.

10. excused the alcoholic's behavior and often condemned the nonalcoholics for being hostile and angry; children could deduce from this that love and caring would come from alcoholics; research, unfortunately, indicates that many ACAs do marry alcoholics to try out their hypothesis.
11. experienced multiple separations and reunions of their parents and learned not to expect any state to continue consistently.
12. continued to have problems, even when the alcoholic stopped drinking. See Tables 7.1 and 7.2 for lists of these problems.

⚔ Family Disease Model

Just as alcoholism is classified as a disease (i.e., it has a known etiology, progressive nature, and known outcome), the alcoholic family is often described in the context of a "family disease." The family members are described as suffering from alcoholism, codependency, and enabling behavior, perpetuating both the alcoholism- and alcohol-related problems. The family is organized around the alcoholic's drinking and the consequences of that drinking. The central organizing principle of the family is focused around the alcoholic's behavior (e.g., Is she drinking? Will she drink? How much will she drink? When and with whom will she drink? Will she get drunk?). The family responds to the alcoholic in a codependent (giving up of self) fashion or enables both alcoholic behavior and drinking. The family disease model describes the family as trying to maintain homeostasis, compensating for the disequilibrium of the alcoholic's behavior and drinking. This results in family members' disconnecting from their own feelings, distorting their perceptions, and invoking the "no-talk, no-feel, no-trust" rule.

Alcoholism/ Drug Addiction— Impact on Marriage

Marriages are at risk when there is a substance-abuse problem. Feelings of betrayal, continuous conflict, chaos, loss, resentments, and pain are constant parts of the marital cycle when one partner is alcoholic/drug-addicted. Ironically, some studies indicate that if spouses drink together and with approximately equal patterns and amounts of use, it may not initially create a problem. However, problems will arise when one partner goes out to drink with friends, or a partner cuts back his or her drinking, enters into treatment, or voluntarily seeks sobriety.

Sexual problems related to substance abuse are very common, confounded by problems of intimacy. John Gottman, author of *Why Marriages Fail* (1995), describes the four horsemen of the apocalypse of marriages—criticism, contempt (nonverbal), defensiveness, and withdrawal. The codependent dance of couples where there is an alcohol or drug problem frequently involves an "in the marriage," "out of the marriage," and "on the fence" attitude toward the marriage and each other. Frequently, all four horsemen are present. There is also a strong ambivalence that the wife of an alcoholic has toward her husband. There is a vacillation between being supportive and understanding and feeling hopeless and withdrawn.

Certainly, recovery not only involves treatment for alcoholics/addicts or problem users but also involves treatment for the spouse.

> Behavioral marital therapy focuses on teaching partners how to communicate with each other, solve problems together and resolve their conflicts. Husbands and wives look directly for ways to break the cycle of criticism, denial and blame that characterizes a chemically dependent family and develop new roles and new ways of interacting that will support recovery ("After Drug Treatment" 1999).

ACAs in Relationship

ACAs Define Self Through Others

ACAs define their sense of identity by the impressions others have of them. ACAs have a strong, often imbalanced need for affirmation from others that they are indeed worthwhile. They approach their world from the outside in versus the inside out stance of self-confident people.

Even though many of my ACA patients have been extremely successful in their professional lives, they still feel inadequate and don't trust their talents, skills, and accomplishments. Many feel that they are charlatans and will be exposed as inadequate persons. They fear that at any time their professional abilities may all be taken away from them. Then they will relive their ultimate fear of being all alone, helpless, abandoned, and rejected; the fears they felt growing up will be played out again. Successful careers and stylish and attractive lifestyles camouflage their poor sense of self, and they are surprised when others don't see through their disguises.

The Disengaged ACA

Growing up in alcoholic families with parents who are unavailable, children often develop patterns of interpersonal disengagement. ACAs may maintain this pattern of disengagement in most interpersonal relationships. Cermak (1984) describes disengaged ACAs as having the following behaviors:

1. Hard-driving, workaholic; always preoccupied by projects and things that have to be done; rarely satisfied with accomplishments; in denial of feelings, relationships take a back seat
2. Defensive, fearful of closeness to others; plays cards close to the vest; unable to deal honestly on an emotional level; longing for relationships; chronic anger
3. Overwhelmed by feelings, buffeted by emotional storms; desperately trying to get other people to behave properly; often unable to work effectively.

Disengaged ACAs exhibit behaviors that on the surface make them seem self-sufficient and self-actualized; in actuality, they are depressed and suffering from deep emotional pain.

Atypical Depression

Another diagnostic category recently associated with ACAs and others who grew up in imbalanced family systems is atypical depression. Atypical depression is an impairment in interpersonal and social skills due to an extreme sensitivity to rejection. Because these individuals are highly sensitive, they overreact, thinking others' remarks, opinions, and/or actions are personal attacks. Many individuals suffering from atypical depression report that this sensitivity began in early childhood and have histories of physical, emotional, and/or sexual violation.

Codependency

Timmen Cermak quotes a metaphor from Charles Alexander: that codependency is "like being a lifeguard on a crowded beach, knowing that you cannot swim, and not telling anyone for fear of a panic." This is the sense of desperation that ACAs feel as they guess at what is normal.

Codependency is "like being a lifeguard on a crowded beach, knowing that you cannot swim, and not telling anyone for fear of a panic."

Cermak, himself an adult child of an alcoholic, defined codependency in diagnostic terms in the hope that codependency would be recognized as a psychiatric disorder. The following are diagnostic criteria for codependent personality disorder:

1. Continual investment of self-esteem in the ability to influence or control feelings and behaviors in the self and others in the face of obvious adverse consequences
2. Assumption of responsibility for meeting others' needs to the exclusion of acknowledging one's own needs
3. Anxiety and boundary distortions in situations of intimacy and separation
4. Enmeshment in relationships with personality-disordered, drug-dependent, and impulse-disordered individuals
5. Maintenance of a primary relationship with an active substance abuser for at least two years without seeking outside support and/or exhibiting three or more of the following characteristics:
   a. Constriction of emotions with or without dramatic outbursts
   b. Depression
   c. Hypervigilance
   d. Compulsions
   e. Anxiety
   f. Excessive reliance on denial
   g. Substance abuse
   h. Recurrent physical or sexual abuse
   i. Stress-related medical illnesses

An individual who has all five criteria of codependency would be diagnosed as having codependent personality disorder. A personality disorder affects all aspects of one's life because pervasive personality traits become inflexible and maladaptive. The results are significant subjective distress and social and occupational impairment. Treatment for codependent personality disorder often involves extensive education, counseling, therapeutic interventions, and sometimes medication to deal with major anxiety and depression.

If you find yourself identifying with some of the diagnostic criteria for codependent personality disorder but not all of them, you might have some codependent traits not a full-blown disorder. If these codependent traits result in significant difficulties in establishing effective, caring, and intimate relationships, they probably need to be investigated.

Boundary Inadequacy

Boundary inadequacy is the inability to set consistent and appropriate boundaries. The result is vascillating or ambiguous boundaries, overly rigid boundaries, and invasive boundaries. As a result, ACAs have difficulty in relationships; often they choose an alcoholic, addict, or a generally dysfunctional partner, or develop codependent relationships. If one were to ask persons with strong codependent traits and difficulties in setting appropriate boundaries to choose persons they were interested in from 100 people—90 of whom are fairly functional and stable—their choices would probably come from the 10 dysfunctional people.

For ACAs, boundaries are often distorted in interpersonal relationships; sometimes they are excessively involved (overattachment) or excessively detached (over-separation).

Overattachment and Overseparation

In their work on chemical dependency and intimacy dysfunction, Eli Coleman and Philip Colgan (1987) focused on overattachment and overseparation in men who grew up in alcoholic families. They identified thoughts, feelings, and behaviors common to both the overseparated and overattached individuals. Table 7.3 lists these thoughts, feelings, and behaviors.

The thoughts of the overattached and overseparated sound like common lyrics to country-western songs. These codependent lyrics include "You should be grateful," "I want so little," "You don't care," "What am I doing wrong?" and "I'm nobody without

---

TABLE 7.3

Overseparation and Overattachment

Overseparation	Overattachment
Thoughts	
You're not good enough.	I'm not good enough.
They want so much.	I want so little.
They give so little.	I give so much.
I'm ambivalent.	You don't care.
If only they would . . .	What am I doing wrong?
I am a rock.	I'm nobody without you.
You should be grateful.	I'm so unappreciated.
Feelings	
Fear, smothering	Fear, abandonment
Self-controlled	Out of control
Indifferent	Needy, burdened
Unsafe with others	Unsafe alone
Trapped	Shut-out
Numb	Desperate
Behaviors	
Is self-protective	Is self-sacrificing
Controls others	Pleases others
Acts to guard feelings	Acts contrary to feelings
Denies	Explains
Is compulsively independent	Is compulsively dependent

From Eli Coleman and Philip Colgan, "Chemical dependency and intimacy dysfunction" in *Journal of Chemical Dependency*, Vol. 1 (1), 1987. Copyright © 1987 by the Haworth Press, Inc. For copies of the complete work, contact Marianne Arnold at The Haworth Document Delivery Service (Telephone 1-800-3-HAWORTH; 10 Alice Street, Binghampton, NY 13904). For other questions concerning rights and permissions contact Wando Latour at the above address.

you." Many people identify strongly with either the overseparated or the overattached column in Table 7.3; others cross over, having both overattached and overseparated characteristics. Overseparated individuals tend to develop relationships with overattached individuals and vice versa. Frequently, ACAs duplicate the kind of relationship their codependent parents had. Just as the disease of alcoholism and drug addiction progresses from generation to generation, so do the patterns of inadequate boundary setting and codependent relationships.

Codependent Dances

The most traditional codependent dance is between alcoholics/addicts and their codependent partners. Alcoholics/addicts and their partners are both codependent; alcoholics/addicts need partners who enable them to continue to use drugs/alcohol and not suffer the full impact of their addiction. Their partners need alcoholics/addicts to avoid their own fears of abandonment and depression. Both of them fear feelings of loneliness, isolation, anxiety, and depression.

The fear of abandonment and rejection is so strong for ACAs that they choose not to develop an individual sense of self. This neglect of oneself while preoccupied or obsessed with changing the partner is codependency. The codependent dances these couples perform have some common features: (1) shame-based styles of communicating and interacting; (2) a denial by at least one partner of dysfunctional and/or codependent behavior; (3) a relationship of bargaining, not an intimate partnership; and (4) shame-based litany of the past. Each partner holds on to unresolved conflicts and continues to use them to shame the other.

✖ Recovery for Adult Children of Alcoholics

An ACA's prognosis for treatment is directly related to the severity of the parental alcoholism and the levels of abuse, violation, and trauma experienced while growing up in the alcoholic/addict family system. The onset of the alcoholism is also a factor in the ACA's recovery. The earlier the alcoholism in the family, and the younger the child when exposed to direct or indirect consequences of the parents' alcoholism, the more extensive the damage, and therefore the deeper the wounds. Impact at early ages can have dramatic developmental consequences (Brown 1988).

Inherited Family Belief Systems

A major recovery issue at the heart of all ACAs' problems is their core belief system. The "process of recovery involves challenging the deepest core beliefs about others and the self that were constructed to preserve core attachments" (Brown 1988). As discussed earlier in this chapter, these core beliefs serve to deny the ACAs feelings and maintain the illusion of their parents' normalcy. ACAs avoid exploring these holes in their belief systems for fear that their swiss cheese system might fall apart. When ACAs can acknowledge how the belief systems acquired from their parents have prevented them from attaining what they want, recovery can begin.

In *Struggle for Intimacy,* Janet Geringer Woititz (1985) devotes an entire chapter to some of the misconceptions, or inappropriate beliefs, that ACAs have when it comes to establishing intimate relationships.

Overview of ACA Recovery

Once ACAs are aware that their belief systems are not serving them, and preventing, blocking, or sabotaging the development of effective relationships, the next step is to develop a more reality-based belief system.

The first step in developing this reality-based belief system is to recognize the dysfunction and trauma of the past and unlock the feelings denied by this dysfunctional belief system.

A trusting therapeutic alliance with a counselor/therapist allows ACAs to feel the loss, grief, and trauma of the past. This difficult process involves (1) giving up the old defense mechanisms and dysfunctional beliefs; (2) feeling; and (3) choosing to honor and integrate those feelings in a new more functional belief system.

Eventually ACAs loosen their defensive controls and develop the ability to respond to different situations and circumstances with flexibility. ACAs can now establish effective boundaries in relationships, stop engaging in dysfunctional behavior and relationships, and establish a core belief system that allows for effective choicemaking and change.

Powerlessness in the Alcoholic Family System

Just as alcoholics/addicts must first admit they are powerless over drugs/alcohol, so must ACAs admit that as children they were powerless to change the alcoholic family system. They were innocent children whose feelings were ignored while living in unhealthy imbalanced situations. Recognizing that as children they were not responsible for their parents' disease of alcoholism frees ACAs to honor their own feelings.

Feeling Awareness

For ACAs who have spent a major portion of their lives denying feelings, the most difficult task of recovery is recognizing and integrating feelings in making decisions, resolving conflicts, and in developing interpersonal relationships.

Jerry, a patient of mine who is a recovering alcoholic and an ACA, quizzically and candidly commented, "Feelings, I am not quite sure what you mean when you ask 'What do you feel?' I don't know what you mean or want from me. When you ask me if I feel sad, or I sound angry, I don't recognize that I am experiencing those feelings until you mention it."

Many ACAs have similar reactions. Unaware of what they feel, they are equally inexperienced in recognizing what others feel. This makes it difficult to effectively communicate with others—especially family members—and to establish sensitive, caring, and intimate relationships.

Identifying Feelings for ACAs

Jael Greenleaf, an ACA counselor in Los Angeles, describes ACAs as having an emotional learning disability. (See Case Studies 7.2 & 7.3) ACAs have learned not to trust their feelings; thus they make decisions based on what they think is appropriate, without integrating what they feel. Feelings are what make us, or define us as, human. The famous television series *Star Trek* gave us Mr. Spock, the cognitive logical unemotional alien, and in the later version of the series, Data, a robot with extensive computer capabilities. Data was often fascinated and marveled at human feelings and emotions and tried to understand them. Mr. Spock does not understand human emotions that may override the logic of a decision. The captain of the *Enterprise* reminds Spock and Data that human emotions are essential and part of the human equation in approaching life.

By being sensitive to what we feel, we can begin to understand our feelings (affective self) and integrate them with what we know (cognitive self). When our affective self is congruent with our cognitive self, the application (whatever action we take) is often more successful. Decisions become easier to make when feelings are balanced with the cognitive side, and there is an interplay of these two sides of our self. Our decisions become more fulfilling, our goals more attainable, and our relationships more effective, when we integrate our feelings. The struggle for the ACA begins with identifying, understanding, and integrating feelings.

A good technique to help ACAs access their feelings is journaling, or writing a feeling diary. Often a counselor asks the ACA to buy a special notebook and keep it nearby—in the car, at work, and at home. Whenever the ACA is aware of an emotional reaction, thought, or feeling, he or she writes about it in the journal. By writing rather than thinking, ACAs soon find that they are accessing feelings that they may not have been aware of previously.

Another method of feeling awareness involves ACAs verbalizing and communicating what they feel directly to others. One method would be using the statement: "I feel _____, when I _____." For example:

"I feel upset when I notice you haven't taken the garbage out, after you said you would."
"I feel confused, and both sad and angry, when I don't get a present for Valentine's Day."
"Right now, I am not feeling close and caring toward you. I do not want to have sex. I am still feeling hurt by the fight we had earlier today. I would prefer talking about it tomorrow when our emotions are not running so deep."

Therapists help ACAs identify and explore a wide variety of feelings (shame, rejection, abandonment, loss, loneliness, isolation, and grief) that were experienced growing up in an alcoholic family system. ACA therapists use various treatment methods to access feelings including guided imagery, gestalt exercises, art therapy, role plays, workbooks, and books and articles on ACA issues (bibliotherapy).

Grief Work

Children who grow up in alcoholic families experience loss, violation, and trauma growing up in imbalanced alcoholic family systems. Many never have an opportunity to mourn what they have lost or missed out on. Mourning is a process of allowing feelings of loss to come to the surface, to be felt, and to be grieved.

An analogy is the improper healing of a cut. In the child's case, an emotionally damaging cut or violation of self has occurred. The cut has healed over but was not cleaned out first; the dirt (leftover unresolved issues and feelings) was not removed. The result is a numbing pain, which is tolerated and denied for years and is

Case Study 7.3
Difficulty in Making Decisions

Norman

Norman, 29, is an adult child of an alcoholic. He grew up in an extremely abusive and physically violating dysfunctional family system. On one occasion in an alcoholic rage, Norman's dad shoved his mom's head through the front window of their living room. Another time, his mom hid his dad's car keys in the garbage because his dad was drunk. They both struggled with the garbage, and she severely cut her hand on the jagged edge of a coffee can. Later, two tall police officers came to quiet them down during another domestic dispute. These were just a few of Norman's memories.

His parents' fighting had a far-reaching impact on Norman and the other children in the family. The fear of abandonment, shame, and rejection caused Norman to act out during his childhood in many destructive ways. He did not achieve at school, despite being very bright and capable.

One day in individual counseling, Norman talked about a trip he took to Reno, Nevada. This trip was a metaphor for his fear of making a career change. After watching for some time at the roulette table with his wife and a friend, he decided to place his bet. Norman placed a two dollar bet on the red and a two dollar bet on the black. He surmised that this was a secure bet. He smiled to himself smugly as the roulette wheel spun and the ball bounded around from number to number. When it landed on a red number, the croupier just pushed his two dollars from the black spot to the red spot, and Norman collected his bet. Despite the odd looks from the croupier, and his friend's efforts to explain why this was a stupid bet, Norman continued to play two dollars on black and two dollars on red simultaneously. After several spins, he stopped betting. He felt entertained and justified that he had played roulette. I didn't hesitate to point out to Norman that the numbers zero and double zero on the roulette wheel are green. If either of those numbers had come up, he would have lost both bets.

This was analogous to what Norman was doing in his conflict about his career. He was betting on his current job for security, but not actively putting himself on the line to find a more fulfilling job. The longer he waited to take action, the more time he was wasting, and the more likely it was that zero or double zero would come up, in the form of either losing his current job due to his dissatisfaction projected to the work setting or not being able to motivate himself to find a better job because he was suffering from feelings of rejection, shame, and abandonment.

Even with this therapeutic insight, Norman waited several months to take any direct action. After a great deal of work, he eventually landed a new job in the field that he really wanted. That job didn't work out but it led to another job. After 2 years of struggle, Norman found himself in a career position that was consistent with his feelings of entitlement and accomplishment; his job affirmed his skills and capabilities.

Discussion

This is a good example of how "playing it safe" for too long can result in significant negative consequences. Norman grew up in a household that was extremely abusive physically, verbally, and emotionally. Norman, like many ACAs, did not act on his passion or feelings. He knew he was unhappy in his job, and he also knew what kind of job he wanted, but he waited too long to take action or make a decision. Change often involves knowing what you feel, knowing what you want, but also having a plan and taking action. Norman was immobilized by fear over negative "what-ifs." What if he couldn't find a new job? What if he got a job and he didn't like it? What if he got fired from his new job? And on and on. This fearful negative cycle of thinking caused him to avoid making a decision, and to stay in an abusive working situation, much like the abusive family he grew up in.

thought to be quite normal. Grief work involves going back and cleaning out this wound by gently and sensitively removing the dirt. By avoiding the feelings and pain accompanying proper healing of this infected wound, individuals are unable to function to a fuller potential. Once their wounds are cleaned, true healing allows ACAs to make more effective choices.

Grief work requires the help of a professional therapist trained and experienced in ACA recovery. The counselor/therapist must be sensitive to the patient's ego strength, general level of functioning, underlying psychiatric issues, and support system. Attempting to do ACA grief work without an experienced professional may cause unnecessary emotional harm by going too deep, too quickly into traumatic issues of the past. A professional trained and experienced in ACA recovery recognizes the pace and depth of the work to be done and shows appropriate judgment in helping patients through this work.

Choice Making

Changing old, imbalanced patterns is possible only if individuals feel they have choices. Discouraging voices of doom and gloom need to be quieted for recovery efforts to be implemented. Self-pity, victim roles, and the poor-me syndrome prevent ACAs from even entertaining a choice to change. The old familial belief system whispers in the ACA's ear: "Change is not possible, so why even try? You'll just waste time and energy and fail, anyway, just as you always have in the past."

Changes involve integration and congruency with feelings and choosing not to respond in dysfunctional, codependent ways. There is the acknowledgment that change is difficult, takes time, may involve pain, and requires support. Sometimes small changes and positive choices can establish the foundation for more significant growth-related choices later. As the Rolling Stones' lyric goes, "You can't always get what you want, but, if you try sometimes, you get what you need."

A variety of therapeutic issues must be explored before the ACA can improve interpersonal relationships. Some of the cognitive and affective therapeutic themes are these:

- Family-of-origin issues (beliefs, roles, rules, and thoughts about relationships)
- Sense of self, or self-concept, and interpersonal interaction, choosing relationships, and maintaining dysfunctional imbalanced relationships
- Boundary setting and decision making in interpersonal situations
- Self-sabotage or destructive behavior, poor impulse control, poor anger and frustration tolerance, and an inability to set and maintain healthy long-range goals

Second-Order Change

Second-order change is a cognitive-behavioral technique to change the way one traditionally responds to situations and interpersonal interactions. Many interactions are mechanical, automatic, even rhetorical. These are first-order interactions. Individuals can choose to respond differently to the first-order cues in communication and interaction. This new response or new order of interaction is second-order change. The following examples illustrate a very common first-order interaction and one possible second-order change. The meta-message, or the underlying true feeling message, is in parentheses. (See Case Study 7.4.)

First-Order—Phone Call from Mom

Mom: Why haven't you called? (Shame on you for not caring about your mom. You probably don't like me. I know I'm just a bother now that I am old.)

Adult child: Well, Mom, I have been very busy with my new job and everything. (Please give me a break, Mom. I'm not in the mood for shame right now. I feel overwhelmed, considering the new job, and other adjustments I am going through. I don't need this right now.)

Mom: Well, I guess your job is more important than your mother. (Double shame on you for not making your mother number one in your life.)

Adult child: Mom, it's not that my job is more important than you. I just didn't get around to calling because I've been so busy at work. (Let me explain. Please, please, understand.)

Mom: You haven't asked me how my back is. (More shame—I don't care about your silly job. I want you to be more concerned with my ailments.)

Adult child: Now, Mom, that isn't fair. You didn't even give me a chance to ask you how you were. (I'm beginning to get angry and lose patience with you. Here we go again. I can't even talk with you without getting angry—self-shame.)

Mom: Now, don't get so upset, dear. (Watch it. This is your powerful supermom, able to abandon and hurt you with the slightest provocation.)

Adult child: [Change in tone] How are you feeling, Mom? I have been worried about you. (I don't want to fight or be abandoned. I'll just give her what she wants. I'm feeling like a helpless child again.)

Mom: Well, you know those doctors want me to come in for some more tests. But I don't think they know what they are talking about. I just don't have any way to get into the hospital, with my back hurting the way it does. (I am helpless. I want you to come home and be with me and take care of me. If you don't, I'll just punish you by suffering.)

Adult child: Mom, can't you get Aunt Joanie to take you in for the tests? (I am worried. I can't come. Maybe I can fix it for you by getting you some help.)

Mom: Oh dear, don't worry about me; I'll be all right. (Worry about me. Shame on you for not coming right away. You ungrateful daughter, I'll just suffer alone.)

Case Study 7.4

Letter to Parents from a Recovering Alcoholic and ACA About the Parents' Alcoholism

Dear Mom and Dad,

It's hard to write a letter like this, so I guess I'll just get right to the point. I'm writing because I'm concerned that you both continue to drink a lot despite the fact that you have both been in ill health recently. And I'm sure that you, Dad, have been warned more than once by doctors that to continue to drink threatens your health.

I've wanted to talk to you both about your drinking for years, but so far I have never been able to break the silence and tell you how truly worried I am about it.

Only you can make a decision to stop drinking. But I feel very strongly that I must tell you both, with love and compassion, how concerned I am, and how much it hurts me to see you continue to damage yourselves through drinking.

I am sure that in your hearts you know that you have a problem, for I have seen you both struggle with it; seen your efforts to control what and when you drink; seen your efforts to cut back. I know I rejoiced during that period when you sobered up entirely for a few months, and you found renewed health and happiness together.

I am also sure you are both aware that the stakes are high; that you are endangering your health as you mix alcohol and various prescription medication, and that drinking can only worsen your struggles with heart disease, diabetes, and the effects of aging.

You know what you have to do. It's so simple, and yet I know from experience how hard it can be. You both so desperately need to stop drinking now, throw out all the booze in the house (even the supply reserved for guests), and get some help staying sober, for you have proven by slipping back into drinking that you cannot do it by yourselves.

I suspect getting help will be the hardest part; it certainly was for me. But it's really the most necessary part of getting better and infinitely better than struggling alone.

Getting help could mean any of the following: Telling Dr. Green that you know you have a problem with alcohol and are tired of struggling with it; that you want to get some counseling or get into a treatment program. Calling AA and attending a meeting together; the nearest AA meeting is right down the street on Maple Rd. Calling the local drug/alcohol helpline and getting a referral to a counselor, social worker, or therapist experienced in working with alcoholics who want to recover.

This letter is not meant to blame or shame or accuse you; it is merely a plea for you to help yourselves for your own sakes, and for the sake of our family. It is an effort to tell the truth about the problem that our whole family has struggled with for so many years.

The truth hurts sometimes. The truth is that all of us have begun to insulate ourselves from your drinking, to control the time and length of our visits, to arrange sober holidays in our own homes, as my sister did this Christmas. We have all shied away from confronting you because it is so painful to see you both caught in this awful disease.

I hope that this letter has not made you angry or resentful. If it has, so be it; but I want you to know that I love you both, and that I want to help you, if there is any way in the world that I can. If you want to talk about this letter, please call me; if not, if it makes you too upset or uncomfortable, we need never discuss it.

Ultimately, there may be an element of selfishness in this letter; because, in the end, I want to be able to look into my heart and say "I tried to help. I told them the truth and encouraged them to get help and save their own lives." For me, it's an important step in dealing with my past and working on my own sobriety.

Case Study 7.4 (*continued*)

Letter to Parents from a Recovering Alcoholic and ACA About the Parents' Alcoholism

Please, for your own sake and the sake of us all, share this letter with each other, and talk about it openly together. I pray that you both will find the strength to quit drinking and get some help together.

Your loving son,

Epilogue

The parents who were sent this letter both got sober. Unfortunately the mother died shortly thereafter. The son spent some quality time with her during the months before she passed away. The father has been in recovery for a number of years now and has remarried. Father and son have quality time together when they visit.

Discussion Questions

Would you write a letter like this to one of your parents about a family issue?
Would you send a letter like this?
What are the "real" healing elements of this exercise?
Suggestion: Write a letter and then identify what the depth & breadth of the problem is.

This dialogue need not be carried out in this first-order manner. The anger, resentments, and shame do not have to be responded to in this traditional codependent dance. The following second-order change occurs after the adult child has done some therapeutic work on the underlying issue of her mother's not wanting to let go of her, for fear of having to work on her (mom's) own issues of loneliness and abandonment.

Second-Order—Change

Mom:	Why haven't you called? (Shame on you for not caring about your mom.)
Adult child:	Mom, boy, I've been wondering about you. How are you doing? (I'm not going to respond to the shaming question. I'll change the focus to you and your reason for calling.)
Mom:	Well, I'm surprised that you asked. Most of the time you're too busy with your job to even call me. (I'll try some more shaming to see if I can get you angry, because I am angry that your job comes before your dear old mom.)
Adult child:	Mom, it's unfortunate that I had to move out of town for this job promotion. I know it's hard on you. By the way, how is Aunt Joanie? (I had to take care of myself. I recognize that you feel abandoned and would prefer that I stay at home, but

	we all have to let go sometime. Why can't you understand like Aunt Joanie?)
Mom:	She's fine. But you know my back has been killing me. The doctors want me to go to the hospital for some more tests, but I hurt too much, and I don't know how I can get there. (Poor me, won't you please come home and help me?)
Adult child:	I know your back has been a problem for quite some time now. It would be nice to find out what the problem is. (I'd like to see you get in for the tests, but I can't help you get to the hospital. If you want some results, you'll have to figure out transportation.)
Mom:	So would I. But I need someone to help me, and Aunt Joanie doesn't drive. (Please, won't you come back home and help?)
Adult child:	Well, there are other ways for you to get a ride to the hospital. I hope you can figure out a way. (I'm not coming, just for this. There are other solutions to the problem and you are capable of figuring it out.)
Mom:	Well, I just don't know if I can do it myself. (Poor me. Shame on you for not helping your poor old mom.)
Adult child:	Well, Mom, I'm sure you'll be able to figure it out. You were always pretty resourceful when we were growing up. I love you. I'll talk to you soon. (You must take care of this yourself. You were very capable raising three children practically on your own, considering Dad's alcoholism. I'm not jumping in to help. I still love and admire you. I am ending this conversation and not giving you an opportunity to feel sorry for yourself.)

You can see the difference in the second-order change. The adult child avoided the shame-based messages and did not get emotionally hooked by displaying anger, rage, or lack of emotional control. Instead, in the second-order model, she focused on the real issues and stayed balanced and in emotional control while maintaining appropriate boundaries.

Changes in Interactions with Family

Robert Ackerman (1978), a noted author, speaker, and counselor specializing in ACA work, tells a story that illustrates the difficulty in changing interactions with family: After working with Ackerman for a few months, one of his patients felt she had made enough progress to share her new therapeutic awareness with her family. She was going home for Christmas (an emotional time for most families, especially alcoholic families) and wanted to talk to her parents about her new insights. Ackerman suggested that she think about what her goal was in sharing her insights. Essentially ignoring his advice, on returning home she told her parents all about her childhood pain resulting from growing up in an alcoholic family and described how this had affected her relationships with men. Initially, her parents were actively listening and seemed to understand. However, the next few days the family returned to the traditional dysfunctional arguments, escalated emotions, and shame-based communications of the past. The daughter had to spend the next few days at a friend's home to survive the rest of the holiday.

At her next therapy appointment, the patient expressed surprise that her parents could engage her in the old dysfunctional dances. She asked, "Why were they still able to push all of my buttons?" Dr. Ackerman, in the wisdom of his years of experience, matter-of-factly said, "They installed the buttons."

The same struggle goes on for most ACA who interact with their families. Some of these families have members still actively using alcohol/drugs or maintaining dysfunctional behavior. It might be necessary for ACA to let their parents know how they feel about their continued use of alcohol/drugs. In some situations, with the help of their therapists, patients have decided to send a letter to their parents who are still using alcohol/drugs. The goal of the letter is to assist ACA in healing and accepting their parents' disease. It is a way for ACA to get in touch with their feelings about their parents' continued use of alcohol/drugs. Patients decide for themselves whether the letter is appropriate for the goal they have in mind, and whether they want to send the letter.

Many ACA must ultimately let go and accept that their parents may never choose to stop using alcohol/drugs. Each patient continues to struggle with personal recovery issues in an ongoing process of self-discovery, supported by others in recovery. At times, it is a process of two steps forward, one step backward, but the process and progress continue.

Group Psychotherapy

Group psychotherapy is the next step once ACA have worked through some of the previously described core issues. Group psychotherapy is a dynamic process in which each group member gets feedback from other group members. Members share their perceptions, feelings, and insights into each other's behavior.

Irvin D. Yalom (1975) describes the following 11 curative factors that make group psychotherapy such an effective process. (See Case Study 7.5)

1. *Instilling hope.* ACA group members see firsthand the growth of other group members. Continued contact with other group members who have improved while doing their work in the group gives ACA hope for their own recovery and confidence in the group process.
2. *Sharing universality.* ACAs realize that they are not alone and that others share common problems. Group therapy reveals that ACA characteristics are universal to those who grew up in alcoholic/addict family systems, as well as imbalanced family systems. ACAs no longer suffer in social or interpersonal isolation. There is the opportunity for affirmation by other group members, who understand them and identify with the issues they have in common.
3. *Imparting information.* Group therapy provides information, education, and training on ACA issues, including family systems, alcoholism/addiction, codependency, and boundary setting in relationships. Both the therapist and other group members offer suggestions, advice, and direct guidance about life problems.

Case Study 7.5

Interpersonal Relationships

Naomi

Naomi was a very attractive, young, and active director of marketing for a major retail clothing manufacturer. She grew up in an alcoholic family and compensated by being extremely successful in all endeavors. She described her mom's sense of self as being directly related to all of Naomi's accomplishments. Unfortunately, Naomi approached interpersonal relationships outside of the family in the same manner and tended to attract friends who mirrored her accomplishments back to her. In group therapy, Naomi began to use this same interpersonal dynamic of trying to control others so they reflected a positive mirror image of her success back to her. Initially, she was worried that the group would ask her to leave when they began to see her self-centeredness. Instead the group was able to make her aware of her imbalanced need for affirmation. The group gave her permission to explore her issues and be herself, while not having to look good all the time. In fact, they enjoyed the Naomi who wasn't always on and saw this aspect of her personality as more relaxed, fun loving, vulnerable, available, present, and worth getting to know.

Discussion

One way to avoid being vulnerable is to be "in control" of most interpersonal interactions. A way to avoid being shamed or criticized is to be "perfect." Naomi was so into control, perfectionism, and image management (e.g., looking good) that pursuing achievement and others' affirmation of her achievements was the dominant way for her to interact with others.

Group therapy reflected back to Naomi this style of interpersonal interaction. Naomi soon realized how lonely she was and began to be more vulnerable in group. She realized that her interpersonal relationships would improve as she became more present and authentic. She began to listen to others and to value relationships for what they were, rather than for the role the other person played in completing a task or achieving a goal.

---

4. *Fostering altruism.* Altruism is the act of giving to others and caring about others' life situations. The group is a place for support, reassurance, encouragement, insight, and sharing, all of which help both the giver and the receiver to grow.

5. *Recapitulating the primary family group.* Recapitulation offers an opportunity for the group to act as a functional family with positive corrective capabilities. Early familial conflicts can be acted out. With the help of the group, ACAs can resolve these conflicts in a functional manner, rather than the previously dysfunctional and rigid manner of the family of origin.

6. *Developing socializing techniques.* Socializing is an obvious curative factor of group therapy. ACAs can explore maladaptive social behavior through honest and caring feedback from group members. Alternative social choices and techniques can be developed with the feedback of the group. ACAs are particularly vulnerable to choosing dysfunctional relationships and maintaining codependent interactions in relationships. The group can alert

ACAs who try to return to codependent ways of interaction and
dysfunctional choice making.

7. *Imitating behavior.* By seeing the reactions and behaviors of others, ACAs
   have numerous new models of behavior.

8. *Sharing interpersonal learning.* The group is a social microcosm of the real
   world. ACAs tend to duplicate the way they approach the real interpersonal
   world in their therapy group. Insights into adult children's interpersonal
   behavior and corrective emotional strategies can be explored in the safe
   environment of the group setting.

9. *Developing group cohesiveness.* The bonding that occurs in therapy groups
   results in a cohesive understanding, which makes the group a safe place to
   go with stressful problems, interpersonal conflicts, difficult decisions, and
   other issues. The group develops a functional interpersonal cohesiveness,
   allowing members to pull for and struggle with the difficult issues in their
   lives.

10. *Sharing catharsis.* The group is a place where ACAs feel safe in expressing
    feelings not safely expressed in other settings. Fears, insecurities, destructive
    thoughts, suicidal ideation, rage, shame, and other emotions are safe to
    express in the group.

11. *Exploring existential factors.* The group helps its members explore meaning
    in their lives. Issues of attachment in relationships, congruency in work
    efforts, and spirituality are all safe for each group member to explore and
    develop. In other words, the functional therapy group explores the human
    condition.

In summary, group therapy is a dynamic process that has a tremendous potential for ACA recovery, especially after ACAs have spent time exploring their issues
in individual counseling.

References

Ackerman, Robert J. 1978. *Children of alcoholics: A guidebook for educators, therapists,
    and parents.* Holmes Beach, Fla.: Learning.

After drug treatment: What happens to the marriage. 1999. *Springbrook Northwest
    Newsletter,* summer.

Black, Claudia. 1982. *It will never happen to me.* Denver, Colo.: M.A.C.

Brown, Stephanie. 1988. *Treating adult children of alcoholics: A developmental perspective.*
    New York: Wiley.

Cermak, Timmen. 1984. Children of alcoholics and the case for a new diagnostic category
    of co-dependency. *Alcohol, Health, and Research World* 8:38–42.

Clinebell, Howard J., Jr. 1985. *Understanding and counseling the alcoholic through religion
    and psychology.* Nashville, Tenn.: Abingdon Press.

Coleman, Eli, and Philip Colgan. 1987. Chemical dependency and intimacy dysfunction.
    Journal of Chemical Dependency Treatment 1:75–91.

Cork, M. 1969. *The forgotten children.* Toronto: Addiction Research Foundation.

Newell, Nancy. 1950. Alcoholism and the father image. *Quarterly Journal of Studies on
    Alcoholism* 11:92–95.

Yalom, Irvin D. 1975. *The theory and practice of group psychotherapy.* New York: Basic
    Books.

Prevention, Intervention, and Treatment

Prevention of Substance-Abuse Problems

❖ Chapter in Review

The early prevention approaches focused primarily on supplying information on the dangers of specific drugs; on warnings of physical, social, and psychological harm; and on punishment for sale, use, and possession. These scare tactics were ineffective, as were other converting programs, which tried to direct, preach, or convince young people not to use drugs. The information presented in these early prevention approaches was often invalid, exaggerated, and overgeneralized, causing young people to question the credibility of the prevention efforts.

The next prevention efforts focused on drug-specific information in the hope that young people would make wise decisions about drugs. Unfortunately, these approaches heightened curiosity and alleviated fears, leading to an increase in drug experimentation, rather than the intended decrease.

The ineffectiveness of scare tactics and drug-specific approaches led to a moratorium on prevention efforts by the government and a review of those features of a prevention program that were effective.

In the 1980s, the thrust of these new prevention strategies shifted from drugs to people, emphasizing educational information, coping skills, personal competence, decision making, refusal skills, and alternative activities.

Alternative activities are successful if they are acceptable, attractive, and attainable.

Today credibility is a basic premise for the effectiveness of any alcohol/drug prevention program. Effective prevention must include youth, be sensitive and include community needs, promote proactivity, and make a longitudinal commitment to long-term prevention efforts. Special programs are also necessary for prevention efforts for at-risk students, people of color, college students, and elders.

Current prevention programs should be aimed at at-risk youth and people of color and other minorities and should be community-based.

Steven Wolin and Sybil Wolin developed a challenge model of resiliency. Daniel Goleman introduced the concept of emotional intelligence. The domains of prevention are primary and secondary defenses. The developmental assets model describes 40 developmental assets in the areas of support, empowerment, boundaries and expectations, constructive use of time, commitment to learning, positive values, social competence, and positive identity.

Alcohol/drug prevention has often been a misunderstood and neglected aspect in addressing the American drug problem. This chapter provides a foundation so that you can apply prevention efforts at home, in school systems, and in the community. Prevention efforts have shifted from scare tactics (dangers and evils of drugs) to emphases on the worth of people and the coping skills needed to avoid a destructive pattern of alcohol/drug dependence. Specific prevention skills outlined in this chapter include goal setting, decision making, and conflict resolution. The goal of prevention, outlined in this chapter, is to develop active, involved, empowered, and capable young people.

For years, society has searched for easy ways to prevent drug dependence and addiction. Initially, frightening movies and horror stories of drug abuse failed to make young people too scared to use drugs. Early efforts to prevent drug use focused primarily on providing the following:

✄ Early Prevention Approaches

- Information on the dangers of specific drugs
- Warnings of physical, social, and psychological harm
- Punishments for sale, use, and possession

Scare tactics proved to be an ineffective prevention strategy. Much of the information was invalid, exaggerated, and overgeneralized, causing young people to question the credibility of the program.

Similar programs were developed and labeled by drug educator Walter M. Mathews (1975) as **converting programs.** These programs used the following tactics to attempt to dissuade young people from using drugs:

1. Directing: Teacher tells students what they must believe, value, and do.
2. Preaching: This was similar to directing, with an added appeal to the students' duty to a vague external authority.
3. Convincing: Teachers appealed to logic where lecturing was the method used.
4. Scaring: Teachers emphasized the dangers of drug use.

Additional converting approaches emphasized admonishment, indoctrination, persuasion, distortion, and fear.

Adolescence is a time of questioning and exploration. The information provided in these approaches was not geared to the sensitivity of young people; it insulted their individuality and ability to make decisions. Adults in authority told them what to do, rather than talking with them. These propaganda approaches did not emphasize communication and open discussion.

The failure of these approaches led to a new prevention strategy of providing factual information about drugs, or **drug-specific approaches.** These approaches emphasized each drug and its pharmacological properties and assumed young people would make responsible decisions about drug use if they knew the negative effects. Inadvertently, these drug-specific approaches heightened curiosity and caused the opposite, alleviating fears of drugs. Many students acquired the knowledge to better attain desired levels of intoxication.

As a result of the failure of scare tactics and drug-specific approaches, the government's Special Action Office on Drug Abuse Prevention (SAODAP) declared a 6-month moratorium in 1973 on all prevention materials development, prevention program implementation, and prevention activities. The moratorium allowed further review of research and determined that, because scare tactics and drug-specific information did not significantly deter drug use, they were ineffective. In 1974, Robert DuPont, then the director of the National Institute on Drug Abuse (NIDA), surveyed drug education programs and concluded that the educators and students believed that the majority of school-based drug education programs were ineffective and should be abolished. In a review of research on school-based drug education programs, Michael Goodstadt (1975) concluded that "there is an almost total lack of evidence indicating beneficial effects of drug education, very few educational programs have been evaluated and almost none have shown any significant improvement in anything other than levels of knowledge; attitudes and drug use have generally remained the same."

In 1974, the prevention branch of the National Institute on Drug Abuse initiated a nationwide, 14-month planning process to develop a national strategy for primary prevention. This planning process involved over 400 prevention specialists in a series of nine planning conferences. In 1975, the institute published the resulting recommendations in *Toward a National Strategy for Primary Drug Abuse Prevention.* The report defined primary drug abuse prevention as "a constructive process designed to promote personal and social growth of the individual to full human potential and thereby inhibit or reduce physical, mental, emotional, or social impairment which results in or from the abuse of chemical substances."

The report established three basic themes for primary prevention: (1) primary prevention must be understood as the development and reinforcement of positive behaviors; (2) primary prevention programs must be responsive in both design and operation to the needs of those they are intended to serve or support; and (3) primary prevention should, wherever possible, use collaborative efforts to utilize the already available capacities and resources of existing human service institutions.

The result of SAODAP's moratorium and prevention planning meetings was a major shift in focus from drugs to the young people and from pharmacological effects to healthy children.

In 1977, NIDA and other agencies developed an interagency report entitled *Recommendations for Future Federal Activities in Drug Abuse Prevention.* This report outlined three major goals for prevention activities:

1. Reducing the percentage of frequent use of the three gateway drugs (tobacco, alcohol, and marijuana) by 15 percent among 8- to 20-year-olds.
2. Reducing the destructive behavior associated with alcohol and other drug abuse by 20 percent among 14- to 20-year-olds, as evidenced by a reduction in overdose deaths, emergency room visits, drug arrests, and other alcohol/drug-related incidents.
3. Retraining attitudes concerning the use of psychoactive substances, especially the gateway drugs, by maintaining current levels of awareness regarding the addictive nature of heroin and alcohol and raising awareness of the addictive nature of tobacco by 50 percent.

✖ Alternative Activities as a Prevention Approach

In Chapter 1, we examined the primary function of alcohol/drugs as serving our natural innate drive to alter our sense of consciousness. Ronald Siegal, in his book *Intoxication,* describes altering one's consciousness as the fourth drive, after hunger, thirst, and sex. The primary goal of alternative activities is to teach people that they are capable of altering their consciousness in a meaningful, longer-lasting, life-enhancing, and satisfying way that is incompatible with alcohol/drug use.

The late 1970s saw a strong movement toward alternative activity programs for young people. The programs usually involved wilderness activities, requiring teamwork, challenge, and risk that developed feelings of competence, skill, and self-worth. Today, many adolescent and adult inpatient and residential chemical dependency treatment programs are including alternative activity program elements as a natural part of the clients' recovery program. This can include rope courses, climbing structures, even what one program calls "equine therapy" (i.e., working with horses).

Alan Cohen (1972), a strong advocate of alternative activities, defines alternatives as pursuits that are valued and truly preferred by individuals and seen as incompatible with drugs. Cohen emphasizes that alternatives are not just a substitution for drugs; they are an integrated and valued part of the person's life.

Alternatives Are Actively Pursued by the Individual

Cohen felt that, for an alternative to be successful, the process of searching for the alternative should be a potent alternative in itself. Individuals are encour-

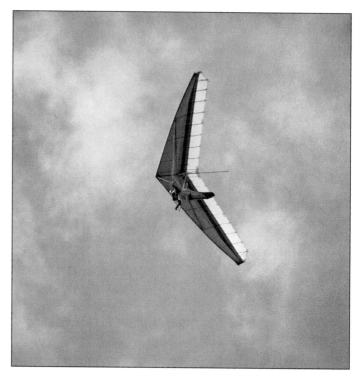

Hang gliding is an alternative activity.

aged to find other activities they can develop, persevere through to mastery, and enjoy. The process of being able to choose ways to get high naturally through one's own interests is truly empowering. It follows that alternatives are more effective if they call for activity, assertion of will or will power, and effort and commitment. Alternatives are less successful if individuals are passive recipients of the activity. This is consistent with the function of drug dependence and alcoholism as a rather passive activity. All alcoholics/addicts have to do is sit back and passively wait for the alcohol/drug to take effect.

Cohen (1972) illustrates this in the example of listening to music: "Passively listening to music is not necessarily a promising alternative to drugs, since one could be passively stoned at the time. Training in active listening and deep study of music is more likely to be frustrating to drug use since the clarity of one's senses and cognition become important in successful completion of the task."

Alternatives Are Acceptable, Attractive, and Attainable

Alternatives must be acceptable and attractive. Any alternative offered must be realistic, attainable, and meaningful. Alternatives must also help people understand themselves and improve their self-image and personal awareness. Dohner (1972) outlined the following characteristics of positive alternatives:

1. They must contribute to the individual's identity and independence.
2. They must offer active participation and involvement.
3. They must offer a chance for commitment.

4. They must provide a feeling of identification with a larger body of experience.

5. Some of the alternatives must be in the realm of the noncognitive and the intuitive.

Alternatives Use Mentors and Role Models

Another essential feature of alternatives is a successful role model or mentor—someone who can guide, facilitate, and encourage the successful attainment of the alternative skill. This person could be a positive parent model, a coach, a teacher, a peer, or anyone else who understands and respects the boundaries in the development of the alternative skill.

Alternatives Integrate Self-Concepts

Alternative activities are effective as preventive tools if they enhance the development of skills associated with improving one's sense of self. Table 8.1 lists Allan Cohen's categories for various alternative activities based on personal attributes and attraction.

Use the alternatives worksheet as shown in Table 8.2 to list your motives and preferred alternatives to alcohol/drug use. Also identify the steps and resources necessary to implement each alternative.

✖ Prevention Approaches of the 1980s

In the 1980s, the new prevention strategy shifted from drugs to people, emphasizing the following:

- Educational information
- Coping skills
- Personal competence
- Decision making
- Refusal skills
- Alternative activities

The goal of these programs was to develop capable young people able to make responsible decisions about alcohol/drugs. The focus changed to understanding the impact of drugs on individuals, rather than understanding the pharmacological properties of alcohol/drugs. The affective aspect focused on the individual's needs, feelings, and emotions about alcohol/drugs.

These new prevention programs develop the following skills:

- Clarifying personal values and ethics
- Improving self-concept
- Learning effective decision making
- Understanding and listening to each other's viewpoints
- Communicating about alcohol/drugs with peers, parents, and others
- Being involved in social and interpersonal activities
- Dealing effectively with feelings of anger, depression, and anxiety

TABLE 8.1

Motives for and Alternatives to the Use of Drugs

Level of Experience	Corresponding Motives	Alternatives to Drugs
Physical	Desire for physical satisfaction, physical relaxation, relief from sickness, more energy, maintenance of physical dependency	Athletics, dance, exercise, hiking, diet, health training, carpentry, or outdoor work
Sensory	Desire to stimulate sight, sound, touch, taste; need for sensual-sexual stimulation; desire to magnify the brain's sensoriums	Sensory awareness training, sky diving, experiencing sensory beauty of nature (lovemaking, swimming, running, mountaineering), *skiing, surfing, massage
Emotional	Relief from psychological pain, attempt to solve personal perplexities, relief from bad mood, escape from anxiety, desire for emotional insight, liberation of feeling, emotional relaxation	Competent individual counseling, well-run group therapy, instruction in psychology of personal development (sensitivity training), *self-help meetings, *emotional support system
Interpersonal	To gain peer acceptance; to break through interpersonal barriers; to communicate, especially nonverbally; defiance of authority figures; cement two-person relationships; relaxation of interpersonal inhibition; solve interpersonal hangups	Expertly managed sensitivity and encounter groups, well-run group therapy, instruction in social customs, confidence training, social-interpersonal counseling, emphasis on assisting others in distress via education, marriage, *participation in organizations and community activities within personal interests
Social (including sociocultural and environmental)	To promote social change; to find identifiable subcultures to tune out intolerable environmental conditions	Social service; community action in positive social change; helping the poor, aged, infirm, young; tutoring handicapped; improving the environment; *Peace Corps work with the homeless, hungry, impoverished, and oppressed
Political	To promote political change; identify with antiestablishment subgroup to change drug legislation out of desperation with the sociopolitical order; to gain wealth or affluence of power	Political service; political action; nonpartisan projects such as ecological lobbying; fieldwork with politicians, and public officials

(continued on next page)

TABLE 8.1 (*continued*)

Motives for and Alternatives to the Use of Drugs

Level of Experience	Corresponding Motives	Alternatives to Drugs
Intellectual	To escape mental boredom; out of intellectual curiosity to solve cognitive problems; to gain new understanding in the world of ideas; to study better; to research one's own awareness for science	Intellectual excitement through reading, discussion; creative games and puzzles; self-hypnosis; training in concentration; synectics training in intellectual breakthroughs; memory training; *seminars, workshops, and conferences; study or discussion groups; work with computers; writing a book or article
Creative-aesthetic	To improve creativity in the arts, to enhance enjoyment of art already produced, to enjoy imaginative mental productions	Nongraded instruction in producing and/or appreciating art, music, drama, crafts, handiwork, cooking, sewing, gardening, writing, singing
Philosophical	To discover meaningful values, to grasp the nature of the universe, to find meaning in life, to help establish personal identity, to organize a belief structure	Discussions, seminars, courses in the meaning of life; study of ethics, morality, the nature of reality; relevant philosophical literature; guided exploration of value systems
Spiritual, mystical	To transcend orthodox religion, to develop spiritual insights, to reach higher levels of consciousness, to have divine visions, to communicate with God, to augment yogic practices, to get a spiritual shortcut, to attain enlightenment, to attain spiritual powers	Exposure to nonchemical methods of spiritual development; study of world religions, introduction to applied mysticism, meditation, yogic techniques; *attending churches with recovery orientation; all activities that enhance spiritual awareness (nature, human connectedness, and activities that deal with existential despair)
Miscellaneous	Adventure, risk, drama, kicks, unexpressed motives, prodrug general attitudes	Outward Bound survival training; combinations of preceding alternatives; pronaturalness attitudes; brainwave training; meaningful employment

From Allan Y. Cohen, "The Journey Beyond Trips: Alternative to Drugs" in David E. Smith and Dr. George R. Gay, Eds., *It's So Good, Don't Even Try It Once: Heroin in Perspective.* Copyright © 1972 Prentice Hall, Inc., Englewood Cliffs, N.J.

* This author's additions are indicated by asterisks.

- Having the ability to relax, play, and enjoy daily activities
- Developing and exploring ways to alter one's sense of consciousness through alternative activities

Agencies originally focused on prevention in secondary schools for adolescents 12 to 17 years of age. It became apparent quickly that in many cases it was already too late to provide preventive education to adolescents. This group required more intervention, skill building, and treatment-related approaches.

TABLE 8.2

Alternatives Worksheet

Level of Experience	Corresponding Motives	Steps and Resources to Implement Alternatives to Alcohol/Drugs
Physical		
Sensory		
Emotional		
Interpersonal		
Social		
Political		
Intellectual		
Creative-aesthetic		
Philosophical		
Spiritual, mystical		
Miscellaneous		

As a result, alcohol and drug curricula and primary prevention activities shifted to kindergarten through the sixth grade. Agencies also developed secondary and tertiary prevention approaches for grades 7 to 12.

A definition of prevention covers three basic categories:

1. **Primary prevention** assumes that the individual has never tried drugs or alcohol and enforces a no-use norm by building positive self-esteem, developing good coping and refusal skills, and providing information on alcohol and drugs.

2. **Secondary prevention** assumes that the individual is in the early stages of use but does not regularly use drugs. Secondary prevention/intervention strategies try to stop drug use by providing drug information, developing decision-making and refusal skills, and improving family communication; it may also include individual counseling.

3. **Tertiary prevention** assumes that the individual is regularly using drugs but has not become a habitual user. Tertiary prevention/intervention includes counseling, drug education, and family therapy. There is a very fine line between the tertiary level of prevention and intervention and treatment services.

�ख School-Based Prevention Curricula—Examples

In 1983, the U.S. Department of Health and Human Services monograph *Drug Abuse Prevention Research* outlined four dimensions of prevention:

1. Course content centers on mental health, drug information, human development, nutrition, ethics, and chemical safety; these courses usually fit into regular social studies, language arts, science, and other subject area curricula

2. Courses on values clarification, problem-solving and decision-making skills, communication skills such as reflection and confrontation, alternative means for meeting needs, group process skills, role-playing, and dramatization

3. Courses that include competencies in human development, interpersonal relationships, personal autonomy, self-esteem, identity, decision-making skills, personal accountability, and accurate attributions of causality

4. Courses that also include general knowledge, conceptual frameworks, implicit assumptions and perspectives that define and describe the way each individual perceives the meaning of self, the nature of the world external to self, and the interrelatedness of things

The following examples of school-based prevention programs reveal typical competencies and coping skills emphasized in such programs. Prevention programs are not limited to alcohol/drug prevention; many health issues are included in school-based prevention programs.

Here's Looking at You—Kindergarten Through Senior High School

One of the most widely used school-based curricula, *Here's Looking at You,* was originally published in 1975. With significant revisions in 1978, 1982, and 1985, it is one of the most highly tested and developmentally sound curricula in the prevention field.

Program goals for students include developing

- Self-concepts to realize they are unique and special persons who are continually growing and changing and who are capable of directing their growth
- Decision-making skills for making responsible choices
- Coping skills so they can cope responsibly with stressful situations

Counseling Leadership Against Smoking Pressure (CLASP)

One of the major efforts of prevention has been the reduction and elimination of cigarette smoking by young people. A variety of successful programs have been developed; one of the most successful is CLASP. The key element of this project is the use of peers as leaders. Peer leaders promote and develop group strategies for coping with peer pressure.

Other antismoking program methods focus on dealing with social pressure, the use of personalized role models and peer opinion leaders, and group commitment to nonsmoking. All of these programs are implemented by the seventh grade.

Cognitive-Behavioral Skills Training

Schinke and Gilchrist (1983), who have done extensive research in the area of pregnancy prevention, developed a cognitive-behavioral model that systematically teaches the skills necessary to enjoy positive lives and to avoid unnecessary risks. Their junior and senior high school model emphasizes the following:

- Social coping skills necessary to handle current problems
- Anticipation and prevention of future problems and conflicts
- Skills in mental health awareness
- Issues of health, social, economic, and physical well-being
- Strategies to enhance skills such as decision making, problem solving, and interpersonal communication in a variety of social situations

Cognitive Interpersonal Skills Training

Spivak and Shuve (1979) developed a program similar to Schinke and Gilchrist's for kindergarten and first grade. The method uses games designed to increase cognitive skills, followed by training in alternative responses to interpersonal problem solving. The concepts taught in this model are the following:

- Creating alternative solutions to problems
- Developing sensitivity to interpersonal problems
- Understanding means-ends relationships

Life Skills Training

The methods used in the *Life Skills Program* are instruction, modeling, rehearsal, and role-playing. Botvin's (1985) program has five major skill areas:

- Enhancing self-esteem by developing goal-setting skills, behavioral change techniques, and positive self-statements
- Resisting persuasive appeals by first identifying persuasive appeals and formulating counterarguments
- Coping with anxiety through relaxation training and mental rehearsal
- Developing verbal and nonverbal communication skills
- Developing a variety of other social skills, such as initiation of social interactions, social communication skills, complimenting, and assertiveness skills

Law-Related Education

Developed by the Center for Action Research, *Law-Related Education* deals with the criminal-justice system. Its goal is to deter the antisocial behavior of young people by increasing their conceptual and practical understanding of the law and legal processes. The program's target populations are kindergarten through sixth grade, and sixth to twelfth grade. The goals of the program are

- To improve citizenship skills
- To enhance the ability to work with the legal system
- To promote favorable attitudes toward law enforcement and the justice system

Skills for Adolescence

As part of the program, students set goals for healthy living. The students also develop projects offering their service to others in the community. This program for grades 6 through 8 focuses on

- Entering the teen years
- Building self-confidence
- Learning about emotions
- Improving peer relationships
- Strengthening family relationships
- Developing critical thinking skills

Skills for Living

A high school program, *Skills for Living* emphasizes self-discipline, responsibility, good judgment, and the ability to interact with others. The curriculum focuses on

- Building self-concept
- Dealing with emotions
- Building constructive relationships
- Preparing for family life
- Building trust and commitment
- Parenting successfully
- Understanding financial management
- Goal setting and life planning
- Developing a personal perspective

Prevention Skills in Decision Making

Many prevention lessons focus on effective decision making. An important aspect of decision making is to help young people identify how they feel about a decision, rather than ignoring feelings that signal a potentially destructive decision. The decision-making model teaches individuals to

1. Explore personal values, feelings, and goals related to a decision
2. Gather information on the subject of the decision (e.g., factual written resources: consumer reports, opinions of others in the field or of those who

have made similar decisions successfully, opinions of others who are valued and supportive)

3. Review alternatives and consequences
4. Evaluate resources, responsibilities, and support as necessary
5. Make a decision
6. Reevaluate the decision and explore feelings about the decision
7. Make necessary adjustments

Empowerment

A term often used in prevention programs is *empowerment*. Many prevention programs emphasize the empowering of the individual. The basic goal of prevention is to empower individuals and prevent the destructive passive choice of alcohol/drug dependence and addiction. Empowerment is a feeling that is developed by being able to

- Say no when that is what one feels and wants
- Establish the core aspects of a sense of self
- Be aware of what one feels and integrate and communicate those feelings to others in establishing goals and making decisions
- Establish and set boundaries, especially in interpersonal and intimate relationships
- Establish integrity in relationships and a healthy, nondestructive, nonsabotaging approach to life

These prevention programs are usually targeted at the general school population, rather than the high-risk students who have already exhibited problem behaviors in and outside of school.

Goal Setting

A model lesson for goal setting would include lessons on (1) setting goals, (2) ranking priorities, (3) making decisions in relation to the goals, (4) persevering in the face of difficult situations, and (5) maintaining effort (motivation) until goals are attained or modified.

Capability Development

Other prevention lessons involve developing capabilities. I had the good fortune many years ago to work with Stephen Glenn at the National Drug Abuse Center in Washington, D.C. Today, Glenn lectures throughout the United States on the family prevention theme of developing capable people. His model for developing capable children includes fostering the following in children:

1. Identification with viable role models
2. Identification with and responsibility for family process
3. Faith in personal resources to solve problems
4. Adequate development of intrapersonal skills (responsibility)
5. Adequate development of interpersonal skills (communication)
6. Well-developed situation skills (demand skills)
7. Adequately developed judgment skills (application)

❈ The 10 Cs of Capability

Another skill-building concept is the ability to be *capable*. A capable person has the 10 Cs, the abilities to

- Resolve conflict
- Make effective choices
- Deal effectively with criticism
- Persevere through times of crisis
- Communicate effectively—understand and be understood
- Deal with competition (rivalry) and competence
- Establish credibility and integrity in an approach to people and life in general
- Express concern and empathy for others
- Be creative

❈ Key Components of a Prevention Program

Address Community Needs

Alcohol/drug prevention should address itself to the needs of the community and interface with community leaders, agencies, and the people. Edward M. Brecher knew community was important when he wrote the following in *Licit and Illicit Drugs* (1972): Stop viewing the drug problem as primarily a national problem to be solved on a national scale. In fact, as workers in the drug scene confirm, the drug problem is a collection of local problems. The predominant drugs differ from place to place and from time to time. Effective solutions to problems also vary; a plan that works now for New York City may not be applicable to upstate New York and vice versa. With respect to education, . . . the need for local wisdom and local control is particularly pressing. Warning children against drugs readily available to them is a risky business at best, requiring careful, truthful, unsensational approaches.

Include Youth in Prevention Planning

A prevention program must take into account the consumer of that program. To develop prevention programs in a vacuum, or from a strictly theoretical base, does not take into account the most important variable—the needs of youth.

Promote Proactivity

A core theme in prevention is to teach young people to move from being passive to being active, or proactive. Being proactive involves taking initiative, anticipating potential problems, and integrating your feelings. Too many young people spend excessive time in passive activities (e.g., watching television, playing computer games).

Parents can teach and model active behaviors and encourage activities that help young people develop a capable, positive sense of self. Proactive choices help develop the child's coping skills and ability to overcome setbacks.

Develop a Long-Term Perspective

Prevention is a long-term strategy. Longitudinal studies over 5 to 10 years are necessary to determine the effects of prevention. Unfortunately, most prevention programs have short-term funding, which limits the evaluation of their true effectiveness. Currently, we focus on the short-range perspective of drug enforcement and interdiction without the balance of a comprehensive prevention strategy to deal with the demand side of alcohol/drugs with youth. Our true hope is that the prevention and family approaches used with 3- to 10-year-olds—the next generation—may break this cycle of problems with dependence and addiction to alcohol/drugs.

In summary, an effective substance-abuse prevention strategy should do the following:

Emphasize cognitive and affective skills that help young people accept responsibility and motivate them to make wise decisions about alcohol and drugs.

Focus on people, not pharmacology, emphasizing educational information, coping skills, personal competence, decision making, refusal skills, and alternative activities.

Develop prevention programs that provide information plus communication, establish credibility, and meet community needs.

Take into account the needs of youth and develop prevention approaches cooperatively with young people in the community.

Develop primary efforts (those who have never used alcohol/drugs), secondary efforts (those in early stages of alcohol/drug use), and tertiary prevention efforts (those in regular stages of alcohol/drug use).

Develop longitudinal commitment to long-term prevention efforts.

Table 8.3 presents additional guidelines for making prevention programs more effective.

Jean Rhodes and Leonard Jason (1988) developed a model that emphasizes the development of **attachments, competence,** and **coping skills** to minimize risk for substance abuse. The more stress the child experiences—without appropriate and strong bonding to parents, attachment to drug-free role models, access to models with a strong sense of self, and good coping skills and resources—the higher the risk of substance abuse.

Based on Albee's social stress model, Rhodes and Jason illustrate two potential tracks, or pathways, that drug use may take: the abuse tract or the coping tract (see Figure 8.1).

�֍ Social Stress Model

FIGURE 8.1 *Two Potential Pathways*

From Rhodes, Jean E. and Leonard A. Jason *Preventing Substance Abuse Among Children,* 1992, Allyn & Bacon.

TABLE 8.3

Guidelines for Making Prevention Programs More Effective

- **Blend school-based and community prevention efforts to effect environmental change.** Community-wide approaches that involve broad participation of all sectors in the development of prevention efforts, including individually focused and environmental and policy focused, are needed.
- **Link prevention programs with the primary mission of schools: academics.** Prevention efforts at schools need to be more fully integrated with academic curricula. The case needs to be made that time spent in schools on prevention programs contributes to academic success.
- **Integrate prevention resource systems to support prevention efforts.** A more integrated approach that crosses disciplines and agencies is needed to maximize available resources. A less categorical approach to prevention is needed in order to address common risk factors. Prevention is about systems and strategies, not more discrete programs.
- **Forge agreement on what is to be prevented as a foundation for program design.** Standards for definitions and terms across prevention disciplines need to be developed in order to avoid contributing to confusion in those looking for guidance.
- **Employ new technologies to support prevention.** Technologies are now available to both reach individuals with prevention messages as well as disseminate information on evidence-based prevention to help communities develop prevention efforts.
- **Increase funding, training, and support for prevention researchers and practitioners.** Prevention works, but questions remain about both what works best in prevention and how communities can implement effective prevention activities.
- **Learn what practitioners, including teachers, are doing at ground level.** Because of the likelihood that practitioners consider program components to be fungible, it is important to know more about which components are essential and in what combinations.

Source: Robert Wood Johnson Foundation, *Prevention 2000* (2000).

Abuse Track

If attachments, coping skills, and resources are not available early, initiation to alcohol/drug use can allay stress during early childhood. If functional coping mechanisms, attachments, and resources are still not available during adolescence, alcohol/drug use may proceed to heavy use. When this pattern continues into adulthood, alcohol/drug abuse occurs.

Coping Track

Low stress, combined with good attachments, coping skills, and resources, leads to abstinence during childhood, abstinence or limited experimentation during adolescence, and reduced risk of problems with alcohol/drugs in adulthood.

Clinicians and researchers have identified a variety of factors that are predictive of later substance abuse by young people. Antisocial behaviors and aggressiveness can predict, as early as the first grade, early alcohol/drug initiation and later substance abuse. Family imbalance, parental problems with alcohol/drugs, and parental dysfunction are also predictive of children having problems with alcohol/drugs.

At-risk youth require a more intensive and modified prevention program than students with no real social and interpersonal problems, who are supported by fairly functional family systems.

Often, teachers and parents cooperatively identify at-risk youth appropriate for the program. Sometimes, key school personnel—teachers, coaches, dean of students, school-nurse, counselor, psychologist—develop a team approach with parents in identifying students at-risk for alcohol/drug problems.

The number of young people who are high risk for developing substance abuse problems is astounding. (See Table 8.4.)

❧ Programs Aimed at At-Risk Youth

TABLE 8.4

American Youth—High Risk for Alcohol Use and Other Problems

1. More than 20 percent (nearly 12.5 million) of all U.S. children (43 percent of Black and 40 percent of Hispanic/Latino children) live at or below the poverty level. Children living in extreme poverty and deprivation are more likely to become enmeshed in delinquent and drug-using behavior, particularly persistent (as opposed to occasional) drug use and delinquent activity.

2. There are 6.6 million children under the age of 18 living in a home with an alcoholic parent.

3. About 85 percent of child abuse cases in 1984 involved a parent-child relationship. In sexual abuse of children, 66 percent of offenders were parents and another 19 percent were other relatives.

4. More than 1 million young people run away from home or are homeless each year, and runaways are at a greater risk for alcohol and other drug problems.

5. One million students drop out of high school each year. One of every four ninth graders will not graduate—the dropout rate reaches 50 percent in some urban areas—and those who drop out are more at risk for developing alcohol and other drug problems.

6. One of eight 17-year-olds in the United States is functionally illiterate. At-risk adolescents with low skills who drop out of school are three times more likely than their more successful peers to become unwed parents. Those youth headed for college are less likely to abuse drugs.

7. More than 1 million adolescents become pregnant annually; half of these young mothers will never complete high school.

8. Nearly 1,900 teens took their own lives in 1984, making suicide the third leading cause of death for young people ages 15 to 24. Up to 80 percent of all adolescent suicides have been reported to be children of alcoholics.

9. In 1985, more than 1.7 million young people ages 14 to 17 were arrested for crimes, not including traffic violations.

10. Epidemiological studies show that one in four American children ages 10 to 17 are at high risk of multiple problem behaviors and negative long-term consequences because of their current behavior involving alcohol and other drug use, failure in school, early sexual activity and risk of pregnancy, and delinquency.

Source: Office for Substance Abuse Prevention 1988.

High-risk youngsters are hard to reach because they resist traditional authority, often have a low literacy level, and may be on the streets instead of in school or in structured community settings.

Their self-efficacy makes them less likely to respond to appeals based on caring about self, such as "take care of your health" or "don't take unnecessary risks that may hurt you." Also, these youth are already drinking and, in some cases, using multiple drugs at early ages. It is too late for refusal skills (saying no). Other obstacles include the following (Office for Substance Abuse Prevention 1988):

- Rejection of help because of fear and lack of trust or perhaps bravado
- Feelings of ambivalence and confusion about alcohol as a result of the many conflicting messages about alcohol use in U.S. society
- Fear by children and youth of being rejected again
- Hopelessness by young people in inner cities about the possibility of ever having a worthwhile future with a decent job and a chance of achieving the "American dream"
- The presence in some inner-city neighborhoods of an open, accessible drug culture without apparent social sanctions and of large sums of money for youth who deal in drugs

Often, the special relationship with a parent, a family member, a teacher, a minister, a coach, or others is what keeps some children on the road to a sober and successful life. Strong religious training is an example of a family ritual that also may save many young people from the streets.

One example of a school-based program for at-risk youth is *Interpersonal Problem Solving*. The program's major focus is on effective problem solving and effective interpersonal skills. Program topics include

- Dealing with authority figures
- Developing empathy
- Standing up for one's rights
- Resisting peer pressure
- Improving behavior in school
- Getting along better with family members

✗ Risk Factors for Substance Abuse

In the early years of alcohol/drug prevention, efforts were primarily focused on generic prevention programs. The thinking was "this is a good thing to promote; maybe it will prevent substance abuse" (e.g., good health habits). These programs were global and aimed at the entire school population. Prevention in the new millennium is targeted at specific at-risk populations, communities of high risk, while focusing on specific risk factors.

J. David Hawkins, Richard E. Catalono, and Janet Y. Miller, in their extensive study "Risk and Protective Factors for Alcohol and Other Drug Problems in Adolescence and Early Adulthood: Implications for Substance Abuse Prevention" (Hawkins, Catalano, and Miller 1992), outline five risk factors for substance abuse and accompanying interventions (see the Appendix). These interventions and risk factors allow prevention efforts to be focused and targeted. Table 8.5 presents factors associated with risk behaviors. Table 8.6 presents factors associated with healthy behaviors.

TABLE 8.5

Factors Associated with Risk Behaviors

Demographic

Less education
Low income
Unemployment

Psychosocial

High level of stressful life events
Poor social support[a]
Poor ethnic identity[b]

Ecological

Exposure to community and interpersonal violence[c]
Poor interactions with health care workers[d]

Individual

Psychological status (e.g., alienation,[e] powerlessness, depression,[f] or post-traumatic stress
   disorder)
Perceptions of levels of stress
Experiences of racism

[a]Neighbors and Jackson, 1984; Gombeski et al. 1982.

[b]Bullough 1967; Abrams, Allen, and Gray 1993; Carter 1991; Munford, 1994.

[c]Sanders-Phillips 1994a, 1994b, 1996a; Cohen et al. 1991.

[d]Freimuth and Mettzger 1990; Harrison and Harrison 1971; James et al. 1984; Perez-Stable 1987; Webb 1984; Makuc,
Fried, and Kleinman 1989; Sanders-Phillips 1996a; Balsheim 1991; Farris and Glenn 1976.

[e]Bullough 1972; Cohen et al. 1982; Hibbard 1985; Morris, Hatch, and Chipman, 1966; Seeman and Evans 1962;
Seeman and Seeman 1983.

[f]Cohen et al. 1991; Leftwich and Collins 1994.

❧ Resiliency

Steven Wolin, M.D., a professor at George Washington University, and his wife, Sybil Wolin, Ph.D., a developmental psychologist, are co-authors of *The Resilient Self: How Survivors of Troubled Families Rise Above Adversity* (1994) and developers of Project Resilience, Washington, D.C.

The Wolins define resiliency as an internal protective factor and the ability to bounce back. In their research on adult children of alcoholics, they found that some children of alcoholics grow up free of drinking because they

- Build on their own strengths
- Develop their own lifestyle and values, which are an improvement over their parents'
- Establish healthy "rituals" in their own family

Applying this knowledge, the Wolins worked with adolescents and young adults from the inner city who grew up in dysfunctional and abusive, alcoholic/addict family systems. They applied their "challenge" model of resiliency, helping these young people realize their own resiliency in attaining healthy growth. They

TABLE 8.6

Factors Associated with Healthy Behaviors

Demographic

High education level
High income
Employment
Positive marital status[a]

Psychosocial

High level of social support[b]
   Emotional support
   Information sharing
   Provision of tangible goods and services
Church participation

Individual

Internal locus of control
Greater self-efficacy regarding the prevention of disease
Positive perceptions of health status
Greater knowledge and positive attitudes about health-promoting behaviors

[a]Cohen et al. 1991; Gottlieb and Green 1984; Rakowski 1988.
[b]Gottlieb and Green 1984; Neighbors and Jackson 1984; Shumaker and Hill 1991.
Source: Glantz, Meyer D., and Christine R. Hartel. Drug Abuse: Origins and Interventions, 1999.

called this "survivor's pride"—a sense that you have been tested and that you have prevailed. (See Figures 8.2 and 8.3.)

Resiliency is described by the Wolins as not getting stuck in the "damage model" but, instead, challenging yourself and celebrating your survival and growth. Resiliency work is about reframing the damage, uncovering strength in a damage- or deficit-oriented story. In the damage model, the individual is seen as helpless, fragile, passive, and trapped. The Wolins emphasize that you need to help the individual understand the damage, express the anger, grieve the past, and move to resiliency.

Resiliency involves deliberation (making a plan). In many abusive family situations, it is a "getaway plan," creating distance from unhealthy situations. Resiliency skills also involve eventually choosing a spouse who is healthy and is developing healthy rituals.

They also describe how, too frequently, therapists perpetuate the victim's trap by

- Maintaining the myth that family problems will inevitably be perpetuated from one generation to the next
- Having the patients deplete themselves by continually blaming their parents for hurting them

Instead, the Wolins describe a more positive therapeutic goal of helping patients get revenge by seeking resiliency: by living healthy, productive lives rather than blaming and finding fault.

RESILIENCY

Resiliency is defined as:

- Mastering your painful memories rather than compulsively rehashing the damage you have suffered

- Accepting that your troubled family has left its mark and give up the futile wish that your scars can ever disappear completely

- Getting revenge by living well instead of squandering your energy by blaming and fault-finding

- Breaking the cycle of your family's troubles and putting the past in its place

FIGURE 8.2
Source: Wolin and Wolin 1994.

RESILIENT ACTIONS

Resilient Actions:

- Find and build on your own strengths

- Improve deliberately and methodically on your parents' lifestyles

- Marry consciously into strong, healthy families

- Fight off memories of horrible family get-togethers in order to establish healthy family times, routines, vacations, celebrations and rituals in your own generation

FIGURE 8.3
Source: Wolin and Wolin 1994.

They describe seven resiliency factors (Wolin and Wolin 1994):

1. Insight—the habit of asking tough questions that pierce the denial and confusion in troubled families
2. Independence—emotional and physical distancing from a troubled family, which keeps survivors out of harm's way
3. Relationships—fulfilling ties to others that provide the stability, nurturing, and love that troubled families do not give
4. Initiative—a push for mastery that combats the feelings of helplessness troubled families produce in their offspring
5. Creativity—representing one's inner pain and hurtful experiences in art forms; "building a new world on the ruins of the old"
6. Humor—the ability to minimize pain and troubles by laughing at oneself
7. Morality—an informed conscience, which imbues the survivor surrounded by "badness" with a sense of his or her own "goodness"

�֍ Emotional Intelligence

In 1995, Daniel Goleman, in his book *Emotional Intelligence,* made a case for a new kind of intelligence, or IQ—an IQ that goes beyond the traditional verbal and performance scales of most IQ tests and redefines what skills make up a successful person. Goleman labels this new IQ *emotional intelligence* and defines it as abilities such as

- Being able to motivate oneself and persist in the face of frustration
- Being able to control impulse and delay gratification
- Being able to regulate one's mood and keep distress from swamping the ability to think
- Being able to empathize and hope

The characteristics of emotional intelligence make one more successful at work, at relationships, at parenting, at coupleship, and at life in general. As we see increases in domestic violence, abuse, physical violence, and alcohol/drug abuse in homes, schools, community, our nation, and throughout the world, we see the importance of emotional intelligence. Managing anger and other moods (depression, fear, worry, and anxiety) is one of the key components of emotional intelligence.

"Of all the moods . . . anger is the mood people are worst at controlling . . . . Anger is the most seductive of the negative emotions, the self-righteous inner monologue that propels along filling the mind with the most convincing arguments to vent rage" (Goleman 1995).

The goals of the emotionally intelligent individual are optimism, motivation, perseverance, and self-efficacy.

✖ Domains of Prevention

Schools, religious and voluntary organizations, the media, the private sector, law enforcement, and health care are the secondary line of defense against drug and alcohol abuse by young people (see Figure 8.4). Families can make a real difference. Secondary approaches have little effect if the home and family environment are not involved and supportive of prevention efforts.

In conducting alcohol/drug educational and skill activities for parents over the past twenty years, I have found that the parents who don't need the information and are already effective parents are the ones that come to every event. The parents who need help are either in denial, too embarrassed or shamed, or too out of control to attend. Until we develop programs that can get these parents to participate, we are fighting an uphill battle.

✖ Prevention Programs and Prevention Emphasis in the New Millennium

Developmental Assets Model

The Search Institute of Minneapolis has developed a research-based framework of developmental assets, or factors that are critical for young people's successful growth and development. The institute's *Healthy Communities—Healthy Youth* programs are part of a national initiative to "motivate and equip individuals, organizations, and their leaders to join together in nurturing competent, caring, and responsible children and adolescents." The institute has identified and measured 40 developmental assets (see Table 8.7). These assets are the foundation that children

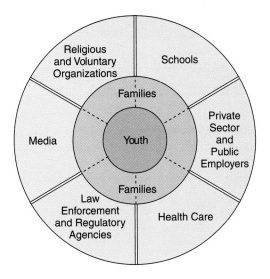

FIGURE 8.4   *A Conceptual Model for Preventive Approaches to Alcohol and Drug Abuse*

From Attorney General John Van De Kamp's Commission of Drug and Alcohol Abuse, 1986, Sacramento, CA
Reprinted by permission of California Attorney General's Office.

and adolescents from many cultural backgrounds need to be responsible, successful, and caring human beings.

"These assets are more than just nice ideas. Research on youth in hundreds of communities finds that these assets are powerful influences on behavior [see Figure 8.5]. Yet, the average 6th- to 12th-grade student experiences only 18 of the 40 assets" (Search Institute 1999). The application of education and skill development of these developmental assets takes place in the schools, with parents and other adults, with young people, with youth serving organizations, in neighborhoods, in communities, in business and industry, in local government, in congregations, in the juvenile justice system, in community care systems, and in community organizations.

School-Based Programs
The Personal Growth Class
Target: Adolescents At-Risk for School Dropout

This school-based program (Thompson et al. 1997) helps adolescents

1. Reduce their involvement in substance use behaviors
2. Improve school performance
3. Improve mood management (e.g., decrease depression, increase anger-management skills)

The two major components of the program are social support and life skills training. The life skills training addresses self-esteem enhancement, decision-making skills, personal control, and interpersonal communication.

T A B L E 8 . 7

Forty Developmental Assets

Type	Asset Name and Definition
Support	1. **Family support**—Family life provides high levels of love and support.
	2. **Positive family communication**—Young person and his or her parent(s) communicate positively, and young person is willing to seek parent(s') advice and counsel.
	3. **Other adult relationships**—Young person receives support from three or more nonparent adults.
	4. **Caring neighborhood**—Young person experiences caring neighbors.
	5. **Caring school climate**—School provides a caring, encouraging environment.
	6. **Parent involvement in schooling**—Parent(s) are actively involved in helping young person succeed in school.
Empowerment	7. **Community values youth**—Young person perceives that adults in the community value youth.
	8. **Youth as resources**—Young people are given useful roles in the community.
	9. **Service to others**—Young person serves in the community one hour or more per week.
	10. **Safety**—Young person feels safe at home, at school, and in the neighborhood.
Boundaries and Expectations	11. **Family boundaries**—Family has clear rules and consequences, and they monitor the young person's whereabouts.
	12. **School boundaries**—School provides clear rules and consequences.
	13. **Neighborhood boundaries**—Neighbors take responsibility for monitoring young people's behavior.
	14. **Adult role models**—Parent(s) and other adults model positive, responsible behavior.
	15. **Positive peer influence**—Young person's best friends model responsible behavior.
	16. **High expectations**—Both parent(s) and teachers encourage the young person to do well.
Constructive Use of Time	17. **Creative activities**—Young person spends three or more hours per week in lessons or practice in music, theater, or other arts.
	18. **Youth programs**—Young person spends three or more hours per week in sports, clubs, or organizations at school and/or in community organizations.
	19. **Religious community**—Young person spends one or more hours per week in activities in a religious institution.
	20. **Time at home**—Young person is out with friends, "with nothing special to do," two or fewer nights per week.
Commitment to Learning	21. **Achievement motivation**—Young person is motivated to do well in school.
	22. **School engagement**—Young person is actively engaged in learning.
	23. **Homework**—Young person reports doing at least one hour of homework every schoolday.
	24. **Bonding to school**—Young person cares about his or her school.
	25. **Reading for pleasure**—Young person reads for pleasure three or more hours per week.

T A B L E   8 . 7   (*c o n t i n u e d*)

Forty Developmental Assets

Type	Asset Name and Definition
Positive Values	26. **Caring**—Young person places high value on helping other people.
	27. **Equality and social justice**—Young person places high value on promoting equality and reducing hunger and poverty.
	28. **Integrity**—Young person acts on convictions and stands up for his or her beliefs.
	29. **Honesty**—Young person tells the truth, even when it is not easy.
	30. **Responsibility**—Young person accepts and takes personal responsibility.
	31. **Restraint**—Young person believes it is important not to be sexually active or to use alcohol or other drugs.
Social Competencies	32. **Planning and decision making**—Young person knows how to plan ahead and make choices.
	33. **Interpersonal competence**—Young person has empathy, sensitivity, and friendship skills.
	34. **Cultural competence**—Young person has knowledge of and comfort with people of different cultural/racial/ethnic backgrounds.
	35. **Resistance skills**—Young person can resist negative peer pressure and dangerous situations.
	36. **Peaceful conflict resolution**—Young person seeks to resolve conflict nonviolently.
Positive Identity	37. **Personal power**—Young person feels he or she has control over "things that happen to me."
	38. **Self-esteem**—Young person reports having a high self-esteem.
	39. **Sense of purpose**—Young person reports that "my life has a purpose."
	40. **Positive view of personal future**—Young person is optimistic about his or her personal future.

Jump Start

Target: African American adolescents, economically disadvantaged, those high on
   sensation seeking

This curriculum (Harrington and Donohew 1997) includes aspects of social-
influence model, social skills training, and alternatives-based programs.

Iowa Strengthening Families Program (ISFP)

Target: A family-based prevention program adapted from the Strengthening
   Families program (Kumpfer 1996), a target intervention for high-risk
   families

The primary goal of Project Family (Spoth and Redmond 1996) is to enhance
family functioning in rural families by teaching parenting skills and other relevant
skills to prevent adolescent substance use and other problem behaviors.

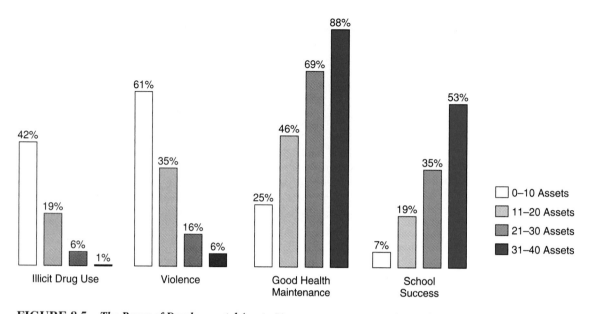

FIGURE 8.5 *The Power of Developmental Assets* The more assets young people experience, the less likely they are to engage in a wide range of risky behaviors, and the more likely they are to engage in positive behaviors.

Based on Search Institute's study of almost 100,000 youth in 312 towns and cities across the United States during the 1996–1997 school year.

Comprehensive Community Prevention Programs
Target: Focus on both the demand and supply aspects of adolescent substance use

Resolving Conflict Creatively Program (RCCP)

The Resolving Conflict Creatively Program (RCCP) is a comprehensive, school-based program in conflict resolution and intergroup relations that provides a model for preventing violence and creating caring and peaceable communities of learning.

RCCP serves 6,000 teachers and 175,000 young people in 375 schools nationwide, including the New York City schools and 12 other diverse school systems.

Schools can play a critical role in encouraging young people to actively contribute to the well-being of others if they provide meaningful opportunities to reconnect students with their communities. To this end, the Resolving Conflict Creatively Program offers schools and communities a model for creating democratic and caring learning communities by developing young people's skills in dealing with emotions, resolving conflict, and honoring differences.

The goals of the RCCP National Center are to use the RCCP model to

- Prepare educators to provide high-quality instruction and effective school programs in conflict resolution and intercultural understanding in a variety of educational settings
- Reduce violence and increase intercultural understanding in school districts across the country

- Transform the culture of participating schools so they model the values and principles of creative, nonviolent conflict resolution and respect for diversity
- Inform school systems, educational leaders, and the general public about the efficacy of social and emotional learning programs and the ingredients that constitute successful implementation
- Provide technical assistance to school systems about long-range, comprehensive program design and implementation

Community Partnership Program (1990–96)

The Prevention Works Through Community project was evaluated by the Center for Substance Abuse Prevention (CSAP). There were 48 communities in the study, and the best evaluations were models in diverse communities—Springfield, Missouri; Lala County, Illinois; El Paso, Texas; South Central Los Angeles; and Knox, Laurel, and Whitley Counties, Kentucky.

These successful community models had several features in common:

- A comprehensive vision, covering all requirements and all aspects of community life
- A wide sharing of this vision, agreed upon by groups and citizens across the community
- A strong core of committed partners at the outset
- An inclusive and broad-based membership, welcoming all segments of the community
- Avoidance of resolution of severe conflict that might reflect misunderstandings about a partnership's basic purpose
- Decentralized units, encouraging participation and action at small-area or neighborhood levels
- Nondisruptive staff turnover of a reasonable rate
- Extensive prevention activities and support for local prevention policies

Healthy People 2010

This project has the support of such people as former president Jimmy Carter and other leaders. The goal is to promote healthy living through prevention interventions and proven clinical services.

The National Cross-Site Evaluations of High-Risk Youth Programs (NIDA 2002a) found that the rate of substance use for high-risk youth participating in their CSAP (Community Substance Abuse Programs) was 12 percent lower at completion of the program than for comparison youth. They also found that this effect lasted—the rate of use for these youth was 6 percent below the rate for the comparison group 18 months later. These prevention programs work and produce lasting results despite the fact that these youth face multiple risk factors in their communities. Connections with positive social environments—schools, family, peers, community, and society—appeared to be important factors in preventing substance abuse. Figure 8.6 depicts this "Web of Influences."

�֍ High-Risk Youth and CSAPs

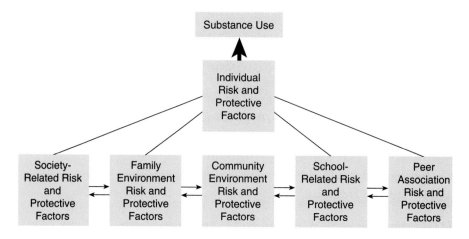

FIGURE 8.6 *The "Web of Influence" on Substance Use*

Source: NIDA 2002a.

✖ Prevention and Special Populations

People of Color and Other Minorities

A variety of factors put people of color and other minorities at risk for substance-abuse problems. Minorities as a group have more unemployment, have less prestigious occupations, and live in poverty and lower socioeconomic conditions. Thus, they experience more feelings of frustration, anger, resentment, and powerlessness. Inadequate education, housing, income, and other factors create additional stress and pressure, which may lead to problems with alcohol/drugs.

For people of color, prevention must go beyond the approaches previously described. One of the biggest problems facing people of color is the crack epidemic in the inner cities, the increase in young cocaine and heroin addicts' giving birth to cocaine- and heroin-addicted babies, and the rise in methamphetamine use.

Prevention for people of color and other minorities must be community based. Residents must conceptualize the problem and jointly develop appropriate strategies.

Community-based prevention programs also must emphasize a systemic strategy to uproot the factors in the system that oppress people of color, such as prejudice and racism, and to implement training in diversity and methods of accessing the system.

Older Adults

Older adults are often forgotten or ignored when it comes to prevention efforts. The lack of any true role experienced by some elders leads to feelings of loneliness, boredom, frustration, rejection, abandonment, anxiety, fear, and depression. When elders complain about these feelings, sometimes the response is to prescribe medication.

Prevention efforts with elders frequently involve training and educational projects to assist them to keep accurate records of their medications or to develop methods to have someone monitor their medication. Elders need to be approached with individuality and dignity. They need to be empowered to develop their own advocacy. Pharmacists, physicians, and other health providers must act in cooperation and be sensitive to each individual case. Drug dosages and regimens must meet individual needs and be sensitive to the elders' ability to maintain their treatment plans.

Monitoring and educating the elder population are necessary prevention strategies. Advocacy for alternatives to medication are also essential, as well as the expansion of senior services. The more active and involved the lifestyles of elders, the healthier are the later years of their lives.

Prevention with elders also involves proactive approaches to healthy activities that promote physical movement (health permitting), interpersonal interaction, and a sense of value and worth. In the years to come, a majority of the population will be elders. Prevention programs and services need to be further developed now to meet the needs of this ever-expanding population.

Young Older-Adults, Older Adults

This category can include a variety of populations. Increases in life expectancy has created new issues for adults.

We have several categories of "older adults." "Young older" are often those in the ages of 55–59, who grew up during the "drug, sex and rock n' roll" era of the late sixties and early seventies. These 55–59 year olds have the highest rate of illicit drug use for older adults (NIDA, 2001). One could speculate a variety of reasons for this— they were smoking marijuana when they were younger, they have more leisure time now to do drugs, and they have more resources/money to buy drugs, etc.

Binge drinking among adolescents and college students has gained much public attention, as outlined in Chapter 3. However binge drinking by older adults has generally been ignored. Older adults aged 65–74 reported a binge episode within the past 3 months, compared to only 5 percent of those 75 years and older. One would speculate individuals 55 to 65 years of age would even report higher levels of binge drinking than those who are 65 to 74, making this age group at risk for both drug and alcohol problems.

More research needs to be done with young-older adults and older adults regarding their patterns of alcohol/drug use and abuse. Issues that may make them more at risk include adjustment to retirement, decreased funds for retirement, general health and nutrition, illness, death of spouses, leisure time, unfulfilled expectations, depression, anxiety, existential issues, etc. We know that as people age, depression and anxiety that was coped with, is much harder to deal with as one ages. All of these factors may contribute to a pattern of increased alcohol/drug use by this population.

Baby boomers will be the largest population of older adults at risk for substance-abuse problems. Their situation is confounded by challenges of retirement, midlife crises, health, interpersonal and family problems (e.g., divorce, empty nest). It is expected that this group will increase their use of drugs and alcohol as they get older.

Neglected older populations will need prevention and counseling programs to help them make the adjustment to older age. Yet few prevention programs currently provide information on retirement, aging, midlife crisis, and other challenges faced by this age group.

College Students

During their first year of college, most students dramatically increase their alcohol/drug use. The MTV spring break party illustrates the pervasive "let loose and get loaded" attitude of young college students.

Alcohol/drug use and abuse is a glamorized way of escape from the pressures of school. The newly acquired freedom of being away at college allows students more opportunities to use alcohol/drugs. The anxiety of adjusting to college and living away from home can result in escalated alcohol/drug use. The functions of alcohol/drugs on college campuses are many—to party, to stay up late and study, to explore a personal sense of self and identity, to facilitate social and interpersonal relationships, and so forth.

Prevention and the Family

Unfortunately, prevention activities take place almost exclusively in school systems. We expect the school systems to prevent this epidemic of alcohol/drug use. The reality is that the families are the real first line of defense against alcohol/drug use by young people.

References

Brecher, Edward M. 1972. *Licit and illicit drugs.* Boston: Little, Brown.

Cohen, A.Y. 1972. *Alternatives to drug abuse: Steps toward prevention.* Rockville, Md.: National Institute on Drug Abuse.

Drug abuse prevention research. 1983. Monograph No. 33. Washington, D.C.: U.S. Depart. of Health and Human Services.

Goleman, Daniel. 1995. *Emotional intelligence: Why it can matter more than IQ.* New York: Bantam Books.

Goodstadt, Michael. 1975. Evaluating drug prevention programs. In *Balancing head and heart: Sensible ideas for the prevention of drug and alcohol abuse,* edited by E. Schaps et al. Lafayette, Calif.: Prevention Materials Institute Press.

Hawkins, J. D., R. Catalano, and J. Miller. 1992. Risk and protective factors for alcohol and other drug problems in adolescence and early adulthood. *Psychological Bulletin* 112(1): 64–105.

Mathews, Walter M. 1975. A critique of traditional drug education programs. *Journal of Drug Education* 5(1): 57–64.

National Institute on Drug Abuse [NIDA]. 2001. *Substance use among older adults.* Washington, D.C.: NIDA, Substance Abuse and Mental Health Services Administration.

National Institute on Drug Abuse [NIDA]. 2002a. *The National Cross-Site Evaluation of High-Risk Youth Program: Preventing substance abuse: Major findings.* Washington, D. C.: NIDA, Substance Abuse and Mental Health Services Administration.

Office for Substance Abuse Prevention. 1988. *Communicating about alcohol and other drugs: Strategies for reading populations at risk.* Monograph 5. Rockville, Md.: Author.

Prevention 2000: Moving effective prevention programs into practice. 2000. St. Michaels, Md.: Robert Wood Johnson Foundation.

Rhodes, Jean E., and Leonard A. Jason. 1988. *Preventing substance abuse among children and adolescents*. New York: Pergamon Press.

Schinke, S. P., and L. D. Gilchrist. 1983. Primary prevention of tobacco smoking. *Journal of School Health* 53:416–19.

Search Institute. 1999. *Ideas for asset building poster*. Search Institute, 700 South Third Street, Suite 210, Minneapolis, MN 55415.

Spivak, G., and M. Shuve. 1979. *The social adjustment of young children*. San Francisco: Jossey-Bass.

Wiscott, Richard, Karen Kopera-Frye, and Ana Begovic. 2002. Later life: Comparing young-old and old-old social drinkers. *Psychology of Addictive Behaviors* 16(3): 252–255.

Wolin, Steven, and Sybil Wolin. 1994. *The resilient self: How survivors of troubled families rise above adversity*. New York: Villard Books.

Motivation and Intervention for Substance-Abuse Problems

❖ **Chapter in Review**

Any attempt to create awareness in others that they might have a problem with alcohol or other drugs is an intervention. Intervention is defined as an action taken by someone to interrupt the progression of problems with alcohol/drugs.

Some defense components of resistance to change are denial, minimization, projection, rationalization, compliance, obsessive focusing, and acting out.

Motivational interviewing is a client-centered approach that uses cognitive therapy, systems theory, and social psychology to aid the patient in taking action toward beneficial change, as well as maintaining change and avoiding relapses once change is implemented.

The stages of motivational interviewing are precontemplative, contemplative, determination, action, maintenance, and relapse prevention.

The "OARS" of motivational interviewing are open-ended questions, affirmations, reflecting, and summarizing. The FRAMES of motivational interviewing are feedback, responsibility, advice, menu, empathy, and self-efficacy.

A formal intervention is a caring, nonjudgmental, behavior-specific effort by the family to get an alcoholic/addict into treatment. Intervention is of benefit to the family because it creates an awareness of the actual dimensions and progressive nature of alcoholism/drug addiction.

✦ Motivational Interviewing

William Miller and Stephen Rollnick (1991) developed a form of intervention known as motivational interviewing. They recognized that formal and informal interventions are effective for many individuals who are in denial of having a problem with alcohol or drugs, but for some individuals the traditional form of intervention doesn't work. Despite the intervention, the individual is not motivated to seek abstinence or recovery from alcohol/drugs.

The same holds true for many individuals who, once in alcohol/drug treatment, either terminated treatment early against medical advice or

didn't respond when confronted by counselors about their denial. Miller and Rollnick espouse a different approach with individuals who are resistant to traditional intervention methods. Some individuals respond negatively to interventions.

Motivational interviewing draws its strategies from a number of disciplines, including client-centered counseling, cognitive therapy, systems theory, and the social psychology of persuasion. The work comes from Miller and Rollnick's contention that there is no one kind of alcoholic or addict or, for that matter, an addictive personality. "This idea of a common alcoholic or addictive personality is supported neither in the original writings of Alcoholics Anonymous, nor by five decades of psychological research" (Miller and Rollnick 1991). It therefore makes sense that alcoholics/addicts need a

---

The names and circumstances of case studies have been changed to maintain anonymity.

variety of approaches to engage them into recovery. Perhaps a different approach might reach those alcoholics/addicts who resist traditional confrontive interventions. Motivational interviewing was therefore designed to help clients build commitment and reach a decision to change.

Miller and Rollnick described motivation as a state of readiness or eagerness to change, and they recognized that motivation may fluctuate over time, situation, and circumstance. They described the basic stages of change and the influences a therapist can make in influencing motivation to change. (See Table 9.1.)

Their approach uses brief, individual counseling, which helps the clients explore and resolve their "ambivalence" about change. Ambivalence is defined as feeling two ways about something, being in conflict between the pros and cons of the status quo (or the pros and cons of changing). Ambivalence is a good description for the conflict many people have about changing, whether it is recovery from alcohol/drugs, unhealthy and self-destructive behaviors (e.g., smoking, overeating), a dysfunctional relationship, a bad work situation, or illegal activities. At the precontemplative stage of change, they are not considering change and may not see or admit problems with

TABLE 9.1

Stages of Change and Therapist Tasks

Client Stage	Therapist's Motivational Tasks
Precontemplative	Raise doubt—increase the client's perception of risks and problems with current behavior. Decrease desirability to status quo, build rapport so you can later provide information about the negative consequences or risks of maintaining the status quo, get to know the client well enough to find out what's important to him or her (what he or she values most). Find something the client did well (maybe it was only being open-minded enough to listen to the counselor's views) and affirm that. Make sure client comes back in the future.
Contemplative	Tip the balance—evoke reasons to change, risks of not changing. Strengthen the client's self-efficacy for change of current behavior. Raise awareness of ambivalence by eliciting and reflecting both sides of the client's ambivalence: the pros and cons of animating the status quo (or the pros and cons of changing, if client prefers to discuss that). Then explore which of these pros and cons mean the most to the client. Try to point out how that status quo is in conflict with the client's deeply held values and how changing might bring the client more in line with those important values.
Determination	Help the client determine the best source of action to take in seeking change.
Action	Help the client take steps toward change. Focus on the plan, what the client is going to do. What is the client willing to do, not willing to do, and ambivalent about doing? People in action still suffer from ambivalence and fear of the unknown, and that ambivalence must be dealt with as you go along. Emphasis on action is on removing barriers to change and problem solving each of these barriers.
Maintenance	Help the client identify and use strategies to prevent relapse.
Relapse	Help the client renew the processes of contemplation, determination, and action without becoming stuck or demoralized because of relapse.

From William Miller and Stephen Rollnick, *Motivational Interviewing: Preparing People to Change Addictive Behavior.* Copyright © 1991 Guilford Press, New York.

the self-destructive behavior (addiction). In the contemplative stage, they are considering change but are ambivalent about it. These are the individuals who waver from day to day and seem easily influenced to go in either direction. When it comes to alcohol/drug abuse and addiction, the alcoholic/addict wants to continue to use alcohol/drugs yet may recognize the risks and negative consequences of use. At the determination stage the individual decides to do something. The action stage is when there has been a recent change or an implemented plan of change. The maintenance stage involves a commitment to a long-term change, where the change has become habit, or part of the person's lifestyle. The relapse prevention stage explores strategies to not return to earlier stages.

Table 9.2 outlines an approach to a nondirective part of motivational interviewing.

Client-Centered Motivational Interviewing

Motivational interviewing is "client centered," which means "that the counselor's top priority—always—is to elicit and understand the client's view. In contrast, more forceful interventions emphasize the views of the significant others staging the intervention" (Dunn 1996).

The motivational interviewing technique is quite different from the intervention model. It is controversial because the active alcoholic/addict wants to continue to drink and will often delay taking action despite significant negative consequences. Many counselors believe that not confronting denial, and giving control back to the alcoholic/addict, will only result in continued destructive, maybe even life-threatening patterns of alcohol consumption. However, the motivational interviewing approach has the perspective that people follow through better and are more committed to recovery if they voluntarily make the decision to choose treatment for themselves. Another controversial aspect of motivational interviewing is the counselor eliciting the client's doubts about recovery, as well as the positive aspects. This helps the counselor reflect back to the client the positive and negative aspects of the decision. Case Study 9.1 presents an example of client-centered motivational interviewing.

Effective Motivational Strategies

There are eight general motivational strategies.

1. Giving *advice.* Well-timed and tempered advice to change can make a difference. Advice should (a) clearly identify the problem or risk area, (b) explain why change is important, and (c) advocate specific change.
2. Removing *barriers.* Address blocks to change, such as resistance to go to AA meetings.
3. Providing *choice.* Few people like to be told what to do. Intrinsic motivation is enhanced by the perception that one has freely chosen.
4. Decreasing *desirability.* Weigh the benefits and costs of change against the merits of continuing as before.
5. Practicing *empathy.* This kind of empathy is not an ability to identify with a person's experiences. Rather, it is a specifiable and learnable skill for understanding another's meaning through the use of reflective listening, whether or not you have had a similar experience yourself.

T A B L E 9 . 2

The "Nondirective" Part of Motivational Interviewing (MI): OARS (Tools for Rowing Along with Your Clients)

"OARS" symbolizes the way motivational interviewing therapists act during a session.

Open-Ended Questions

Can't be answered with "yes" or "no"
Keep resistance down
Build trust rapidly
Encourage client to talk about what's important to him or her
Reveal what's "delicious" to clients
Help therapist find the "carrot" for change

Affirmations

Very hard to use genuinely; requires much practice
Build self-esteem
Show respect
Reduce treatment dropout rates
Get a "winning streak" going for clients (clients who succeed come back for more success)

Reflecting

Takes practice; sounds phony at first
Is like throwing "empathy darts" while client holds up the target
Client will always let you know if you're accurate or not.
Very satisfying for both to be accurate
More than just paraphrasing the client's message content; also reflects underlying feelings
Happens after every few sentences spoken by clients
About three of every four statements by MI therapist is a reflection (how do you get anything done?)

Summarizing

Gathers together what client said, so it can be heard again (especially the positive change talk)
Shows client what's been accomplished during the session
Can help therapist close one topic and move on to another
Can help end sessions on good terms

Whenever you are stuck, you can fall back on this style of being with your client, until you figure out what your directive strategy is going to be. Without adding the directive motivational interviewing techniques, OARS will only help you row about in circles (but at least you're not sinking. . .).

6. Providing *feedback.*
7. Clarifying *goals.* Help the client to restate the goal in realistic or attainable terms.
8. Helping *active.* Express actively and affirmatively your interest in your client's change process.

Case Study 9.1

Contemplative and Action Stages

Don

Don knew he had a problem with alcohol/drugs. He took some action by attending AA meetings, yet he still didn't want to stop drinking. He would maintain abstinence for limited periods of time (30–100 days) but then would lapse into drinking. Despite negative consequences at home and at work, and having gone through two inpatient programs, he still was not committed to recovery. He tried to convince himself that he wasn't really an alcoholic, yet he soon found himself in alcoholic binges. Each time he relapsed, he seemed motivated to get sober and work at a program of recovery, yet, despite attending AA, attending outpatient counseling, even working with a sponsor, he was ambivalent about recovery. At the suggestion of his sponsor, he attended several different AA meetings. After attending an AA meeting at a local mission for the homeless, he wondered if he had to "hit bottom" by losing his job, family, and home to stop drinking. The very next day, he talked to an old-timer at another AA meeting who told him, "Maybe things have to get really bad before you get better." He was then convinced that he had to continue to drink until things got worse, before he would stop. In his ambivalence, he called his sponsor with this new idea and was told, "You'll come up with any excuse to continue drinking." His resolve to seek recovery was so ambivalent and such a struggle that he could easily be influenced to go either way—recovery or self-destruction.

Don talked to his outpatient counselor about this conflict during a one-on-one session, and the counselor effectively used motivational interviewing techniques to help Don resolve this ambivalence, so he could move closer to action. The counselor focused more on Don's ambivalence about committing to AA, rather than the global issue of ambivalence about recovery in general.

Counselor:	It's good to see you again, Don. Tell me how have you been doing for the past few weeks, so I can get caught up? [open question]
Don:	Not great, if you really want to know. I haven't drunk or used in over four weeks now. In fact, I'll be 30 days sober tomorrow. But, big deal, I'm more screwed up than ever. I don't mean to sound sorry for myself, but I just feel lousy. And I know I've got to do something, but I don't know which end is up.
Counselor:	Congratulations on making it to one month! You've been working hard and it hasn't been a picnic for you. [affirmation acknowledging client's progress and empathic statement]
Don:	[silent]
Counselor:	But things are tough, and you aren't getting the rewards of feeling better yet. [accurate reflection] Tell me what you mean when you say you're more screwed up now than ever? [open question]
Don:	I was talking with my sponsor yesterday, and he told me he's worried about me. He thinks I'm gonna go out and drink again. He says I'm subconsciously planning a relapse.
Counselor:	What do you think he means? [open question]
Don:	He says I'm looking for an excuse to go back out and drink. He said he wasn't sure I had enough willingness to get active in AA like he wants me to. And he told me I'm just setting myself up for a drink.
Counselor:	And this is all making you feel screwed up?

Case Study 9.1 (*continued*)

Contemplative and Action Stages

Don

Don:	Yup. Really bad.
Counselor:	There were three things that you just mentioned: your sponsor, your degree of involvement in AA, and your chances of drinking again. Does any one of those three stand out for you? [summary and open question]
Don:	I don't know what you mean.
Counselor:	Well, first you said you feel really screwed up right now, and then I was hearing you mention three things: your sponsor, AA, and a possible relapse. Which one do you think has got you the most screwed up?
Don:	Oh, I don't know. I know my sponsor's right. If I keep finding excuses to stay away from AA, and not get involved, I know I'll relapse, like I did that last time. I know what I gotta do, but I can't make myself get into it.
Counselor:	So you agree with your sponsor and you share his worry about relapse? [reflection]
Don:	Yeah, I know he's right. [Don stares at the floor.]
Counselor:	And you said you know what you need to do, but you can't get going. [reflection]
Don:	Yeah.
Counselor:	You've already thought this over and figured out what it is you need to do. [affirmation]
Don:	[silent]
Counselor:	That's a pretty good start for somebody who feels more screwed up than ever.
Don:	Big deal. It's not helping me any if I don't *do* anything. [Counselor decides to further explore Don's ambivalence about AA by asking about the pros and cons of AA, as Don sees it. The counselor begins with a summary reflection.]
Counselor:	You were telling me that you're afraid of relapsing if you don't take certain actions, yet you can't seem to get yourself to take those actions. And being stuck that way is making you miserable.
Don:	Right.
Counselor:	Will you let me in on what those certain actions are? [open question acknowledging Don's power to talk or not talk about it]
Don:	It's the same old stuff. I gotta get a home group that I go to all the time and get involved in service.
Counselor:	And you feel two ways about choosing a home group. First of all, what are some of your objections to getting one?
Don:	I don't like joining groups because it's corny or something.
Counselor:	Okay. What else?
Don:	I don't want to have to go to the same group every week because I get tired of the people there.
Counselor:	Okay, some groups seem corny to you and you get tired of some people. What else?

(continued on next page)

Case Study 9.1 (*continued*)

Contemplative and Action Stages

Don

Don: I don't know; that's all I guess.

Counselor: O.K., what about the other side of the coin? What are the most positive things you might get from choosing a home group?

Don: Well, it might help me stay sober.

Counselor: How?

Don: Just by staying close to a group. They get to know you and, if you start to drop off meetings, somebody might ask you if you're okay.

Counselor: So people get to know you and care enough to say something to you to help you get back on track, and you might not mind hearing it because you know them, right?

Don: Yes.

Counselor: So people can help you stay on track. What else might be positive for you if you decided to get a home group?

Don: Well, they say people get to know your story and you get to know everybody there pretty good, because you hear their stories as well.

Counselor: So if you spend more time with your home group you could get to know them better than the people in other groups if you just "shop around" from group to group.

Don: Right.

Counselor: Almost as if each person in your home group were a separate TV show that you tune into each week to see how things are going with them. Kind of entertaining.

Don: Yeah, I never thought of it that way before.

Counselor: [summarizing] On one hand, you're not much of a joiner and you might get tired of seeing some people every week. But, on the other hand, you could get to know those people better and actually get some support, even enjoyment from being around them each week. Maybe even get so you look forward to going each week?

Don: I suppose so, although I don't think I'd ever feel really comfortable there. The way it is now, I just go to whatever meeting I feel like. But I never look forward to meetings, because I know I'm just gonna bolt right after it is over.

Counselor: [reflecting, then trying to tip the balance in favor of change] Sounds a little lonesome. As you look at the balance, pros and cons of getting a home group, Don, do any of those pros or cons stand out as more important to you?

Don: [arguing for change] Yeah, making friends. It might be nice to get to know some people who don't drink. I never got that far last time I quit drinking. I stayed away from my old drinking buddies, but I also stayed away from people in AA.

Counselor: People are a big deal to you. And you think you might find some that you like if you were to hang around one meeting long enough. Well, Don, the

(continued on next page)

Case Study 9.1 (*concluded*)

Contemplative and Action Stages

Don

decision is totally in your hands. It's understandable that you haven't acted yet, considering that you basically feel two ways about getting a home group. But being stuck where you're at doesn't sound comfortable either. Based on what you've told me, it sounds like getting people in your life that you like and may even begin to trust might make your sobriety nicer. But what do you think?

Summary—Counselor tried to move client from contemplation into preparation and action, regarding the specific behavioral issue of getting a home AA group.

[Counselor turns over the responsibility for the decision to Don and then asks if he's ready for action—i.e., getting a home group. If the answer is no, the counselor affirms the work that Don did in acknowledging both sides of the painful issue and lets the issue rest for now, closing the topic on good terms, to be returned to later. If the answer is yes, they proceed with discussing an action plan for getting a home group and removing barriers to doing so.]

Motivational Interviewing is a non-directive approach. Miller & Rollnick use the mnemonic of OARS to describe non-directive counseling. You can "row along with your clients if you O—ask Open-ended questions, A—provide affirmations, R—reflect on client verbalizations, S—summarize what client says. (See Table 9.2.)

Active Ingredients of Effective Brief Counseling

Miller and Rollnick (1991) have developed the mnemonic of FRAMES* to remind counselors of the effective ingredients for motivational interviewing and brief counseling: FRAMES—feedback, responsibility, advice, menu (i.e., a list of choices), empathy, self-efficacy (i.e., you can do it). (See Figure 9.1.)

The general principles of motivational interviewing (see Table 9.2) are the following:

1. *Express empathy.* Acceptance facilitates change; skillful reflective listening is fundamental; ambivalence is normal.
2. *Develop discrepancy.* Awareness of consequences is important; a discrepancy between present behavior and important goals will motivate change; the client should present the arguments for change.
3. *Avoid argumentation.* Arguments are counterproductive; defending breeds defensiveness; resistance is a signal to change strategies; labeling is unnecessary.

---

*From William Miller and Stephen Rollnick, Motivational Interviewing: Preparing People to Change Addictive Behavior. Copyright © 1991 Guilford Press, New York.

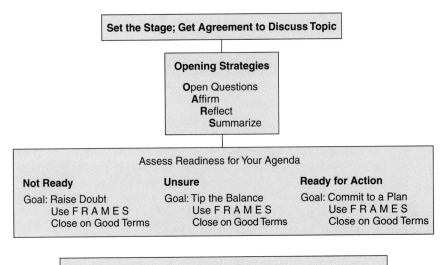

FIGURE 9.1   *One of Many Ways to Do a Brief Intervention*

Source: Miller and Rollnick, *Motivational Interviewing,* 1991.

4. *Roll with resistance.* Momentum can be used to good advantage; perceptions can be shifted; new perspectives are invited but not imposed; the client is a valuable resource in finding solutions to problems.
5. *Support self-efficacy.* Belief in the possibility of change is an important motivator: the client is responsible for choosing and carrying out personal change; there is hope in the range of alternative approaches available.

✖ Change

The focus of motivational interviewing is influencing the individual to develop a motivation to change. The whole subject of change is fascinating and complicated. People change for very personal and individual reasons. Many people can go for years, even a lifetime, wanting to change, intending to change, even verbalizing a desire to change, without taking the action necessary to change.

Why will any given person stop drinking or taking drugs, eat healthier, exercise regularly, commit to a task, pursue a passion, or to get out of an imbalanced situation or relationship? The answer is different for each person. Some people will put up with a lot before they are forced to make a change. Others will make difficult changes, despite tremendous obstacles, risks, and personal sacrifice, because they feel or know it is what they have to do. In the alcohol/drug recovery field, we often refer to the experience of "hitting bottom—the point where the consequences of drinking or taking drugs are so bad that the individual decides to do something about their drug/alcohol use. The consequences of their addictive behavior have become so demeaning, so shaming, and so foreign to their perception of themselves that users are motivated to take action to do whatever it takes to stop using alcohol or other drugs.

Some people stop using because the negative cycle and negative consequences have gone on for too long. They decide that they are "sick and tired of being sick and tired."

Change can occur when others influence, directly or indirectly, the motivation to change. Friends, teachers, family members, mentors, or significant others can help the individual to see the need for change and help support change. Certainly counselors play a pivotal role in helping these individuals explore their perception of their alcohol/drug use, and the need for change. For some users, hearing the same thing from different people, in a timely manner, causes them to consider making a change. What motivates one individual to change, might be quite different for another. Others might make a change because their job is in jeopardy, or because they have been touched in a heartfelt way by someone they love. The counselor is challenged to push the right "button" for each individual.

Change may be gradual or it can seem sudden and abrupt. William Miller, lead author of *Motivational Interviewing,* describes this process of collaboration and gradual influence to motivate the client to explore healthy change. In *Quantum Change* (2001), Miller and coauthor Janet C' de Baca, describe a more sudden and immediate kind of change. A "quantum change" is a personal transformation that has some key elements:

- *Vivid*—identifiable, distinctive experiences during which the transformation occurred, or at least began
- *Surprising*—not comprehensible as ordinary responses to life events
- *Benevolent*—involves loving kindness
- *Enduring*—it is a permanent transformation
- *Involves conflict*—a rupture in the knowing context

Miller and C' de Baca (2001) quote Bill Wilson, the co-founder of Alcoholics Anonymous, as he describes his "quantum change":

> Slowly the ecstasy subsided. I lay on the bed, but now for a time I was in another world, a new world of consciousness. All about me and through me there was a wonderful feeling of Presence. A great peace stole over me and I thought, "No matter how wrong things seem to be, they are all right.

Whether change occurs gradually or suddenly, the outcome is the same—personal transformation.

Everything one does to create awareness of an alcohol/drug problem is an intervention. The slightest suggestion to a friend, colleague, or family member that he or she may be drinking/drugging too much is an intervention. Everyone is different. Those who are at early stages of substance abuse without a family history of alcoholism/addiction may very well pay attention to your observations. If enough people are bringing the drink/drug problem to the person's attention, he or she might decide to do something about it. On the other hand, there are individuals who, if they were hit over the head with a two-by-four, wouldn't recognize their substance abuse problem.

⚔
Intervention

Resistance is a natural part of the change cycle. Whether it is an adolescent who resists cleaning up his or her room or an adult who delays paying his or her taxes, resistance is embedded in our nature. For some, it is laziness, and procrastination, probably related to family-of-origin issues. But most people resist doing something that may bring discomfort or dysphoria or that is just downright uninteresting. Resistance comes out in the various defense mechanisms used by people to avoid taking action on a problem behavior (e.g., substance abuse).

Common Defense Components of Resistance to Change (Choppel)

1. *Denial*—most common
   Counselor tip: look for the usefulness of the defense to person, what he or she is avoiding and why wait to point out denial, premature disclosure can "turn off" the client (i.e., you are judging them)
2. *Minimization*—used to maintain self-esteem (e.g., "My drinking/drugging never had an impact on my children, since I drank outside of the house")
   Counselor tip: suggest client get feedback from valued and reliable other sources, rather than getting into a tireless debate with client
3. *Projection*—has important protective function, may cover deeper disturbance
   Counselor tip: be sensitive to self-blame and guilt, and the client feeling shamed by any suggestion of criticism; preface feedback with "some people might think"
4. *Rationalization*—clever answers used to avoid responsibility and maintain frozen feelings
   Counselor tip: avoid your own frustration and anger in trying to get through to a highly intellectualizing client
5. *Compliance*—hidden form of resistance, may cover up magical expectations
   Counselor tip: recognize the potential of provoking rebellion at some point
6. *Conflict avoidance*—problems handling feelings of anger and disappointment, need to be liked and approved
   Counselor tip: provoking client to deal with conflict too much may be a hazard
7. *Obsessive focusing*—all-or-none thinking, may be overly self-critical or, overly critical of others, may be perfectionistic
   Counselor tip: understand the person's situation while suggesting that he or she "lighten up"
8. *Acting out*—lacks awareness of feelings, impulses communicated by behavior, most provocative of defenses
   Counselor tip: direct to needed change, stay out of harm's way (i.e., be careful not to put self in jeopardy)

Interventions at Various Stages of the Alcohol/Drug Use Continuum

Alcohol/drug intervention is any action taken by someone to interrupt the progression of problems with alcohol/drugs. This definition can be expanded to any attempt to help someone from further developing problems with alcohol/drugs. At each stage of alcohol/drug use (i.e., initial contact, experimentation, integrated use, excessive use, addiction), intervention attempts may prevent progression to the next, more damaging stage of alcohol/drug use. This may take the form of an employer expressing concern about an employee's job performance or a teacher talking with parents and letting them know their child is tired and falling asleep in class. There have been a variety of intervention programs in the school system. One such program helps teachers develop core teams (usually involving the school nurse, an administrator, a coach, a dean, etc.), which identify students with behaviors, attitudes, and problems that may indicate alcohol/drug problems. All of these approaches are interventions. Whether it is a conversation expressing concern about alcohol/drug use or a formal intervention, the common goal is to let the individual know that we are concerned about him or her.

In Chapter 4, the various stages of alcohol/drug use are described—nonuse, initial contact, experimentation (situational and circumstantial), integrated use, excessive use (periodic and continuous), and addiction. At each of these stages, there are opportunities for intervention. If one can effectively intervene at earlier stages and interrupt the progression to later stages of alcohol/drug use, the negative consequences may be avoided. Obviously, the later stages of alcohol/drug abuse require more concerted efforts, such as a formal intervention.

The following suggestions illustrate various interventions for children at each stage of the alcohol/drug use continuum.

Stage 1—Nonuse Interventions
- Parental, peer, and other support to maintain nonuse
- Emotional support during difficult times, conflicts, developmental tasks, and emotionally charged events that may make the individual at-risk try alcohol/drugs
- Affirmation and support in activities that promote a good sense of self and alternative activities to alcohol/drug use
- Focus on refusal skills and dealing with peer pressure
- Education and implementation of effective parenting, communication skills, and other alcohol/drug prevention skills

Stage 2—Initial Contact Interventions
Two common problems at this stage are overreaction and underreaction. As a parent, you don't want to be an alarmist and overact in rigid, shaming, and blaming ways to a child's initial contact with alcohol/drugs. You also don't want to ignore the use, disregard the significance, and minimize the impact on the child. As a result,

- Become more aware of the child's behavior and signs of alcohol/drug use.
- Talk with other parents about the child's behavior in their homes.
- Once aware of initial contact, talk with child (i.e., break the no-talk rule); don't ignore the fact that your child used or avoided the opportunity to discuss his or her use of alcohol/drugs.
- If your child has used, let him or her describe the situation, without being judgmental, blaming, or negative.

- Express concerns about safety (e.g., Was your child with friends that he or she could trust? Was it a safe place if problems occurred? Was your child in physical or psychological danger?).
- Without being negative and an alarmist, or lecturing, let the child describe his or her own perception of safety.
- Discuss at-risk factors of alcohol/drug dependence and addiction (especially if there is a family history of alcoholism and/or drug dependence).
- This may be an opportunity to reevaluate other aspects of the child's life (e.g., school, friends, activities).
- This may be an opportune time to explore other family problems and seek an assessment from a counselor who specializes in alcohol/drug recovery and family systems.

Stage 3—Experimentation Interventions
- Focusing on communication and exploration of values, attitudes, and feelings about alcohol/drugs
- Teaching and modeling skills in decision-making, conflict resolution, goal setting, and so on
- Teaching and modeling skills in coping with conflicts, dealing with authority figures, and controlling destructive impulses
- Providing information about chemical dependency and addiction
- Providing information about at-risk factors if there is a family history of chemical dependency (e.g., if one parent has or had problems with alcohol/drugs, the child has a four times higher risk of developing problems with alcohol/drugs; if both parents have or had a problem, there is an eight times higher risk for the child to develop problems with alcohol/drugs)
- Identifying, assessing, and perhaps counseling for problems in the family, at school, and so on
- Educating about alcohol/drug prevention and family systems

Stage 4—Interventions at the Integrated Stage
- Identification and communication of concerns and negative consequences as a result of integrated alcohol/drug use
- Expression of concern—in a caring, nonjudgmental way—regarding the well-being of the individual using alcohol/drugs
- Point out the individual's denial of an alcohol/drug problem
- Assessment by a trained chemical dependency family counselor to assess alcohol/drug use and family dynamics
- If problems are identified, work on these issues in counseling (i.e., family members attend Alanon; take educational classes on chemical dependency, parenting, and family systems; and attend regular counseling)

Stages 5 and 6—Interventions at the Excessive Use and Addiction Stages
All of the previous strategies are appropriate at both the excessive and addictive stages. However, the longer and more pervasive the problems with alcohol/drugs, the more difficult and intense the level of intervention.

- Alcohol/drug assessment, including regular urinanalysis for drugs and blood alcohol tests
- Intensive outpatient counseling for chemical dependency and family issues
- Strong boundary setting and consequences for violation of family rules and alcohol/drug use
- Formal alcohol/drug intervention
- Inpatient/residential treatment for chemical dependency
- Involvement in AA and other self-help meetings, including active involvement in 12-step work with a sponsor

Table 9.3 describes the do's and don'ts of dealing with someone who has an alcohol/drug problem.

TABLE 9.3

Do's and Don'ts of Dealing with Someone Who Has an Alcohol/Drug Problem

1. Deal with your emotions.

If possible, try to be calm, balanced, and caring. This may be difficult; however, remember that, if you lose control, you lose.

Do Not

Try to talk with someone while he or she is under the influence of alcohol/drugs; if your child or spouse comes home late at night under the influence of alcohol/drugs, wait until the morning to discuss it.

Threaten to make ultimatums unless you have had time to think them through (e.g., Is it realistic? Can you follow through? What is the impact of the ultimatum on other family members?). Threats said in anger can be unrealistic, inflexible, and abusive. Idle threats or constant threats that are not followed through are meaningless in changing behavior. Threats only set up a lack of consistency, poor trust, and lack of credibility.

Lose your temper, rant and rave, or lose control. It might temporarily make you feel good to let out your frustration and anger, but it does not help the child or adult in addressing the alcohol/drug problem.

Do

Express a willingness to get help and resolve the problem. This is usually in the form of counseling.

Communicate your concern and feelings (e.g., fear, worry, love) without trying to control or lecture the alcohol/drug user.

Set boundaries that are reasonable (to promote appropriate behavior and consistent family rules).

Follow through with consequences for boundaries that were violated.

2. Communicate with behavior-specific examples, rather than generalizations and secondhand or speculative information.

Do Not

Ask why the person is using alcohol/drugs. "Why" questions are often blaming questions, as if asking, "How could you do this to your mother and me?"

Use words such as *drunk, loaded, wasted.* Instead, describe specific behaviors you observe (e.g., slurred speech, staggered gait, etc.).

Generalize about alcohol/drug use. Be specific about alcohol/drug use, if possible (e.g., "I saw you drink five glasses of wine and snort two lines of cocaine").

(continued on next page)

TABLE 9.3 (continued)

Do's and Don'ts of Dealing with Someone Who Has an Alcohol/Drug Problem

Use sarcasm, ridicule, and other behaviors that may shame or embarrass the alcohol/drug user. This only perpetuates resentments and often results in later passive-aggressive behavior.

Do

Seek professional counseling to help with family communication about alcohol/drug problems. Seek out a counselor experienced in alcohol/drug treatment and family systems.

3. Trust what you see (behaviors), not what the addict/alcoholic or problem user says.

Do Not

Expect that things will get better on their own. Often, the problem alcohol/drug user will decrease his or her use when he or she suspects that you may do something. Alcoholism and drug addiction are progressive diseases that only get worse over time unless the individual is motivated to change.

Expect that the problem alcohol/drug user will recognize his or her use as a problem. Denial is often the case.

Assume that the alcoholic/addict will be rational and logical. Instead, he or she may exhibit self-deception and delay getting help.

4. Avoid being distracted from the real issue—the individual's abuse of alcohol/drugs.

Do Not

Spend time or physical and emotional energy on distracting wild goose chases (e.g., finding out who gave the person alcohol/drugs or blaming the school system or other parents). These are all secondary issues. The primary issue is that your child or family member may have an alcohol/drug problem.

Compare the alcohol/drug problems of others that are more involved in alcohol/drug use. This is a form of rationalizing away the problem. Expressions such as "kids will be kids," "he or she will outgrow this," and "most people drink/drug this way" tend to discount the real dimensions of alcohol/drug dependence.

Get distracted by excuses for alcohol/drug abuse (e.g., "I'm experiencing a great deal of pressure right now" or "It's because my girlfriend just broke up with me"). The fact is the person has a problem with alcohol/drugs and is vulnerable to relapse when normal, stressful events happen again.

(continued on next page)

Obstacles to Interventions

There are many obstacles that prevent families from getting help for alcohol/drug problems. Getting the family member with the alcohol/drug problem into treatment may not be realistic unless these obstacles are first addressed. Some common obstacles to families getting help are listed in Table 9.4.

The Olympic Story

On an extremely hot summer day in 1984, I attended the Olympic Games in Los Angeles. Like most spectators that day, I tried to find a shady area on the lawn outside the stadium while awaiting the afternoon field events. While we watched Carl Lewis qualify for the long jump, a quiet, unsettling nervousness ran through the crowd in anticipation of the finish of the first women's marathon in Olympic history. The wide

T A B L E   9 . 3   *(c o n c l u d e d)*

Do's and Don'ts of Dealing with Someone Who Has an Alcohol/Drug Problem

4. Avoid being distracted from the real issue—the individual's abuse of alcohol/drugs. (continued)

Do Not

Take responsibility for the total problem. Avoid self-blaming statements (e.g., "I'm an awful parent" or "I should have _____; then he or she wouldn't have an alcohol/drug problem"). Self-blame serves only to distract from the issue at hand—the fact that your child or family member has an alcohol/drug problem and needs help. You cannot go back and change the past; you can only work on the future.

Do

Seek treatment for the addicted person and the entire family. The sooner you do this, the better is the prognosis.

5. Seek professional help for alcohol/drug assessment, education, prevention, intervention, and treatment.

Do Not

Isolate from others and hide the family alcohol/drug problem. The longer you hide the problem from others to avoid feelings of shame and embarrassment, the more damage occurs to your family system.

Get advice from people who may have an alcohol/drug problem themselves or individuals who deny the problem. This only reinforces denial.

Attempt to counsel the family member who has the alcohol/drug problem yourself. This will inadvertently end up being another form of enabling behavior.

Do

Attend Alanon, Codependency Anonymous, and other self-help meetings and develop a relationship with a sponsor. This will help you develop a support system necessary to make changes.

Attend educational presentations, classes, and conferences that focus on parenting, family systems, prevention, alcohol/drug recovery, intervention, codependency, and other personal growth issues.

Find a counselor who specializes in alcohol/drug treatment, family systems, and codependency. For more information on choosing a counselor, see Chapter 11.

Take care of yourself and continue with your own recovery, regardless of whether the family member who has the alcohol/drug problem gets help.

---

screen monitor at one end of the stadium broke the boredom and heat by showing Joan Benoit with a significant lead in the marathon. The men's 800-meter qualifying race drew our interest, distracting us from the heat of the afternoon.

The slow, methodical repertoire of the shot-putters was in full progress when the wide video screen came alive with Joan Benoit maintaining a significant lead. The crowd began to buzz with excitement. The shot-putters were caught by surprise as the more than 40,000 people in the coliseum began to applaud Benoit. The ensuing 30 to 40 minutes were like a New Year's Eve party as the crowd counted down the minutes until Benoit entered the stadium for the final two laps of her 26-mile ordeal. We were all standing, watching both the video screen and the western entrance to the coliseum. Finally, the moment came: the crowd exploded in cheers as Benoit entered and began her last two laps around the track. As she circled the track, each section of the stadium stood, cheering and waving little American flags. It was truly a wave of human emotion and pride affirming her accomplishment: the first women's

T A B L E   9 . 4

Obstacles to Reaching Parents and Families

- Denial of family dysfunction/imbalance and alcohol/drug problems
- Skepticism about alcohol/drug messages that don't fit parents' own experience
- Assumption by parents that children's alcohol/drug use will be O.K.
- Distorted, depressed view of life by dysfunctional families
- Fear of being stigmatized or labeled as dysfunctional
- Fear of loss of confidentiality
- Narcissism of parents
- Lack of insurance resources for parenting/counseling services
- Lack of energy/time by parents
- Distrust of the system
- Lack of credible message sources for cultural/racial minority groups
- Lack of concern/respect for experts' opinions about alcohol/drugs
- Lack of awareness of community resources, discomfort with middle-class settings
- Overwhelming need for services for basic survival
- Cultural mores

Source: Office for Substance Abuse Prevention 1990.

Olympic marathon winner was an American. This was the crowd's hope and, for some, their only reason for attending the Olympics that day.

A few minutes later, I became aware of another struggle. A Swedish runner was approximately the sixth runner to enter the stadium. Benoit had already finished the race, and the crowd was still alive with energy. Its focus soon shifted to the Swedish runner, who, on entering the track, was staggering. She took two steps forward, then two steps sideways, then another step forward. Clearly, she had hit the wall and was suffering from oxygen deprivation. As she advanced on the track, each section of the crowd rose and cheered her on. The human wave was in slow but full motion as the section where I was sitting stood up and cheered her on. As she began her second and last lap around the track, a medical team, dressed in their whites, ran alongside her. The thought struck me: what if we were all cheering and encouraging her to her death? The woman was clearly suffering, yet we applauded her to continue on despite the possibility of bodily harm. Fortunately, she did finish the race without any permanent physical damage. A physician in attendance told me that within a few hours her vital signs and physical functioning were back to normal. However, what if she had not been that fortunate?

This raises some important questions. Should there have been a medical intervention to assess her condition? In the heat of the race, do runners have a proper frame of physical and mental reference to decide if they are capable of continuing? Do we have a responsibility to intervene when someone is in danger of harming himself or herself?

This brief scenario from the 1984 Olympics illustrates one situation in which we might intervene. Other sports, on recreational to professional levels, also illustrate situations when there may be a need for intervention. Boxing, football, weight lifting, even team sports such as soccer, basketball, and baseball may require interventions to safeguard players. The use of protective equipment, rules that lower the risk of serious and/or permanent injury, and other advances minimize unnecessary harm to athletes, yet some athletes choose to disregard their own health to enhance performance. As pointed out in Chapter 3, they use steroids, painkillers, stimulants, and other drugs to attain a competitive edge. Advances in sports medicine are being applied as an intervention and preventive approach to injuries, in an attempt to stop serious long-term damage. Another situation where we might intervene is when individuals have alcohol/drug problems and may harm themselves or others.

Intervention Services

The concept of alcohol/drug intervention began in the 1960s, when Vernon Johnson—at that time a pastor—felt frustrated when he was unable to help spouses of alcoholics. Deciding to abandon the traditional approach of waiting until the alcoholic/addict hit bottom, he tried a strategy that he later called intervention (Johnson 1986).

Webster's Tenth New Collegiate Dictionary defines *intervene* this way: "to occur, fall, or come between points of time or events." Alcohol/drug intervention is a process that prevents, alters, or interrupts the progression of the disease. The intervention is a process of getting involved or stepping into a situation in an attempt to interrupt the disease and to get the individual into alcohol/drug treatment. Persons who intervene choose to talk about the issue of alcohol/drug dependence that is destructive to the individuals, their families, and friends. Due to the alcoholic/addict's strong denial system, a trained interventionist with an expertise in chemical dependency treatment must lead or facilitate the intervention.

Intervention services are offered by most chemical dependency inpatient and residential treatment centers. Trained chemical dependency counselors also specialize in conducting interventions. The choice of the interventionist is a critical element in determining the success of an intervention. Local, state, and national alcohol/drug help lines are excellent referral sources for finding trained and experienced interventionists.

Intervention Approaches

There are a variety of approaches to the alcohol/drug intervention, including formal and informal chemical dependency interventions, in which each interventionist has his or her own style of conducting the intervention. The principles described in this chapter form a basic framework within which most interventionists work.

Professional Intervention Assistance

Whatever the format or style, conducting an intervention without professional guidance is often doomed to failure, no matter how powerful the individual. Untrained, grandstanding individuals who coerce someone into chemical dependency treatment often cause further resistance by the individual needing help. Do not use this information to try to conduct an intervention on your own; consult a professional interventionist for help.

Intervention as a Caring Response

The most important aspect of an intervention is that it is a caring effort designed to interrupt the disease of alcoholism and drug addiction. Individuals involved in an intervention can be effective only if they maintain a caring, behavior-specific approach and support each other within the basic guidelines of their intervention group.

Goals of Intervention

The primary goal in developing an intervention is to get the addicted person to recognize that he or she has an alcohol/drug problem and to get that person into appropriate chemical dependency treatment. Treatment is usually a minimum 21- to 28-day inpatient or residential program.

Secondary goals of the intervention are to

1. Provide an opportunity for those who care about the alcoholic/addict to express concern about the impact the alcoholic/addict's dysfunctional behavior has had on them
2. Provide information on alcohol/drug addiction and family patterns of interaction, such as enabling behavior, to the significant others (parents, spouses, family members, employers, and peers)
3. Promote the development of a healthy family system and provide resource information for family members to continue working on their issues

Family Interventions

Interventions are 100 percent effective in that, regardless of whether the alcoholic/addict decides to get help and go to treatment, family members go on with their recovery. The family has begun a process of change. The growth that the family members experience in developing an intervention can empower them to continue to be true to their feelings and to their own individual recovery, whether or not the alcoholic/addict decides to seek treatment. Via the intervention process, the family members learn about the disease of alcohol/drug addiction. They recognize their own enabling behavior and the role they play in the dynamics of the disease. The intervention may be the first time in a long time that the family members have interacted by functionally discussing their feelings. It may be the first time they have candidly discussed the impact the alcoholic/addict's alcohol or drug use has had on each of them.

Candidates for Intervention

Using a formal intervention process on adolescents, or young adults who are developmentally still at the adolescent stage, is usually ineffective. Adolescents often feel violated by the process of intervention. Because they are still exploring their own issues of identity and boundaries, they feel that it is unfair for family members to be planning an intervention without their knowledge. Adolescents fail to recognize or acknowledge that all previous direct efforts have not been effective in getting them to listen and understand the true dimensions of their problems.

Interventions are far more effective in getting individuals into treatment, when addicts recognize that their behavior has been a problem. The addict who still values and respects members of the intervention group is the best candidate. In some situations, addicts have alienated so many people that only job-related people are left. This relationship with an employer or business associates might be the integral element that makes some addicts good candidates for intervention.

Stages of Formal Intervention

The four basic stages of a formal intervention are assessment, preintervention, intervention, and postintervention. The rest of this chapter describes these stages with many examples and a case study.

Assessment

Families consider an alcohol/drug intervention because a family member recognizes that the family needs to do something about the person with the alcohol/drug problem. Likely, people have approached the addict about getting help on numerous occasions. Despite their efforts, the addict still chooses not to recognize the problem or get help. The alcoholic/addict's goal is to continue drinking or drugging.

A family member begins the intervention process by contacting a professional who conducts interventions. The interventionist schedules an appointment with family members to assess the alcohol/drug problem and to determine if an intervention is appropriate.

An experienced interventionist is trained to assess alcohol/drug problems. In the initial assessment sessions, several family members, friends, colleagues, and even the employer describe what they know about the alcohol/drug use of the person being assessed for the intervention. Individuals seeking to intervene on a family member with an alcohol/drug problem are often at a late stage of frustration with the alcoholic/addict's dysfunctional and destructive behavior. Many look at the intervention as a last-ditch alternative. Despite the family's urgency to conduct an intervention, the interventionist conducts a proper assessment to determine if the person really does have an alcohol/drug problem.

The key element of the assessment is eliciting *behavior-specific information* and avoiding hearsay and generalized information. The interventionist needs specific times, dates, and firsthand knowledge of the actual level of consumption of alcohol and drugs. Some assessment questions are "What makes you think the individual has a problem with alcohol/drugs?" "What have been the consequences of this individual's alcohol/drug use?" The interventionist asks family members to explain or clarify the

Frequency of use, amounts used (dose and routes of administration), and set and setting of use

Patterns of use—binges, periods of nonuse, and cycle of use

History of negative consequences—overdoses, medical complications, and physical and emotional harm

Periods of abstinence, if any, and methods used
Any medical conditions that affects alcohol/drug use
Use of coffee, cigarettes, and medications and other addictions
Difficulties with the criminal-justice system
Financial problems and interpersonal problems

Family members at the assessment sessions are asked to describe specifically what they know about the addict's use of alcohol and drugs and resulting dysfunctional and destructive behavior. The assessment clarifies the dimensions of the problem with alcohol/drugs. The family, and others present, usually recognize, confirm, and validate their own worst fears—the individual has an alcohol/drug problem.

Another extremely important aspect of the assessment is to determine whether the person you are going to intervene on is able to listen and understand. Someone who is going to physically attack, verbally explode, or rage at others at the intervention is not appropriate for an intervention. During the assessment stage, interventionists often ask the family members and others present, "How does the person you are planning to intervene on deal with anger?" "What do you think his or her reaction is going to be to the intervention?" These questions should elicit responses that determine if the individual is violent and if there have been some physical violations in the past. Sometimes individuals can be paranoid and/or delusional, especially if they have been using cocaine, crack, or free base. Obviously, you do not want to do an intervention if there is a high risk that the individual will be violent or unable to listen and understand. One alternative is to videotape the intervention and give it to the addict.

Some people have a negative reaction to the concept of an alcohol/drug intervention. They believe that it is an invasion, or a violation, of the individual and his or her right to use alcohol/drugs. For the intervention to be effective, it must be planned without the knowledge of the person being intervened on. Some individuals have difficulty with this behind-the-scenes aspect. Once the interventionist has assessed that an intervention is warranted, members of the intervention group must decide whether they are comfortable proceeding with the intervention.

Case Study 9.2 illustrates the perils of initiating an intervention without first doing a proper assessment.

Preintervention

The preintervention stage consists of all the sessions necessary to prepare for the actual intervention to take place. The ingredients essential for a successful intervention include (1) the commitment and participation of meaningful and significant others (family members, friends, relatives, peers, and children); (2) a proper assessment by the interventionist; and (3) specific, nonjudgmental information about the individual's alcohol and drug behavior.

In preparation for the intervention, preintervention sessions develop a cohesive group of significant others—a group that has the goal of getting the alcoholic/addict into appropriate treatment.

The interventionist begins developing this group by educating the members, giving them information about the dynamics of chemical dependency. The education emphasizes the progressive nature of the disease of alcoholism/drug addiction, which affects the entire family.

Case Study 9.2

Intervention Without Proper Assessment

J. R.

J. R., an aspiring vice president in a developing company, contacted an interventionist and re-quested an intervention for another vice president in the same company. The family members of the person with the supposed alcohol problem believed that Roger had been drinking reg-ularly but were not sure that he had an alcohol problem. Insisting that his coworker's drink-ing was a problem, J. R. was unable to come up with any behavior-specific examples of in-creased alcohol use. Despite the limited information and secondhand generalizations, the interventionist decided to go ahead with the intervention. The result was disastrous. Roger did not have an alcohol problem and quickly identified sabotage by his colleague, who desired his sales territory. Needless to say, Roger was justified in proceeding with litigation against the interventionist for not conducting a proper assessment.

The group members then develop their scripts and role-play the intervention. Role-playing allows the group to anticipate the reactions of the person they are go-ing to intervene on. The group members can then redevelop their intervention to make it more effective.

The alcoholic/addict is a master in distracting the intervention group from the goals of the intervention. When each family member communicates generalizations and judgments, the alcoholic/addict picks at their statements and distracts the group, thus weakening their ability to get the alcoholic/addict to commit to treatment. Therefore, the members of the intervention group must develop and communicate be-havior-specific examples of the alcoholic/addict's dysfunctional and self-destructive behavior.

The following examples illustrate generalized statements, followed by the al-coholic/addict's distracting statements. The appropriate behavior-specific statement follows each set of generalized and distracting responses.

Example 1

Generalized and blaming statements: "Boy, you were really wasted at the party picnic and got violent. You were drunk and loaded on cocaine."

Alcoholic/addict distracting statements: "What do you mean wasted? You were drinking just as much as I was. Weren't you? Boy are you hypocritical. You use cocaine."

Behavior-specific statements: "John, I'm here because I care about you. On Saturday, July 4, 1991, at the company picnic, I saw you drink five beers from 1 to 3 P.M., then snort six lines of cocaine, which was followed by two more beers. You sat down in the outfield during the softball game and fell asleep. When I went over to wake you up, you threw a punch at me, right in front of the head of our company. You left the field. I found you a half hour later, with a six-pack in the back of your car. Two of the cans of beer were already empty. I am worried about you. I'm afraid you are going to lose your job. You've been like a brother to me. I pray that you will get help. I know it's the alcohol and drugs."

Example 2

Generalized and blaming statements: "You are an awful husband and father. You are always using drugs and drinking too much. Last night you were drinking and snorting cocaine all night. You scared the kids to death that night by yelling so loud at them, like a madman."

Alcoholic/addict distracting statements: "You think you are such a great mother? I remember the time you. . . ."

Behavior-specific statements: "John, I'm your wife and I'm here because I care about you. On Friday night, November 3, I went to the church meeting. When I came home at 10:15 P.M., I smelled alcohol on your breath and clothes. There was an empty gram bottle of cocaine on the kitchen table and three lines of cocaine still on the mirror. There were 12 empty beer cans on the living room floor and the kids were hiding in their closet upstairs. When I went into their room, they ran to me, shaking and out of control. That night I had to sleep with them because they were so frightened. The next day, they told me you threw beer cans at them and told them you would kill them if they didn't stop bothering you. I love you, John; I know it's the alcohol and drugs. I would like all of us to get help."

Each person involved in the intervention uses the following script format to avoid generalized, blaming statements:

"I'm here because I care about you. You are my _____. I *care* about you."
"I saw _____" (describe the behavior-specific incidents that occurred)
"I feel _____" (embarrassed, hurt, frightened, worried, ashamed, etc.)
"I know it's the drugs." (or the alcohol or cocaine)
"I want you [us] to get help."

Script Example

"John, I'm here because I *care* about you. We've been friends a very long time. During Christmas, I *saw* you snort half a gram of cocaine. In the next hour, you drank four beers. I *felt embarrassed* when you were trying to kiss your niece. I *felt ashamed. I saw* the hurt on your wife's face. I *know it's the cocaine. I know it's the alcohol. I want you to get help.*"

Some interventionists prefer the words "I want you to get help." Others prefer "I want us to get help" because everyone in the family is going to get help to stop enabling the alcoholic/addict's use of alcohol/drugs.

During the preintervention, the intervention group members determine

1. When the intervention will take place
2. Where the intervention will take place—usually a neutral setting such as the interventionist's office is best
3. Who will bring the person to the intervention
4. Their scripts, role-play the intervention, and determine the most effective way of communicating their message
5. In which order each member will talk during the intervention

6. Who is going to ask for a commitment to listen from the person being intervened on

7. That arrangements have been made with the alcohol/drug treatment program; insurance and other details have been completed; and a bed is reserved at the treatment center starting on the day of the intervention

8. All contingencies, so that the individual can go directly to the treatment program; bags have been packed and are in the car; and a family member drives the addict directly to the treatment program.

Every detail is planned, even the seating arrangement. The actual intervention session will start and flow as planned. The family members will be prepared to continue their own recovery, regardless of the addict's decision. The session will not escalate into an uncontrollable situation. The family will approach the intervention as a process, rather than a static event. Bear in mind that, if the preintervention sessions have gone well, the interventionist is available to help the family members during the intervention, but most often he or she plays a minimal, facilitating role.

Intervention

Each intervention is unique. However, they all have the same common ingredients for success, such as a nonjudgmental tone and behavior-specific caring responses by family and friends. The following is an example of an intervention.

Audrey is an attractive, energetic 33-year-old. She owns a very successful travel agency. She is the single parent of two children: Andy is 12 years old and Bridget is 7 years old. Audrey is dynamic, aggressive, and—the most critical feature—an alcoholic.

Audrey's sister Mary, 39, is concerned enough to seek intervention for her sister. Both sisters grew up in an alcoholic family system. Their father died of alcoholism when Mary was 16 and Audrey was 9 years old. Those involved with the intervention are the following:

Mary—Audrey's older sister
Ann—a very successful businesswoman, Audrey and Mary's mother
Roger—Mary's son, Audrey's nephew, a 20-year-old student at the University of
      Washington
Andy—Audrey's 12-year-old son

Mary has taken Audrey to the interventionist's office under the pretense that they have been having some family counseling sessions for her son Roger. She said they wanted Audrey to participate in one session. All the family members are present at the office, waiting for Audrey and Mary to arrive.

Mary: Audrey, this is Dr. Fields. [Shakes hands.] Just sit right here. Audrey, we are all here because we care about you. We are concerned about you and the children. We would like to be able to talk to you about our concerns. We would each like to say some things. We need your commitment to listen to us and not to respond until we are finished. You will have an opportunity to respond then. Will you promise to first listen to us and not talk until we are finished?

Audrey: But, I thought we were here for Roger.

Mary: We are here for you, Roger, and all the family members.

Audrey: Yeah, but you didn't let me know what this was about.

Mary: Audrey, we wanted you to come. Will you just hear us out? Then you can have your chance.

Audrey: I, I . . . don't . . . yeah, I guess so. O.K., I'll listen to what you have to say.

[Establishing ground rules allows each family member to talk without being distracted by the addict's ambiguous arguments. Having the addict agree to listen and not talk back is an essential ingredient for the intervention to be successful. Even though Audrey has been deceived in getting her to the intervention, she knows or suspects what the meeting is about. She is curious and is even challenging the group to try to affect her.]

Roger: Thank you. You've been like a big sister to me, even though you are my aunt. You have provided a lot of opportunities to me. You've taken me on vacations and introduced me to all sorts of people, activities, and even jobs that I never would have had access to. I care about you a great deal. You've been a tremendous influence and I am very proud of you. I am here because I love you.

Lately, however, I find that I'm not so proud of you anymore. I'm worried about you. I'm worried about Andy. I'm worried about Bridget. At your birthday party on January 7, you came home smelling of alcohol. You had three margaritas within an hour. I saw you in the kitchen, downing two doubles, as if they were water. You stumbled out of the kitchen and fell and cut your lip.

Audrey: That was my birthday party. Don't you understand?

Roger: You promised you would listen. After you cut yourself, when Andy, Bridget, and I came into the kitchen to help, you screamed and yelled at us to get away. Andy was so frightened he hid in his room and Bridget couldn't stop crying. They said they were so frightened that you were going to hit them again.

This isn't the first time this has happened. The same thing happened when we went down to Mexico. You had four drinks at the airport bar and four drinks on the flight. I was so embarrassed when you were flirting with the man next to you. The kids were embarrassed when you were kissing him and when you yelled at me for interfering. When we got to our hotel, the first thing you did was to order more booze.

In February, I was at the travel agency and you went into the bathroom. You invited me in and you had some lines of cocaine that you offered me. I saw you do 10 lines of cocaine and then come out and act as if everything was O.K. You made six trips to the bathroom in the hour that I was there.

Audrey: I didn't do that much. As if you are so innocent!

Roger: You promised that you would listen and not interrupt. I was with you the night you got arrested for driving under the influence of alcohol. The kids were frightened sitting in the back seat. Despite my arguing with you, you insisted on driving. I was so frightened that we all would be killed. I went along because I felt guilty that you would kill yourself and the kids. I tried to take the keys away from you, but you wouldn't let me. I was so angry with your boyfriend, Al, for insisting that you were O.K., when you couldn't even walk straight. I was so angry with you when the police arrested you in front of your children. But I was more upset with myself for allowing myself to get drawn into the whole situation.

Audrey, despite all of this I love you and the children and I want you to get help.

Audrey: What kind of help?

Roger: [No response, head tilted down to ground, feeling emotionally spent.]

Ann: Audrey, you were a beautiful child; I gave birth to you. I love you a great deal. You were always so fun loving, energetic, and interested in so many things. We went shopping the other day, last Wednesday, and you had four beers at lunch, after you said you would cut back. You told me that you were just wired. You were agitated, nervous, jittery. Audrey, I'm frightened for you. When we came home from the travel agency last Friday, you smelled of alcohol. You were driving erratically. I was afraid we would get pulled over and you'd be arrested again. When I told you that you were in no condition to drive, you yelled at me to stop nagging.

Audrey: You, you're always telling me what to do. You're always bothering me. You're always involved in my life, telling me how to parent my kids.

Ann: That day, I saw you drink three beers before we left the agency.

Audrey: You guys are in this together. I don't even know why I'm here.

Roger: You said you'd listen.

Audrey: How can I listen to you if you keep on getting together? How could you guys get together behind my back to do this?

Ann: We're here because we care about you. We love you. I know it's the drugs. I know it's the alcohol. I want us to get some help.

Mary: We've grown up together. We've always been close. I love you. I care about you. Last week, we went out to Morgan's restaurant. You drank five margaritas within an hour and a half. You were snorting cocaine in the bathroom. You left the restaurant with two men whom you didn't know. I am really frightened for you. The next day you called me and told me you had a problem with alcohol and wanted help. Two days later, on Sunday, when I asked you about getting help, you said that you were doing much better and were getting your act together.

	It was only a week later, that Friday night, when you were back at Morgan's. I saw you drink three doubles in an hour. You insisted that I stay. It was too hard to stay and watch you order another drink. I'm afraid that you are hurting yourself. I worry about you. I want my younger sister back. I want you to get help.
Andy:	[Tears rolling from his eyes] Mommy, I am afraid when you drink and use drugs that you will hurt me. I am afraid that you will hurt Bridget. I want you to go get help. Will you?
Audrey:	[Hugs Andy] Yes, I'll get help. I love you and don't want you to be frightened.
Mary:	We have reserved a bed at the treatment center and Roger will drive you there.
Audrey:	You mean you want me to go right now?
Mary:	Yes.
Audrey:	But what about the appointments at the agency?
Mary:	I've arranged for Natalie to come in and manage the agency while you are gone.
Audrey:	But what about the meeting with the accountant on Thursday?
Ann/Mom:	I can cover the meeting, since I know all about the new bookkeeping system.
Audrey:	What about clothes?
Mary:	I packed some of your things in a suitcase. Anything else you want I can get to you tomorrow.
Audrey:	Can the children come and visit?
Mary:	After the first week, there are regular family visits and a family counseling program. We chose this program because it specializes in providing counseling for young children.
Audrey:	I guess you thought of everything.
	[In reality, the family did think of everything. Any potential form of denial was anticipated, so that Audrey and her family could get the help they needed.]

In the event that Audrey did not agree to go into treatment, the family had prepared another bottom-line script. The purpose of the bottom-line script is to let the addict know that, if she refuses to go into treatment, the family is not going to continue to enable her alcohol/drug use, as they have in the past. In implementing the bottom-line script, family members have to be willing to follow through with their bottom lines. Otherwise, there is no point in stating them. For example, if Audrey had refused to go into treatment, the bottom-line stage of the intervention would have followed:

Roger:	Audrey, I care about you. You've been a person that I greatly admire. I love you a great deal. I'm frightened about the alcohol and drugs. I'm fearful that you'll hurt yourself or the kids. If you don't go into treatment, I can no longer come over to the house. I won't see you until you get help. It's too difficult for me to see you killing yourself.

Ann/Mom: Audrey, I love you. You are a wonderful, caring mother. I see you teaching the kids to read and doing wonderful, creative things with them. You'll always be my daughter. If you don't get help I'm going to have my lawyer start the process of declaring you unfit. It hurts me to do this, but I can't allow the children to be abused the way they are. I know it's the alcohol and drugs, and I want us to get help. [Ann cries.]

Mary: We've been more than sisters. We've been best friends. If you don't get help, I'll help Mom get the children in a safe environment and away from the alcohol and drugs. I'm afraid for the children and their future. Please get help.

The bottom-line script is implemented only if the individual refuses to get treatment. If the individual still refuses treatment after the bottom line, the intervention is over, and the family members implement the bottom line.

Postintervention

The trauma and emotion of the intervention affects all of the family members and friends involved in the intervention. Immediately after a successful intervention, families are often relieved and hopeful. However, the road to family recovery has just begun. The family should get together with the interventionist within a month, prior to the end of the 30-day inpatient program attended by the person who was intervened on. This gives the family members an opportunity both to reflect on their original commitment to the intervention and on their own enabling behavior and to reiterate their commitment to recovery.

References

Alcoholics Anonymous. 1976. *The history of how many thousands of men and women have recovered from alcoholism.* 3d ed.: World Services.

Johnson, Vernon E. 1986. *How to help someone who doesn't want help.* Minneapolis: Johnson Institute Books.

Miller, William, and Janet C'de Baca. 2001. *Quantum change: When epiphanies and sudden insights transform ordinary lives.* New York: Guilford Press.

Miller, William, and Stephen Rollnick. 1991. *Motivational interviewing: Preparing people to change addictive behavior.* New York: Guilford Press.

Disorders Co-occurring with Substance Abuse

❖ **Chapter in Review**

The term *co-occurring disorder* refers to the condition of having both a psychiatric diagnosis and a chemical dependency diagnosis.

This chapter describes the problems related to mood disorders and chemical dependency, with specific emphasis on major depression, dysthymia, atypical depression, bipolar disorder, and mood-cycling disorder.

What differentiates these various types of affective (feeling) disorders are their severity, duration, frequency, and precipitating factors. Common vegetative signs of a mood disorder are disrupted sleep, difficulty with appetite and weight regulation, decreased cognitive functioning (including problems with concentration, memory, and problem solving), decreased libido or sex drive, lack of motivation, decreased energy (anergia), and difficulty experiencing pleasure (anhedonia).

This chapter also explores the co-occurring disorder of personality disorders and chemical dependency. Most personality traits have both adaptive and maladaptive qualities or features. When personality traits are persistently maladaptive and lead to chronic difficulty in interpersonal, occupational, and social functioning, there is a personality disorder. The two major personality disorders most frequently associated with chemical dependency are antisocial personality disorder and borderline personality disorder.

⚔ Definition of a Co-occurring Disorder

The terms *dual disorders, comorbid disorders,* and *co-occurring disorders* have been used interchangeably to describe the condition of having both a psychiatric diagnosis and a chemical dependency diagnosis. The symptoms produced by psychiatric disorders and chemical dependency can overlap. The concept reminds us of this overlap in symptoms and highlights the need to make an accurate diagnosis, so that appropriate treatment can be provided.

Until recently, counselors in the mental health and chemical dependency fields took a somewhat provincial outlook. Each has accused the other of

minimizing the importance of his or her own perspective. In many ways, the situation has become like the story of the blind men asked to describe an elephant. Each described it according to the body part he could touch but without regard to the remaining, unseen portions of the beast. Recent years have witnessed the emergence of a greater understanding and acceptance of the dual disorders or co-occurring disorder concept. Increasingly, members of both fields are educating themselves about each other's areas of specialty.

Clinically, we think of patients as existing on a continuum between purely psychiatric disorders at one end and purely chemical dependency problems on the other. Most patients lie somewhere between the extremes. An evaluation would take into account the relative position on the continuum. Today, it is rare to find a patient who has purely one condition, either psychiatric or chemical depen-

Some material in this chapter has been adapted from Field and Vanderbelt 1992a, 1992b. The names and circumstances of case studies in this chapter have been changed to maintain anonymity.

dency. Many psychiatric patients are affected by alcohol/drugs, and many patients with alcohol/drug problems have psychiatric symptoms.

It is common to see prevalence rates of substance abuse ranging between 40 and 60 percent of any psychiatric population. A report of a commission of mental health providers in New York State estimated that, of the 75,000 individuals hospitalized in New York each year for psychiatric conditions, close to 40,000 admissions "involve persons with dual disabilities or a serious psychiatric illness and an alcohol and/or drug abuse condition" (Bauer 1987).

A more recent, community-based survey of 20,291 people found that 53 percent of the surveyed drug abusers and 39 percent of the alcohol abusers had at least one mental illness, and 29 percent of the mentally ill in the survey abused either alcohol or drugs (Regier et al. 1990). Kenneth Minkoff, M.D., associate professor of psychiatry at Harvard and a proponent of the integrated model of disorders, believes that co-occurring disorders are an expectation, not an exception.

The evolution of the co-occurring disorders concept has paralleled our expanded understanding of the biological nature of both alcoholism and certain mental disorders. The 1990s was labeled the "decade of the brain," as we learned more about brain functions and their relation to affect. Research suggests that the causes of mental illness such as schizophrenia, depression, anxiety disorders, and affective disorders are substantially, if not primarily, biological. Genetic research of families with a history of alcoholism has supported the biological nature of alcoholism. There is a higher rate of alcoholism and other drug abuse in the families of patients with affect and mood disorders and vice versa. Quite possibly the genetic traits that predispose one to depression or other mental illness may be the same or similar genetic traits for chemical dependency.

The two major co-occurring disorders covered in this chapter are (1) affective (feeling) disorders and chemical dependency and (2) personality disorders and chemical dependency.

The Difference Between a Depressive Mood and a Depressive Disorder

✣ Affective (Feeling) Disorders and Substance-Use Disorders

It is common to feel down, sad, or even depressed after experiencing disappointment, frustration (blocked goal), setback, or trauma. Feelings of sadness, melancholia, grief, and loss are normal aspects of life. Working through the grief or loss is an essential feature of growth. However, when these depressive feelings persist beyond the common period of time to work through them, an affective disorder may be developing.

It is also normal to feel bad or low in early recovery from abusing alcohol and other drugs. Some of this is due to withdrawal from the chemicals but, even after withdrawal, problems in mood may persist. Chemical dependency causes financial, civil, criminal, interpersonal and family problems in the lives of many alcoholics/addicts—all of which can cause lasting pain. However, what is going on if the depression continues beyond normal alcohol/drug recovery?

Everyone experiences symptoms of depression from time to time. When symptoms become severe and persistent, however, diagnosis of an affective (feeling) disorder could be warranted. As researchers and clinicians have used various systems of classifying depression over the years, they have increasingly recognized the different types and subtypes of depression. What differentiates various types from one another is their **severity, frequency, duration,** and **precipitating factors.**

Affective disorders are different from the normal emotions of feeling down or sad. The following questions may help distinguish common depressive feelings from an affective disorder:

Severity: How deep is your depression? How low do you feel? Are you suicidal or self-destructive?
Frequency: How often do you feel depressed?
Duration: How long does the depression last? Are there periods when you are not depressed?
Precipitating factors: What triggers your depression? Do you know what is causing your depression?

Regardless of what causes depression initially, once it has been present for long enough it locks in and takes on a life of its own. This is another way of saying that the brain changes physiologically in response to internal or external events that have persisted for a sufficient time. After the physiological changes have taken place, a number of biological, or physical, signs of depression emerge. These *vegetative signs* include disturbances in the basic biological functions that the brain regulates. Vegetative signs of depression include the following:

- Disrupted sleep patterns
- Difficulty with appetite and weight regulation
- Decreased cognitive functioning (including problems with concentration, memory, and problem solving)
- Decreased libido, or sex drive
- Lack of motivation, decreased energy (anergia)
- Difficulty experiencing pleasure (anhedonia)

Denial and Depression

The psychological aspects of depression bring with it feelings of shame, as outlined in Chapter 6. Many individuals are extremely frightened to be labeled depressed, labeled manic-depressive (with bipolar disorder), or labeled with other affective and mood-cycling disorders. The denial of these feeling disorders is often self-medicated with the use of alcohol/drugs in an attempt to avoid the shame. Despite the fact that a vast majority (99 percent) of individuals suffering from affective disorders can be helped, only one in three depressed individuals seeks help. It is estimated that over 10 million people suffer from depressive illness, and 2 million people suffer from bipolar disorder. Serious depressions are "whole body" disorders affecting body, feelings, thoughts, and behaviors (U.S. Department of Health and Human Services 1987). Most people view themselves as weak and inferior in not having the will power to overcome depressive illness. This is much like the denial of the disease of alcoholism and drug addiction. In fact, depressive disorder is a disease much like alcohol/drug addiction in that it has a known etiology, gets progressively worse

> ### Case Study 10.1
>
> *Major Depression and Addiction*
>
> #### Elaine
>
> Elaine is a 53-year-old divorced woman with two previous psychiatric hospitalizations for severe depression. These were treated successfully with antidepressant medication. She returned to her psychiatrist after a 10-year absence due to progressively worsening depression for 2 months. Further questioning revealed that she had experienced anxiety symptoms last year and her gynecologist had prescribed diazepam (Valium). She took the medication in low doses as prescribed until sustaining a neck injury in an automobile accident 5 months ago. At that time, the doctor prescribed narcotic pain medication. Initially, she took the pain medication as prescribed but later took the medication in increasing doses. She found that her pain and anxiety symptoms were manageable with the higher doses and she simultaneously increased her daily dose of Valium, taking a moderate to heavy dose at night to help her overcome her physical discomfort and to improve sleep. Her escalating use of the medication surprises her, since she had never used similar drugs in the past and had avoided alcohol and street drugs because of religious beliefs. She is troubled by a growing preoccupation with suicide and fears that she may commit suicide, as her mother and maternal grandmother did. A physical exam by her internist later in the day revealed slightly elevated blood pressure, sweaty palms, and slightly dilated pupils.
>
> #### Discussion Questions
>
> What are the signs of depression?
> What role do you think age played in this case?
> Can you describe a case that is similar to this and identify signs?
> Give some examples of maladaptive behaviors as a result of depression.

over time, and has significant negative consequences if untreated. Case Study 10.1 presents an example of an individual who suffers from both depression and substance addiction.

Categories of Mood Disorders

Some common affective disorders are

- Major depression
- Dysthymic disorder (a low-grade depression)
- Atypical depression (depression related to sudden loss)
- Organic depression
- Bipolar disorder, formerly referred to as manic-depressive illness (severe mood swings)
- Cyclothymic (mood-cycling) disorder (a less severe form of mood swings)

Case studies in this section give you an understanding of the dynamics of the affective disorder and chemical dependency. In some case studies, chemical dependency

TABLE 10.1

Antidepressant Medications

Generic Name	Trade Name
amitriptyline	Elavil
amoxapine	Asendin
bupropion	Wellbutrin
citalopram (SSRI)	Celexa
desipramine	Norpramin, Pertofrane
doxepin	Adapin, Sinequan
clomipramine	Anafranil
fluvoxamine (SSRI)	Luvox
fluoxetine (SSRI)	Prozac
imipramine	Tofranil
isocarboxazid (MAOI)	Marplan
maprotiline	Ludiomil
mirtazapine	Remeron
nefazodone	Serzone
nortriptyline	Aventyl, Pamelor
paroxetine (SSRI)	Paxil
phenelzine (MAOI)	Nardil
protriptyline	Vivactil
sertraline (SSRI)	Zoloft
tranylcypromine (MAOI)	Parnate
trazodone	Desyrel
trimipramine	Surmontil
venlafaxine	Effexor

Source: *Medications,* Dept. of Health and Human Services, NIMH, publ. No. 02-3929, Revised April 2002.

is the primary diagnosis. Other case studies demonstrate that, even after sobriety, the underlying affective disorder still persists and requires treatment.

Many mood disorders are treated with antidepressant medications. Table 10.1 lists generic and trade names for many such medications. Table 10.2 shows categories of antidepressants. Medications specifically for treatment of substance-use disorders are listed in Table 10.3.

Major Depression

This depressive syndrome may occur as a single episode or as repeated episodes over the years. This diagnosis generally connotes a severe depressive episode with fairly clear onset and accompanying vegetative signs. Individuals suffering from major depression exhibit difficulty in the most basic of tasks (e.g., getting out of bed, brushing their teeth).

Episodes of major depression typically last from 6 to 12 months and then clear sometimes even without treatment. However, an episode can last significantly longer.

TABLE 10.2

Examples of Medications for Depression

Type or Class of Medication	Examples of Chemical Names	Examples of Brand Names	Typical Dose Ranges
Selective serotonin reuptake inhibitors (SSRIs)	Fluoxetine	Prozac	20–80 mg/day
	Paroxetine	Paxil	20–50 mg/day
	Sertraline	Zoloft	50–200 mg/day
	Citalopram	Celexa	20–60 mg/day
Bicyclics	Venlafaxine	Effexor	75–225 mg/day
	Mirtazapine	Remeron	15–45 mg/day
Heterocyclics	Trazodone	Deseryl	150–400 mg/day
	Maprotiline	Ludiomil	75–150 mg/day
	Bupropion	Wellbutrin	200–300 mg/day
Tricyclics (TCAs)	Amitriptyline	Elavil	75–300 mg/day
	Imipramine	Tofranil	75–200 mg/day
	Desipramine	Norpramin	75–300 mg/day
	Nortriptyline	Pamelor	75–100 mg/day
Monoamine oxidase inhibitors (MAOIs)	Phenelzine	Nardil	15–90 mg/day
	Tranylcypromine	Parnate	30–60 mg/day

Source: Daley and Moss 2002.

TABLE 10.3

Pharmacotherapy of Substance-Use Disorders

Type of Chemical Dependence	Class of Drug	Examples of Chemical Names	Examples of Brand Names	Typical Dose Ranges
Opiate dependence	Narcotic replacement maintenance	Methadone	Dolophine	40–160 mg/day
		Levomethadyl (LAAM)	ORLAAM	60–90 mg/day
	Narcotic antagonist maintenance	Naltrexone	Revia	50 mg/day
	Mixed replacement/ antagonist	Buprenorphine	Buprenex	8–32 mg/day
Alcohol dependence	Alcohol Anticraving	Naltrexone	Revia	50 mg/day
	Aversive therapy	Disulfram	Antabuse	250 mg/day
Nicotine dependence	Nicotine Anticraving	Bupropion	Zyban	150–300 mg/day
	Nicotine replacement maintenance	Nicotine	Nicorette (gum)	36–48 mg/day
			NicoDerm (patch)	15–21 mg/day
			Nicotrol (nasal spray)	8–40 mg/day

Source: Daley and Moss 2002.

T A B L E 1 0 . 4	

Diagnostic Criteria of Major Depressive Disorder

A. At least five of the following symptoms have been present during the same two-week period and represent a change from previous functioning; at least one of the symptoms is either (1) depressed mood or (2) loss of interest or pleasure. (Do not include symptoms that are clearly due to a physical condition, mood-incongruent delusions or hallucinations, incoherence, or marked loosening of associations.)

  1. Depressed mood (or can be irritable mood in children and adolescents) most of the day, nearly every day, as indicated either by subjective account or observation by others

  2. Markedly diminished interest or pleasure in all, or almost all, activities most of the day, nearly every day (as indicated either by subjective account or observation by others of apathy most of the time)

  3. Significant weight loss or weight gain when not dieting (e.g., more than 5% of body weight in a month), or decrease or increase in appetite nearly every day (in children, consider failure to make expected weight gains)

  4. Insomnia or hypersomnia nearly every day

  5. Psychomotor agitation or retardation nearly every day (observable by others, not merely subjective feelings of restlessness or being slowed down)

  6. Fatigue or loss of energy nearly every day

  7. Feelings of worthlessness or excessive or inappropriate guilt (which may be delusional) nearly every day (not merely self-reproach or guilt about being sick)

  8. Diminished ability to think or concentrate, or indecisiveness, nearly every day (either by subjective account or as observed by others)

  9. Recurrent thoughts of death (not just fear of dying), recurrent suicidal ideation without a specific plan, or a suicide attempt or a specific plan for committing suicide

B. 1. It cannot be established that an organic factor initiated and maintained the disturbance.

  2. The disturbance is not a normal reaction to the death of a loved one (uncomplicated bereavement). *Note:* Morbid preoccupation with worthlessness, suicidal ideation, marked functional impairment or psychomotor retardation, or prolonged duration suggest bereavement complicated by major depression.

C. At no time during the disturbance have there been delusions or hallucinations for as long as two weeks in the absence of prominent mood symptoms (i.e., before the mood symptoms developed or after they have remitted).

D. Not superimposed on schizophrenia, schizophreniform disorder, delusional disorder, or psychotic disorder.

From American Psychiatric Association: *Diagnostic and Statistical Manual of Mental Disorders*, Fourth Edition, Revised, Washington, D.C., American Psychiatric Association, 1994.

Episodes of depression that are longer in duration require adequate and careful attentiveness and sensitivity to potential suicide attempts. (See Table 10.4.)

Case Study 10.2 takes a look at a familiar storybook character who suffers from depression.

Dysthymic Disorder

Dysthymic disorder is a mood disorder of longer term than major depression but is a lower-grade depression. Patients with dysthymic disorder frequently comment that they have never felt completely happy or that, if they do achieve a period of feeling

Case Study 10.2

Eeyore Syndrome

The donkey, Eeyore, in the children's story *Winnie-the-Pooh,* could be clinically described as suffering from major depression or dysthymic disorder.

When Eeyore is asked by Pooh and other characters in the story, "Would you like to go swimming today?" Eeyore answers, in his low, depressed voice in a number of negative statements, "No, I'm so tired today and it's too far to walk to the swimming hole," or "I might get sun burned on a sunny day like today," or "It's too hot and I might get overheated."

Eeyore worries about everything. Instead of enjoying being with his friends, he isolates himself. Instead of enjoying the activity (swimming) and a beautiful summer day, he can't see anything positive. He is constantly in the black cloud of depression, even though it is a bright, sunny day.

Discussion

Remember, two major signs of depression demonstrated by "Eeyore" are:

- anergia (a lack of energy for activities that one would normally be motivated to do—e.g. swimming on a sunny summer day)
- anhedonia (an inability to gain pleasure from something that normally would be pleasurable—e.g. playing/swimming with friends).

---

well, it is relatively short-lived. Anxiety symptoms, headaches, and muscle tension are frequent, in addition to symptoms of depression. (See Table 10.5.) Patients with dysthymic disorder come to assume that their own baseline mood is normal; they are frequently surprised that they actually do experience improvement with treatment. Only 25 percent of patients with major depression receive adequate diagnosis and treatment; it is very likely that the percentage is even lower for dysthymic disorder, given the less intense and less notable degree of symptoms. Case Study 10.3 presents an example of dysthymic disorder.

Atypical Depression

Atypical depression is not a common condition, as the symptoms and duration of symptoms are different from those of major depression or dysthymic disorder.

Atypical depression is frequently the diagnosis for many adult children of alcoholics. Usually, a patient with atypical depression experiences intense and sudden depressions in response to interpersonal loss or threatened interpersonal loss. We may, in fact, be talking about a condition similar to that described by James Masterson (1976) as abandonment depression.

This condition is common in patients who may also have severe personality disturbances, such as borderline personality disorder. Psychodynamically, a sudden severe depression in response to feelings of loss, rejection, and/or abandonment may be related to a childhood loss so traumatic that it triggers this depression when feelings of loss are activated in present-day situations.

TABLE 10.5

Diagnostic Criteria for Dysthymic Disorder

A. Depressed mood (or can be irritable mood in children and adolescents) most of the day, more days than not, as indicated either by subjective account or observation by others, for at least two years (one year for children and adolescents)

B. Presence, while depressed, of at least two of the following:
1. Poor appetite or overeating
2. Insomnia or hypersomnia
3. Low energy or fatigue
4. Low self-esteem
5. Poor concentration or difficulty making decisions
6. Feelings of hopelessness

C. During a two-year period (one year for children and adolescents) of the disturbance, never without the symptoms in A for more than two months at a time

D. No evidence of an unequivocal major depressive episode during the first two years (one year for children and adolescents) of the disturbance. *Note:* There may have been a previous major depressive episode, provided there was a full remission (no significant signs or symptoms for six months) before development of the dysthymia. In addition, after these two years (one year in children or adolescents) of dysthymia, there may be superimposed episodes of major depression, in which case both diagnoses are given.

E. Has never had a manic episode or an unequivocal hypomanic episode

F. Not superimposed on a chronic psychotic disorder, such as schizophrenia or delusional disorder

G. It cannot be established that an organic factor initiated and maintained the disturbance—e.g., prolonged administration of an antihypertensive medication.

From American Psychiatric Association: *Diagnostic and Statistical Manual of Mental Disorders,* Third Edition, Revised, Washington, D.C., American Psychiatric Association, 1987.

Atypical depression is also different because these patients may not report a loss of appetite and insomnia but, instead, experience an increase in appetite and sleep. Perhaps this is also indicative of the frequent problems in body image, binge patterns of eating, and other eating disorders that these clients exhibit. Patients with atypical depression may increase alcohol/drug use in a similar manner.

Case Study 10.4 presents an example of atypical depression.

Organic Depression

Depression may also occur as a result of organic factors, such as brain tumors, head injuries, nutritional deficiencies, physical illness, or alcohol/drug use. Many chemically dependent patients have nutritional deficiencies as a result of decreased intake, malabsorption, and poor eating habits. Alcohol is especially high in calories with poor nutritional value. Other drugs disrupt the appetite (e.g., cocaine reduces appetite) and create problems in nutrition. After initial recovery from alcohol/drug use, depression may continue for a while due to nutritional causes. However, once a normal diet and vitamin therapy have been reimplemented, organic (nutritional) depression should improve.

Head injuries are fairly common, especially in end stage alcoholics, and may contribute to cognitive deficits as well as mood disturbances. Pancreatic cancer is

Case Study 10.3

Dysthymic Disorder

Duane

Duane is a 39-year-old married male who completed inpatient treatment for alcoholism and cocaine dependence nearly 3 years ago. Since then he has maintained sobriety while regularly attending his aftercare counseling sessions and cocaine and Alcoholics Anonymous meetings. He has also been involved in individual and group counseling to deal with the effects of growing up in an alcoholic and emotionally abusive family system. Despite these efforts, he continues to experience symptoms of low energy, periods of irritability, and an inability to have fun without a great deal of effort. His therapist has referred him for a psychiatric evaluation.

Most notable in Duane's history is that earlier he was abstinent from alcohol and drugs for approximately 4 to 5 months. During that time, he experienced the same depressive symptoms. Besides alcoholism, his family history includes several relatives with depression. A recent physical exam was unremarkable.

Discussion

Explain why his relapses might occur after four to five months.
As his counselor, what would you recommend to cope with the depression?
What kinds of physical, emotional and interpersonal activities might help this client?
What kind of cognitive-behavioral approaches might be taken?

Case Study 10.4

Atypical Depression

Gail

Gail is 28 years old, single, and an accountant. She is extremely shy and often feels uncomfortable in social situations. She is 7 years sober and attends AA meetings regularly. Gail cries easily whenever she is involved in conflict. She suffered a number of losses in her childhood, including the loss of her father, who was reported missing in action in the Vietnam War. Around the same time, Gail's maternal grandmother, to whom Gail was extremely close, died while sleeping in the same bed with Gail. Gail has also had to deal with the issue of having been sexually abused at 12 years of age.

After Gail began counseling, her self-confidence improved. But she still felt sad, so she got an evaluation from a psychiatrist experienced in alcohol and drug recovery. The psychiatrist recommended an antidepressant. After 2 weeks, Gail felt tremendous relief and realized that she had been struggling with depression for quite some time.

Discussion Questions

Can you describe the stages of grief (DABDA)?
How does grief get complicated by an "atypical" depression?
What would you recommend for Gail's shyness?

also more common in the alcoholic population and can look identical to major depression clinically.

Prolonged use of opiates, benzodiazepines, alcohol, sedative hypnotics, and especially stimulant drugs can produce depression. Users of cocaine and amphetamines typically experience a crash at the end of a binge pattern of cocaine use. This occurs because of the depletion of the neurotransmitter that the stimulant drug causes to be released in greater than normal quantities.

Bipolar Disorder

The first bipolar disorder described and understood was the classic manic-depressive illness. Manic-depressive illness consists of repeated depressive episodes over the years; these episodes are typically briefer than those in a major depression. In addition, a manic-depressive has less frequent but equally intense highs, or manic episodes. Characteristics of the manic phase of the disorder include the following:

- Euphoria
- Irritability
- Racing thoughts
- Decreased need for sleep
- Excessive spending
- Grandiosity
- Pressured speech
- An increased preoccupation with sexuality, religious, and/or philosophical themes

A manic episode may also include delusional beliefs and disorganization of thinking. Highs may not always involve euphoria; many patients simply become much more irritable, bizarre, and erratic in their behavior. Case Study 10.5 presents an example of bipolar disorder.

Descriptions offered by people with bipolar disorder give valuable insights into the various mood states associated with the illness (NIMH, 2001):

Depression: I doubt completely my ability to do anything well. It seems as though my mind has slowed down and burned out to the point of being virtually useless. . . . (I am) haunt(ed) . . . with the total, the desperate hopelessness of it all. . . . Others say, "It's only temporary, it will pass, you will get over it," but of course they haven't any idea of how I feel, although they are certain they do. If I can't feel, move, think or care, then what on earth is the point?

Case Study 10.5

Bipolar Disorder

Gustav

Gustav is a 45-year-old salesman with a history of binge drinking and erratic job performance. He goes on 2- to 3-week binges every spring and uses alcohol only socially at other times. He feels remorseful about these binges. In the weeks preceding a binge, he typically is quite productive, energetic, and successful in making sales. Gustav comments that his springtime burst in earnings helps compensate for his lackluster winter performance, when he typically feels lethargic and moody. In the past, he has used cocaine intermittently during the winter months to help brighten his mood. His finances have not allowed him to do cocaine in recent years. His occupational history is notable for multiple sales jobs across the country. He has made a number of impulsive springtime moves to pursue hot job possibilities. He does not find this unusual because his father, uncle, and brother all have similar histories. Closer questioning reveals that, during the springtime bursts of increased sales activity, he has less need for sleep, a feeling of euphoria, and an increased philosophical preoccupation. Coworkers have commented on his high energy level and rapid speech. He has no history of previous psychiatric treatment.

Gustav's history reveals a patient with a bipolar disorder who binge drinks when he is high. There is a seasonal component to his mood swings, as he experiences manic symptoms in the springtime and symptoms of depression in the winter. Notably, he has a family history of similar mood swings and a personal history of minimal alcohol or drug use when he is not high. He is a good candidate for treatment with a mood-cycling agent, such as lithium, and would benefit from counseling on how to manage his impulses to drink. He should use available resources for support, such as AA.

Discussion Questions

Why is this client/patient so difficult to treat?
What would you recommend for treatment?
How would you "engage" this client in counseling?
Would you get permission and talk to family members for counseling with Gustav?
What problems and sabotaging do you anticipate in counseling Gustav?

Hypomania: At first when I'm high, it's tremendous . . . ideas are fast . . . like shooting stars you follow until brighter ones appear. . . . All shyness disappears, the right words and gestures are suddenly there . . . uninteresting people, things become intensely interesting. Sensuality is pervasive, the desire to seduce and be seduced is irresistible. Your marrow is infused with unbelievable feelings of ease, power, well-being, omnipotence, euphoria . . . you can do anything . . . but somewhere this changes.

Mania: The fast ideas become too fast and there are far too many . . . overwhelming confusion replaces clarity . . . you stop keeping up with it— memory goes. Infectious humor ceases to amuse. Your friends become frightened . . . everything is now against the grain . . . you are irritable, angry, frightened, uncontrollable, and trapped.

TABLE 10.6

Examples of Medications for Bipolar Disorder

Phase of Treatment	Class of Drug	Examples of Chemical Names	Examples of Brand Names	Typical Dose Ranges
Acute mania/ hypomania	Mood stabilizers	Lithium	Lithobid	600–1800 mg/day
		Valproate	Depakene	250–750 mg/day
		Carbamazepine	Tegretol	400–800 mg/day
	Typical antipsychotics	Haloperidol	Haldol	Dependent on symptoms and response
		Fluphenazine	Prolixin	
		Chlorpromazine	Thorazine	
	Atypical antipsychotics	Resperidone	Resperidol	Dependent on symptoms and response
		Olanzapine	Zyprexa	
		Quetiapine	Seroquel	
Bipolar depression	Combined mood stabilizers and antidepressant drugs	See chapter on depression for listing of antidepressant medications		
Maintenance phase	Long-term mood stabilizers	Lithium	Lithobid	See above
		Valproate	Depakene	
		Carbamazepine	Tegretol	

Source: Daley and Moss 2002.

A variety of bipolar disorders have somewhat different patterns. Some patients experience recurrent depressive episodes with smaller and less intense manic episodes (hypomania) in between. During a hypomanic episode, a patient might typically experience all of the preceding symptoms except for the psychotic symptoms, such as disorganization of thinking, delusional material, and bizarre behavior.

Patients with bipolar disorder are typically plagued by mood instability; they may experience mood swings as frequently as daily. Patients who have significant mood swings, more than four times per year, are said to have a rapid cycling bipolar disorder. A growing accumulation of evidence suggests that some of these rapid cycling bipolar disorders may actually be a variation of epilepsy. Some of these patients may respond favorably to the medication that had previously been used only for epilepsy.

Table 10.6 lists common medications for bipolar disorder.

Mood-Cycling Disorder

The frequency of the cycling and the amplitude of the highs and lows are aggravated by alcohol/drug use. A relatively low-grade mood-cycling pattern may become much more aggravated with the use of alcohol/drugs, and the symptoms may become more clinically apparent.

Patients who otherwise have no psychotic symptoms, such as delusions, hallucinations, or disorganization of thinking, and have a mood-cycling disorder may develop psychotic symptoms, given the extra push from alcohol/drug use. (This is especially apparent with cocaine, amphetamines, hallucinogens, and even marijuana use.) Again, this stresses the importance of taking a thorough alcohol/drug history with each patient.

Personality Traits vs. Personality Disorder

In describing people's personalities, we may think of traits that describe the way people behave, experience life, and interact in relationships. Personality is an important dimension that defines who we are. "Each of us is known not only by his or her physical features, occupation, and family background, but especially by what is called personality" (Nace 1990).

The American Psychiatric Association (APA) defines personality as "the ingrained pattern of behavior that each person evolves, both consciously and unconsciously, as the style of life or way of being in adapting to the environment" (APA 1984).

Most personality traits have both adaptive and maladaptive qualities or features. For example, being logical and organized are valuable traits in a computer programmer. But always being ruled by logic and being compulsively organized can also be maladaptive, since these traits may limit one's capacity to be emotionally expressive. On the other hand, a creative and artistic person might not be as suited to a situation or an occupation that requires logical, politically correct, and decisive action. We all have a mix of personality traits, which define us as individuals. When personality traits are persistently maladaptive and lead to chronic difficulty in interpersonal, occupational, and social functioning, there is a personality disorder.

The fourth edition of the *Diagnostic and Statistical Manual of Mental Disorders* (APA 1994), known as the *DSM-IV*, recognizes 11 personality disorders and divides them into three clusters, or groups (see Table 10.7):

Cluster A is a group characterized by odd and eccentric traits and may lead to psychiatric conditions, such as delusional disorder or schizophrenia.

✤ Personality Disorders and Substance-Use Disorders

TABLE 10.7

Personality Disorders

To qualify for a personality disorder diagnosis, an individual's traits and behaviors must be longstanding and must cause significant impairment in social or occupational functioning or subjective distress. The following are the 11 DSM III-R personality disorders.

Cluster A	Cluster B	Cluster C
Paranoid	Antisocial	Avoidant
Schizoid	Borderline	Dependent
Schizotypal	Histrionic	Obsessive-Compulsive
	Narcissistic	Passive-Aggressive

From American Psychiatric Association: *Diagnostic and Statistical Manual of Mental Disorders*, Third Edition, Revised, Washington, D.C., American Psychiatric Association, 1987.

Cluster B is a group characterized by behavior that is erratic, emotional, or dramatic. This cluster has the strongest association with substance abuse, particularly antisocial and borderline personality disorder.

Cluster C is a group characterized by feelings of fear and anxiety. Substance abuse occurs in this group, but not as frequently as in Cluster B.

Personality Disorder vs. Chemical Dependency Disorder

The difficulties in differentiating between a personality disorder and an alcohol/drug disorder are often confounded by a common overlap in behaviors associated with each disorder. "Some behaviors that are symptomatic of particular Axis II disorders (manipulativeness, exploitativeness, dishonesty) may be integral or sometimes even adaptive aspects of addicted behavior, particularly among individuals who use illicit drugs" (Weiss 1996).

Personality-disordered individuals may be attracted to alcohol/drugs to self-medicate feelings of discomfort, anxiety, depression, anger, grief, and even shyness. V. M. Hesselbrook and associates (1983) reported that 52 percent of a sample of male alcoholics had a current or lifetime diagnosis of antisocial personality disorder.

Kleinman and colleagues (1990) found that, of 76 lower-social-class cocaine abusers, 71 percent had at least one personality disorder and 40 percent had two or more. The four most common personality disorders identified were

- Antisocial personality disorder—21 percent
- Passive-aggressive personality disorder—21 percent
- Borderline personality disorder—18 percent
- Self-defeating personality disorder—18 percent

Weiss and Mirin (1986), in their study of an upper-middle-class addict population, found borderline personality disorder and narcissistic personality disorder to be the most common diagnoses.

Craig (1988) used the very sensitive Millon Clinical Multiaxial Inventory and found that, of 121 opiate addicts from the Chicago area, all of them (100 percent) had at least one personality disorder and 27 percent had more than one. The most common diagnoses were

- Antisocial personality disorder—22 percent
- Narcissistic personality disorder—18 percent
- Borderline personality disorder—16 percent
- Dependent personality disorder—16 percent.

This surprising result brings up the question of to whether drug abuse and addiction lead to behaviors that are characteristic of personality disorders. Edward Kaufman, author of *Psychotherapy of Addicted Persons* (1995), points out that the characteristic inherent in substance abusers—such as unstable and intense interpersonal relationships; inappropriate, intense, out-of-control anger; affective instability; and physically self-damaging acts—can all meet the diagnostic criteria for borderline personality disorder and other personality disorders. Widiger et al. (1986) state that there is good evidence that many substance abusers who are diagnosed as having borderline personality disorder are really "pseudoborderline."

Case Study 10.6
Depression and Withdrawal Symptoms

Evan

Evan is a 27-year-old male who is receiving inpatient treatment for his cocaine dependency. He was referred for a psychiatric evaluation because of his current severe depression symptoms. He had been freebasing cocaine for 2 to 3 months prior to admission to the treatment unit 3 days ago. Now he is feeling severely depressed and experiencing cocaine cravings.

Evan has no history of depression and no family history of psychiatric disorders. During childhood, he experienced hyperactivity and had mild learning disabilities. He notes that since beginning drug use in his mid teens, he has preferred stimulant drugs ("they calm me down"). He has received inpatient treatment for cocaine dependence once previously and had 2 years of complete abstinence before relapsing several months ago. During his clean time, he experienced no mood difficulties but continued to feel somewhat hyper.

Evan is a patient who experiences severe depression as part of cocaine withdrawal. There is no reason to suspect an underlying problem with depression, given his personal and family history. He would benefit from a short course of treatment with desipramine, an antidepressant that is particularly effective for treating acute depression and cocaine cravings during cocaine withdrawal. Such treatment typically lasts for 2 to 4 weeks.

Discussion Questions

> What relapse prevention strategies might you suggest for Evan (see Chapter 11 for relapse prone behaviors)
> Could Evan be diagnosed with ADHD? What symptoms indicate this?
> What do you think Evan's prognosis is for recovery?
> What would he need to do to increase the probability that he would sustain recovery and sobriety?

It is clear from the research that personality traits and personality disorders play a major role in substance abuse. The extent and depth of the role personality plays in substance abuse is confounded by the old "chicken or egg" question. Did the personality disorder cause substance abuse, or did substance abuse lead to behaviors that resemble the criteria for a diagnosis of a personality disorder? Case Study 10.6 presents an example of an individual who suffers from depression when withdrawing from an addictive substance. Case Study 10.7 describes personality problems for an individual who is addicted to alcohol.

Antisocial Personality Disorder
Antisocial Personality Disorder and Chemical Dependency

Antisocial personality disorder (ASPD) is estimated to be found in 2 to 3 percent of the male population. Of all the personality disorders, the strongest relationship with substance abuse is with antisocial personality disorder. ASPD has been found in 15 percent of alcoholic men, as compared were a 4 percent lifetime prevalence in

Case Study 10.7

Alcoholism

Charlie

Charlie is a 53-year-old married engineer at a local aerospace company. He has a long-standing, but progressively worsening, history of irritability, nervousness, and difficulty sleeping. Charlie is under the care of Dr. Greenhorn, a physician just out of his internal medicine residency. Dr. Greenhorn assumed the practice of Charlie's previous physician and golfing buddy, Dr. Barleycorn.

Dr. Greenhorn reviews the previous medical record and notes difficulties with stomach irritation and ulcers, elevated triglyceride and cholesterol levels, and persistent complaints of decreased libido, or sex drive. Charlie requests some of the sleeping pills that Dr. Barleycorn had prescribed. Further questioning reveals a history of regular heavy drinking, which began when Charlie and Dr. Barleycorn were fraternity brothers. This heavy drinking behavior persisted over the years. Charlie typically drinks three or four mixed drinks or glasses of beer per weeknight and six or seven drinks per night on the weekends. He can recall going 2 to 3 days without alcohol during a church retreat several years ago. At that time, he felt very shaky and irritable. Physical examination reveals a moderately enlarged liver, and laboratory studies reveal elevated liver enzyme levels and mild anemia.

Discussion Questions

Do you think his personal relationship with his physician is a problem? If so, explain why.

Why do you think Charlie has sleeping problems?

What would you recommend?

---

nonalcoholic men (Helzer and Pryzbeck 1988). Hesselbrook, Meyer, and Kenner (1985) found ASPD to be the most common additional diagnosis in a hospitalized sample of more than 200 male alcoholics—49 percent met the diagnostic criteria for ASPD. The diagnosis is predominately attributed to men, whereas borderline personality disorder is primarily found in women. The ratio of men to women with antisocial personality is approximately 8 to 1. In contrast, the ratio of women to men is 8 to 1 for borderline personality disorder.

Childhood Precursors of Antisocial Personality Disorder

Conduct disorders and attention-deficit hyperactive disorder (ADHD) in children are precursors of both substance abuse and antisocial personality disorder. Early assessment, intervention, and counseling with these young people and their families are recommended to address current problems and to prevent future problems.

Denial, Alcohol/Drugs, and Antisocial Personality Disorder

The shame attached to identifying one's personality traits as causing problems in life and in relationships often results in denial. It is easier to blame others for conflicts, problems, and personality issues than to take responsibility. A major feature of a personality disorder is that the individual may not consider the personality trait that is causing conflict as undesirable. The individual might attribute others' complaints about them as the fault of others—"The hell with them if they can't take a joke."

The traditional denial defense mechanisms of rationalization and minimization are used to deny the true dimensions of a personality disorder. Integrity, honesty, and responsibility are discounted in the self-centered behavior of the ASPD.

Difficulty *regulating behaviors* (poor impulse control, recklessness, and a failure to anticipate consequences) and *affect intolerance* (the inability to recognize, regulate, and tolerate emotions) lead to substance abuse (Khantzian 1981).

Nace and associates (1983) described alcohol/drugs as providing immediate gratification followed by regressive behaviors. These regressive behaviors include the following:

- *Impulsivity*—cannot delay gratification; has stimulus-bound decreased frustration tolerance; is impatient; overreacts to situations; is inconsistent
- *Self-centeredness*—is stubborn and defiant; lacks empathy; exhibits grandiosity; either overvalues or undervalues self; sees things in either/or, rather than shades of gray; can't compromise; exhibits perfectionism, sees self as unique
- *Passivity*—is withdrawn; is isolated; feels helpless; is "mentally lazy"; avoids self-revelation
- *Affect intolerance*—has difficulty in recognizing feelings; fears feelings; has decreased ability to endure or regulate painful emotional states

Some questions that may identify antisocial personality traits are the following:

- Do you exaggerate your achievements and talents?
- Are you preoccupied with thoughts of great success, power, brilliance, beauty, achievement, or idealized love?
- Do you often want a great deal of attention and admiration?
- Do you have a tendency to dominate conversations and activities (perhaps "showing off")?
- Do you expect special favors but feel you don't have to return them?
- Do you sometimes feel surprised and angry that people do not do what you want them to?
- Do you ever take advantage of others so that you can get what you want?
- Do you sometimes disregard the rights or personal boundaries of others?
- Do you alternate between thinking too much and too little of a person?
- Do you sometimes feel you don't care enough about other people's pain and feelings?
- Do you change jobs frequently? Have you changed jobs three or more times in the past five years, but not because of the kind of job or because of economic or seasonal fluctuations?
- Have you been unemployed for six months or more during a period of five years, when you might have been able to work?
- Have you walked off jobs at various times without having another job already lined up?

- If you have children, do you feel you adequately provide food, safety, and shelter for them?
- Have you spent money on drugs, alcohol, or personal items that probably should have been spent on *necessities?*
- Have you committed repeated thefts or engaged in illegal occupations (fencing, selling drugs, prostitution, pimping, etc.)?
- Have you had multiple arrests or been convicted of a felony?

Extreme difficulties in relationships with your spouse or partner could also indicate antisocial personality traits. The following are some further questions to consider.

- Have you been separated (whether legally married or not) or divorced several times?
- Have you had 10 or more sexual partners in one year?
- Do you sometimes feel that you are overly irritable and aggressive?
- Have you frequently been involved in physical fights or assaults?
- Have you ever physically abused your spouse or children?
- Have you failed to plan ahead for the future or have you been extremely impulsive?
- Have you lied repeatedly, used aliases, or "conned" others to get what you wanted?
- Have you frequently driven while drunk?

TABLE 10.8

Diagnostic Criteria for Antisocial Personality Disorder

A. There is a pervasive pattern of disregard for and violation of the rights of others occurring since age 15, as indicated by three (or more) of the following:
    1. Failure to conform to social norms with respect to lawful behaviors as indicated by repeatedly performing acts that are grounds for arrest
    2. Deceitfulness, as indicated by repeated lying, use of aliases, or conning others for personal profit or pleasure
    3. Impulsivity or failure to plan ahead
    4. Irritability and aggressiveness, as indicated by repeated physical fights or assaults
    5. Reckless disregard for safety of self or others
    6. Consistent irresponsibility, as indicated by repeated failure to sustain consistent work behavior or honor financial obligations
    7. Lack of remorse, as indicated by being indifferent to or rationalizing having hurt, mistreated, or stolen from another
B. The individual is at least 18 years.
C. There is evidence of conduct disorder with onset before age 15 years.
D. The occurrence of antisocial behavior is not exclusively during the course of schizophrenia or a manic episode.

From American Psychiatric Association, *Diagnostic and Statistical Manual of Mental Disorders,* 4th ed. (1994) Washington D.C.

Case Study 10.8

Antisocial Personality Traits

Tony

Tony is a 24-year-old construction worker. He says he began working after leaving high school at the age of 15. As a child, he was hyperactive, and his behavior problems caused him to perform poorly in school. Thus, school was frustrating for Tony and his teachers.

Tony told lies, stole, and fought with other children. His family took him to a counselor (a behavioral specialist) after Tony repeatedly set fires. During one school year, Tony was treated with Ritalin, a medication that helps children calm down and stay focused, and he did better in school. But during summer vacation he stopped taking the medication and refused to resume taking it the next fall.

Since dropping out of high school, Tony has held a number of jobs. Usually he gets fired because he fights with his coworkers or doesn't show up for work; this irritates Tony, who feels victimized. Although his employment—or lack of it—has caused financial problems, Tony admits that he has lied and not paid his bills. He tells friends, creditors, and bill collectors, "The check is in the mail," or "I'll send the payment as soon as. . . ." Although he has a relationship with a woman, he has also had several one-night stands with other women he has met at bars. He has snorted and smoked cocaine, often squandering his money while partying with friends and women he picks up. His parents have bailed him out financially several times. Tony's attitude was "They have the money, so they should be able to help me out."

After two DUIs, Tony was referred to a chemical dependency program as part of a deferred prosecution. He is now slowly working on both his chemical dependency and his personality problems.

Discussion Questions

What is your prediction for Tony's sobriety?
What would help Tony stay sober?
Do you think Tony could be "rigorously honest"?

The *DSM-IV* diagnostic criteria for ASPD are shown in Table 10.8. Case Study 10.8 presents an example of the problems an individual with ASPD can create for himself and others.

Borderline Personality Disorder and Chemical Dependency

The second most common personality disorder that has a high incidence of substance abuse is borderline personality disorder. A number of studies have reported co-occurring substance abuse and borderline personality disorder—43 percent (Koenigsberg et al. 1985), 28 percent (Johnson and Connelly 1981), and 13 percent (Nace, Saxon, and Shore 1983).

In Chapter 6, we described abandonment depression as the common factor in borderline personality disorder. As previously mentioned, the term *abandonment depression* was coined by James Masterson to describe a personality disorder that has six key elements: (1) feelings of emptiness and void; (2) hopelessness and helplessness; (3) panic; (4) guilt; (5) suicidal depression; and (6) homicidal rage.

Someone suffering from abandonment depression probably had a highly stressful separation from parent(s) or a primary caregiver early in life (18 months to two years of age). The separation could have been caused by natural events (death, separation, divorce, health, etc.), or the parent(s) might not have been emotionally available.

Some common questions that may help identify abandonment follow. Did you have parents or guardians who

- Were not open or available to you physically and emotionally?
- Attacked you verbally or physically or blamed you for many of their problems?
- Gave mixed messages, called *double binds,* saying one thing but meaning something else?
- Had unreasonably high expectations or standards for you or had ambiguous expectations of how you should behave, what you should do, and how you should feel?
- Did not show you warmth or sensitivity, did not make you feel secure or safe, or did not pay much attention to your feelings, concerns, and conflicts?
- Discounted your sense of self or violated your physical and psychological boundaries, such as by committing physical, emotional, or sexual violations?
- Disparaged, blamed, or rejected you if you had any difficulty with developmental tasks?
- Disregarded, ridiculed, blamed, or teased you?
- Jokingly or seriously threatened to abandon or leave you?
- Made you feel that your fears were unwarranted or inappropriate?
- Did not understand you or were insensitive to your needs and desires?

Patients with borderline personality disorder have a marked instability of mood and often form intense interpersonal attachments. They typically feel abandoned and rejected during instances of real or perceived interpersonal loss. Many borderline patients engage in repeated self-destructive or suicidal acts during episodes of intense depression and despair. Theoretical explanations of the origin of this personality disorder range from developmental to biochemical explanations. In all probability, the condition is a result of both nature and nurture (i.e., inadequate bonding and parenting during early years and a genetic predisposition). Most clinicians agree that borderline patients have a great deal of difficulty regulating their degree of attachment to others. They want the closeness and trust that intimacy brings but fear the dependency, vulnerability, and possible rejection that may occur. Not surprisingly, these patients have a high incidence of chemical dependency as they attempt to blunt the intensity of their emotions by using alcohol/drugs. They are especially prone to becoming dependent on addicting prescription drugs, such as benzodiazepines. Their impulsivity, frequent thoughts of suicide, and substance abuse make them especially at risk when prescribed psychiatric medication. Many psychiatric medications are lethal when taken in amounts only 5 to 10 times the usual dosage, especially if the individual is already toxic with alcohol or drugs.

Abstinence from alcohol/drugs is essential in treating borderline patients, as their already fragile mood stability is quite sensitive to alcohol/drugs. Such patients generally need psychotherapy. When medication management is indicated, doctors

TABLE 10.9

Examples of Medications for Borderline Personality Disorder

Class of Drug	Examples of Chemical Names	Examples of Brand Names	Typical Dose Ranges
Typical oral antipsychotic	Haloperidol	Haldol	4–75 mg/day
	Fluphenazine	Prolixin	1–10 mg/day
	Chlorpromazine	Thorazine	100–400 mg/day
"Atypical" oral antipsychotics	Clozapine	Clozaril	200–600 mg/day
	Resperidone	Resperidol	2–6 mg/day
	Olanzapine	Zyprexa	5–10 mg/day
	Quetiapine	Seroquel	150–750 mg/day
	Ziprasidone	Geodon	40–160 mg/day
Selective serotonin reuptake inhibitors (SSRIs)	Fluoxetine	Prozac	20–80 mg/day
	Paroxetine	Paxil	20–50 mg/day
	Sertraline	Zoloft	50–200 mg/day
	Citalopram	Celexa	20–60 mg/day
Bicyclics	Venlafaxine	Effexor	75–225 mg/day
	Mirtazapine	Remeron	15–45 mg/day
Heterocyclics	Trazodone	Deseryl	150–400 mg/day
	Maprotiline	Ludiomil	75–150 mg/day
	Bupropion	Wellbutrin	200–300 mg/day
Monoamine oxidase inhibitors (MAOIs)	Phenelzine	Nardil	15–90 mg/day
	Tranylcypromine	Parnate	30–60 mg/day
Mood stabilizers	Lithium	Lithobid	600–1800 mg/day
	Valproate	Depakene	250–750 mg/day
	Carbamazepine	Tegretol	400–800 mg/day

Source: Daley and Moss 2002.

commonly prescribe antidepressant or mood-cycling agents. Which medication the patient receives depends on the clinical symptoms that are most troublesome (more on treatment of dual disorders appears in Chapter 11). Medications commonly prescribed for borderline personality disorder are listed in Table 10.9.

Do you have a pattern of unstable and intense personal relationships? For instance, does your attitude about your relationships keep changing? Do you idealize or romanticize your friends? Do you put them down, manipulate them, or often use them to meet your own needs? Do you find yourself treating some friends very well and some very poorly? Do you have intense anger that is not really justified? Or do you lack control of your anger? Are you concerned about your self-image, your gender identity, your long-term goals or career choice, your friendship patterns, your values, or your loyalties? (If you are concerned, you might have thoughts like these: *"Who am I?"* or *"I feel just like my sister when I'm good."*) Do you have deep mood swings? Are you depressed when alone? Do you try very hard to avoid being alone? Do you feel empty or bored most of the time?

TABLE 10.10

Diagnostic Criteria for Borderline Personality Disorder

A pervasive pattern of instability of interpersonal relationships, self-image and affects, and marked impulsivity beginning by early adulthood and present in a variety of contexts, as indicated by five (or more) of the following:

1. Frantic efforts to avoid real or imagined abandonment
2. A pattern of unstable and intense interpersonal relationships characterized by alternating between extremes of idealization and devaluation
3. Identity disturbance: marked and persistently unstable self-image or sense of self
4. Impulsivity in at least two areas that are potentially self-damaging (e.g., spending, sex, substance abuse, reckless driving, binge eating)
5. Recurrent suicidal behavior, gestures, or threats or self-mutilating behavior
6. Affective instability due to a marked reactivity of mood (e.g., intense episodic dysphoria, irritability, or anxiety usually lasting a few hours and only rarely more than a few days)
7. Chronic feelings of emptiness
8. Inappropriate, intense anger or difficulty controlling anger (e.g., frequent displays of temper, constant anger, recurrent physical fights)
9. Transient, stress-related paranoid ideation or severe dissociative symptoms

Source: American Psychiatric Association: *Diagnostic and Statistical Manual of Mental Disorders,* Fourth Edition, Washington, D.C., American Psychiatric Association, 1994.

Table 10.10 lists the *DSM-IV* diagnostic criteria for borderline personality disorder. Case Study 10.9 illustrates the dual disorder of borderline personality disorder and substance addiction.

❈ Treatment of Disorders Co-occurring with Substance Abuse

Treatment of co-occurring disorders means addressing both the mental illness and the substance abuse. Treating one and ignoring the other will only result in relapse. American Psychiatric Association (2000) Practice Guidelines for the Treatment of Psychiatric Disorders include these:

1. Establish and maintain a therapeutic alliance with the client.
2. Manage the client's psychiatric (or substance use) symptoms and monitor the status of these over time.
3. Provide education regarding the disorder(s) and treatment.
4. Determine the need for medications and other specific treatments.
5. Develop an overall treatment plan.
6. Enhance adherence to the treatment plan.
7. Help the client and family adapt to the psychosocial effects of the disorder(s).
8. Promote early recognition of new episodes and help identify factors that precipitate or perpetuate these episodes.
9. Initiate efforts to relieve and improve family functioning.

Case Study 10.9

Borderline Personality Disorder

Francine

Francine is 26 years old and single. Her alcoholic parents divorced when she was 3 years old. She lived with her mother, who drank heavily and had a series of live-in boyfriends. Her mother was physically and emotionally unavailable and spent a great deal of time at bars. Her mother's boyfriends physically and sexually abused Francine. To try to cope, Francine began using alcohol in mid adolescence. She was also sexually promiscuous. She was involved in shoplifting and occasionally went on eating binges. Today, she acknowledges that she drinks to blunt emotional pain.

As an adult, she has had intense relationships with men. When a relationship breaks up, her rage and anger have been equally intense. Francine cannot cope with rejection in relationships and says she feels "empty inside" when she thinks she has been abandoned. Her sudden shifts in mood and her occasional threats of suicide have alienated boyfriends and other friends.

Although she drinks alcohol to lessen the intensity of her feelings, it ultimately causes deeper depression and leads to impulsive, self-destructive behavior. Several times, when her relationships have broken up, Francine has taken overdoses and cut her wrists.

Francine ended a previous therapy after three or four sessions—she said the therapist was getting "too close" and she felt too vulnerable. But she is once again in counseling and is making progress in dealing with her addiction and the personality traits that have caused problems.

Discussion Questions

What is the prognosis for Francine?
What would help her to maintain recovery and sobriety?
Do you think her problems in relationships are important? Explain.
Do you think she would benefit from all women AA meetings and/or a women's
    therapy group? Why? Explain.

10.   Facilitate access to services and coordinate resources among different service providers.

Working with co-occurring disorders requires a strong team approach and good communication among mental health caregivers (case counselor, psychologist, psychiatrist, group counselor, etc.) so that the client doesn't "fall between the service gaps." This supportive team approach also can counter recurrent sabotaging by client and family members, treatment and medication noncompliance, and inconsistency in care and messages to the client and their family (i.e., it avoids triangulation).

One can clearly understand why depressive disorders may lead to suicidal ideation and suicide. The combination of depression and alcohol/drug use places patients at an even higher risk for suicide. Self-destructive acts that otherwise might be contemplated and dismissed are frequently acted on impulsively by those who are intoxicated

✖ Affective Disorders and Suicide

and disinhibited. In earlier chapters, we discussed alcoholism and drug addiction as a kind of death wish. Disaster might also occur when a depressed, forgetful patient is drinking and inadvertently takes an overdose of antidepressant medication. The antidepressants, especially the tricyclic antidepressants, are lethal when mixed with alcohol.

The vicious psychological pattern of affect (feelings) plus shame can also contribute to suicidal ideation and actions—for example,

depressive feelings + shame = feelings of despair

Shame is exemplified as "I shouldn't feel depressed; I'm weak to have these feelings. I feel unable to control my feelings and there must be something inferior about me."

This cycle continues to the next stage of

feelings of despair + shame = suicidal ideation

The shame takes the form of thoughts such as "I'm not worthy. There is no hope; things won't change; I don't have any choices. Things are so painful and never change; they only get worse. There is nothing to get any pleasure or joy from life."

The next and often fatal stage is

suicidal ideation + shame = suicide

It is no wonder that initial or normal feelings of sadness, or melancholia from unresolved trauma from childhood, is avoided and not grieved. The individual suffering from depressive illness is fearful that any negative experience will start this cycle in motion of depression to self-destruction. As a result, feelings of sadness and emotional pain are often self-medicated with alcohol/drugs. One can see the importance of supportive counseling for depressed patients in addition to the appropriate use of antidepressant medication.

References

American Psychiatric Association [APA]. 1984. *Psychiatric glossary.* Washington, D.C.: American Psychiatric Press.

American Psychiatric Association [APA]. 1994. *Diagnostic and statistical manual of mental disorders.* 4th ed. Washington, D. C.: Author.

Bauer, Anne. 1987. Dual diagnosis patients: The state of the problem. *Information Exchange (TIEUNES)* 9(3, July): 1–4, 8.

Craig, R. J. 1988. A psychometric study of the prevalence of DSM-III personality disorders among treated opiate addicts. *International Journal of the addictions* 23(2): 115–24.

Daley, Dennis C., and Howard B. Moss. 2002. *Dual disorders: Counseling clients with chemical dependency and mental illness.* 3d ed. Center City, Minn.: Hazeldon Foundation.

Fields, Richard, and Russell Vandenbelt. 1992a. *Understanding mood disorders and addictions* [pamphlet]. Center City, Minn.: Hazeldon Educational Materials.

Fields, Richard, and Russell Vandenbelt. 1992b. *Understanding personality problems and addiction* [pamphlet]. Center City, Minn.: Hazeldon Educational Materials.

Helzer, J. E., and T. R. Pryzbeck. 1988. The co-occurrence of alcoholism with other psychiatric disorders in the general population and its impact on treatment. *Journal of Studies on Alcohol* 49:219–24.

Hesselbrook, M. N., R. E. Meyer, and J. J. Kenner. 1985. Psychopathology in hospitalized alcoholics. *Archives of General Psychiatry* 42:1050–55.

Hesselbrook, V. M., E. G. Shaskan, and R. E. Meyer. 1983. Summary of bio/genetic factors in alcoholism. *NIAAA Research Monograph Series* 9:159–66.

Johnson, R. P., and J. C. Connelly. 1981. Addicted physicians take a closer look. *Journal of the American Medical Association* 245:253–57.

Kaufman, Edward. 1995. *Psychotherapy of addicted persons.* New York: Guilford Press.

Khantzian, E. J. 1981. Some treatment implications of the ego and self-disturbance in alcoholism. In *Dynamic approaches to the understanding and treatment of alcoholism,* edited by M. H. Bean and N. E. Zinberg. New York: Free Press.

Kleinman, P. H., A. B. Miller, and R. B. Millman. 1990. Psychopathology among cocaine abusers entering treatment. *Journal of Nervous and Mental Disease* 178:442–47.

Koenigsberg, H. E., et al. 1985. The relationship between syndrome and personality disorder in DSM-III: Experience with 2,462 patients. *American Journal of Psychiatry* 142(2): 207–12.

Masterson, James. 1976. *Psychotherapy of the borderline adult: A developmental approach.* New York: Brunner/Mazel.

Nace, E. P. 1990. Substance abuse and personality disorder. In *Managing the dually diagnosed patients: Current Issues and Clinical Approaches,* edited by D. F. O'Connell [Special issue]. *Journal of Chemical Dependency Treatment* 3(2): 183–98.

Nace, E. P., J. J. Saxon, and N. A. Shore. 1983. A comparison of borderline and nonborderline alcoholic patients. *Archives of General Psychiatry* 40:54–56.

National Institute of Mental Health [NIMH]. 2001. *Bipolar disorder.* NIMH Publication No. 01-3679, Washington, D.C.: Dept. of Health and Human Services.

Regier, Darrel A., et al. 1990. Comorbidity of mental disorders and alcohol and other drug abuse: Results from the Epidemiologic Catchment Area (ECA) Study. *Journal of the American Medical Association* 19:2511–18.

U.S. Department of Health and Human Services. 1987. *Helpful facts about depressive illnesses* [DART pamphlet]. Rockville, Md.: National Institute of Mental Health.

Weiss, R. D., and S. M. Mirin. 1986. Subtypes of cocaine abusers. *Psychiatric Clinics of North America* 9:491–501.

Weiss, Roger. 1996. Personality parallels. *Professional Counselor Magazine,* January/February, pp. 15–16, 40–41.

Alcohol/Drug Treatment and Relapse Prevention

❖ **Chapter in Review**

Self-help meetings are the most widely used and successful approach to alcohol and drug recovery.

Government-supported chemical dependency treatment programs from 1970 to 1980 consisted primarily of therapeutic communities, outpatient methadone clinics, outpatient drug-free programs, and university-affiliated research centers. The cocaine epidemic of the 1980s changed the course of chemical dependency treatment, as did managed care in the 1990s.

Richard Rawson's model describes the five stages of alcohol/drug recovery:

> 0–15 days—withdrawal
> 16–45 days—honeymoon
> 46–120 days—the wall
> 121–180 days—adjustment
> 181+ days—resolution

Each of these stages has its own behavioral, cognitive, emotional, and relational symptoms.

Early phases of alcohol/drug recovery focus on issues of stabilization and safety. As recovery progresses, the individual focuses more on affect (feeling), recognition, and modulation. The advantages of family treatment and family system work are outlined in this chapter, as are the beneficial curative factors of group psychotherapy.

There is a tremendously high relapse rate following alcohol/drug treatment. Training patients in relapse prevention is an integral component of the recovery program; it was often neglected in early chemical dependency treatment approaches.

Recognizing that specific times, places, things, and people can trigger alcohol/drug cravings is an important component of chemical dependency relapse training. It has also been demonstrated that drug relapse is induced by a return to alcohol use.

Two key points made in this chapter are, first, that alcohol/drug recovery is an ongoing process and no one is cured due to the ongoing nature of the disease of alcoholism/drug addiction and, second, that chemical dependency treatment is often as good as the counselor or treatment program itself, assuming that the patient is motivated to achieve recovery.

Other relapse factors are the importance of structure and pitfalls to too much structure, health and physical well-being, and cognitive, emotional, and spiritual well-being.

An outline is presented of common troublesome behaviors attributed to many co-occurring-disorders with patients and the boundaries the counselor needs to establish with these clients. We focus on four categories of these patients—the dependent clingers, the demanders, the manipulative help-rejecters, and the self-destructive deniers. Special considerations for co-occurring-disorders patients range from education, cognitive-behavioral approaches, and medication compliance to family involvement.

Approximately 1 million people in the United States currently are receiving treatment for drug or alcohol addiction (NIDA 2002). This final chapter gives a balanced overview of alcohol/drug treatment while placing major emphasis on relapse prevention. Sobriety and abstinence from alcohol/drugs is an ongoing process. Recovery is a lifelong process involving not only alcoholics/addicts but also their entire family systems.

This chapter highlights treatment issues and approaches for specific alcohol/drug and co-occurring-disorders. You are encouraged to explore referenced material, take counseling courses specific to alcohol/drugs, and pursue supervised internships for more in-depth counseling skill development.

It's appropriate to start this chapter on treatment with the most widely used approach for recovery from alcoholism and drug addiction—self-help groups.

✖ Self-Help Meetings

Alcoholics Anonymous

Alcoholics Anonymous (AA) was founded in the early 1930s by Bill W., a stockbroker, and Bob S., a surgeon. Both of these men found that willpower alone was not enough to keep them from using alcohol. After admitting to each other their common disease and shared frustration with alcohol recovery, they discovered that they could help one another remain sober through mutual support. They soon discovered that others had the same experiences in struggling with recovery from alcoholism, and the movement was begun. Small groups of alcoholics met on a regular basis to share their experience, strength, hope, and support for one another. In 1938, the basic principles of AA were first outlined as the now famous Twelve Steps. (See Table 11.1.)

Alcoholics Anonymous has been the most successful program of recovery to date. There are AA meetings every day in almost every city and town in the United States. Throughout other parts of the world, more than 90 countries have AA meetings. The fellowship crosses all religious and racial barriers; the only requirement for membership is a desire to stop drinking.

"There are no dues or fees for AA membership; they are self-supporting through their own contributions. AA is not allied with any sect, denomination, politics, organization, or institution; does not wish to engage in any controversy; neither endorses nor opposes any causes. Our primary purpose is to stay sober and help other alcoholics to achieve sobriety" (Alcoholics Anonymous 1978).

Advantages of AA as a Recovery Model
Lawson, Peterson, and Lawson (1983) identified the following key factors that contribute to the success of AA as a recovery model:

1. Mutual sharing by members, which provides solutions to alcohol-related problems and helps alleviate guilt by showing members that others have acted irrationally also

TABLE 11.1

The Twelve Steps

1. We admitted we were powerless over alcohol—that our lives had become unmanageable.
2. Came to believe that a Power greater than ourselves could restore us to sanity.
3. Made a decision to turn our will and our lives over to the care of God as we understood Him.
4. Made a searching and fearless moral inventory of ourselves.
5. Admitted to God, to ourselves, and to another human being the exact nature of our wrongs.
6. Were entirely ready to have God remove all these defects of character.
7. Humbly asked Him to remove our shortcomings.
8. Made a list of all persons we had harmed and became willing to make amends to them.
9. Made direct amends to such people wherever possible, except when to do so would injure them or others.
10. Continued to take personal inventory and, when we were wrong, promptly admitted to it.
11. Sought through prayer and meditation to improve our conscious contact with God as we understand Him, praying only for knowledge of His will for us and the power to carry that out.
12. Having had a spiritual awakening as the result of these steps, we tried to carry this message to alcoholics and practice these principles in all our affairs.

The Twelve Steps are reprinted with permission of Alcoholics Anonymous World Services, Inc. Permission to reprint the Twelve Steps does not mean that AA agrees with the views expressed herein.

AA is a program of recovery from alcoholism—use of the Twelve Steps in connection with programs and activities that are patterned after AA but that address other problems does not imply otherwise.

2. Provision of a regular support group of individuals working toward the goal of abstinence
3. Frequent and regular meetings to help members structure their time
4. Availability of AA as an adjunct to other treatments, such as counseling and psychotherapy
5. Absence of membership fees and nondiscrimination by race, sex, or socioeconomic status
6. Establishment of comprehensive goals covering the emotional, behavioral, and spiritual life of the members

A number of studies have found favorable treatment outcomes from participation in AA (e.g., Armor, Polich, and Stambul 1978; Bateman and Peterson 1971; Browne-Mayers, Seeley, and Brown 1973; Kish and Herman 1971). In 1965, a study by Robson, Paulus, and Clark found that 71 percent of regular AA attendees improved and 57 percent improved from attending no more than 10 meetings.

Despite these figures, treatment programs that are exclusively AA-oriented without the incorporation of other treatment methods and modalities have been less effective. Costello and associates (1976) found that the effectiveness of intermediate care was doubled (18 to 36 percent) when the unit converted from an exclusively AA-oriented model to a program with many treatment methods, AA being one of them.

Resistance to Attending AA and Other Self-Help Groups

For a variety of reasons, individuals in early alcohol/drug recovery often resist attending self-help meetings. Some of the reasons they give are the following:

1. Difficulty with the concept of a higher power, or references to God
2. Lack of tolerance by self-help members, at times, to
   a. Use medication for affective or feeling disorders and other psychological conditions
   b. Help understand that there are different types of alcoholism
   c. Reject treatment (therapy and other treatment modalities)
3. People are uncomfortable in group settings and are concerned with the group's maintaining strict confidentiality
4. The disruptive influence of people (especially court-referred) who don't have a true desire to be sober

Despite these drawbacks, which can be overcome, AA and other self-help meetings have been a positive and extremely beneficial source of inspiration and hope for millions of recovering alcoholics/addicts.

Application of Self-Help to Other Problems

Other standard self-help meetings that have adapted the AA 12-step model for a variety of problems, include the following:

NA—Narcotics Anonymous
CA—Cocaine Anonymous
MA—Marijuana Anonymous
Al-Anon—for family members of alcoholics
Narcanon—for family members of drug addicts
Alateen and Alatot—for teenagers and youngsters of alcoholics
ACA—for Adult Children of Alcoholics
FA—Families Anonymous
OA—Overeaters Anonymous
CODA—Co-Dependents Anonymous

There are self-help meetings for survivors of incest and sexual abuse; meetings for those addicted to gambling or compulsive sexuality; and meetings to help those having problems with spending and those grieving the loss of a child. There are even self-help groups for people suffering from similar physical, psychological, and emotional conditions. In California, while working in a community mental health center, I ran across a group for people suffering from bipolar disorders. The group appropriately called itself the "Ups and Downs Group." Whatever the condition, the self-help model is being applied as a successful treatment modality, especially when it is

TABLE 11.2

The Recovery Directory (National Telephone Numbers Included Where Available)

Adult Children of Alcoholics	Overeaters Anonymous
Adult Survivors of Child Abuse	Partners of Survivors of Incest Anonymous
Al-Anon/Alateen (800) 344-2666	Phobics Anonymous (619) 322-COPE
Alcoholics Anonymous	Prostitutes Anonymous (818) 905-2188
Chemically Dependent Anonymous	Racism and Bigotry Anonymous
Chronic Fatigue Immune Disease Syndrome Anonymous	Recovering Couples Anonymous (314) 830-2600
Cocaine Anonymous	Self-Help Group Information (800) 222-5465
Co-Dependents Anonymous (602) 277-7991	Self-Mutilators Anonymous
Debtors Anonymous	Sexaholics Anonymous
Emotions Anonymous (612) 647-9712	Sex and Love Addiction Anonymous
Emphysema Anonymous (813) 391-9977	Sexual Addiction Hotline (800) 321-2066
Gamblers Anonymous (213) 386-8789	Shame Anonymous
Incest Survivors Anonymous (213) 428-5599	Shoplifters Anonymous (800) 848-9595
Marijuana Anonymous (800) 766-6779	Smokers Anonymous
Nar-Anon Family Group (213) 547-5800	Survivors of Incest Anonymous
Narcotics Anonymous	Survivors Reaching Out (916) 967-0424
Nicotine Anonymous	Workaholics Anonymous

From Joan Ellen Zweben, Ph.D., in *Psychotherapy and Substance Abuse: A Practitioner's Handbook,* Arnold M. Washton, Ph.D., editor, Guilford Press, N.Y., 1995.

integrated with a variety of other treatment modalities. Alcohol/drug self-help meetings are the most widely used modality for recovery from alcoholism and drug addiction. Table 11.2 lists a directory for several self-help groups.

Rational Recovery

Rational Recovery (RR) was started by Jack Trimpey in 1986 as an alternative to Alcoholics Anonymous and other self-help meetings. The principles of RR are based on the rational-emotive approach developed by Albert Ellis, Ph.D. The major focus of rational recovery is on changing the way people think and feel about themselves and their use of alcohol/drugs. "In RR, we learn to take control of our emotions so that we are not compelled to reach for an anesthetic when we are feeling bad" (Trimpey 1996). Trimpey, a clinical social worker in California, wrote *The Small Book* (1985), which attacked the principles of the AA *Big Book*. Unfortunately Trimpey's book is too intent on bashing AA, rather than outlining another alternative for people who have problems with AA meetings or principles.

In 1990, Trimpey set up a for-profit organization, Rational Recovery Systems, Inc. Many people had problems with the incongruity of a self-help meeting that had a for-profit motive. In 1993, a new organization, RRSN (Rational Recovery Self-Help Network), was developed as a nonprofit organization, with new bylaws and elected officers. Trimpey also developed Addictive Voice Recognition Training (AVRT) in 1993–94. Many psychologists who were involved in the original Rational Recovery groups developed a new organization, called SMART Recovery. SMART

Recovery is based on rational-emotive behavioral therapy and cognitive-behavioral approaches.

F. Michler Bishop's article "Rational-Emotive Behavior Therapy and Two Self-Help Alternatives to the 12-Step Model" (1995) outlines in more detail the history and dimensions of these approaches. The article describes some of the common tenets of these approaches as the following:

1. People are largely responsible for their behaviors, including addictive behaviors.
2. A person can recover; that is, a person can gain control over his or her addictive behaviors.
3. Lifetime membership is not required; many people can recover in a year or two.
4. Labeling of all kinds is discouraged; a person does not have to call himself or herself an alcoholic to begin to recover.
5. Alcoholism may or may not be a disease; however, a person has to find a way to cope and take responsibility for his or her life in any case.
6. The value of a person is not linked to his or her behavior, addictive or otherwise. A person will not be a better person if he or she gives up alcohol or some other addictive behavior; he or she may be a happier person, a person who has better relationships and can keep a job, but behavioral change does not affect the "goodness" of the self.
7. A person is not necessarily, ipso facto, "in denial" if he or she does not accept the basic AA tenets.
8. A person is not doomed to a life of alcoholism if he or she does not accept help from AA, a rehabilitation clinic, a hospital, and so on. People can recover on their own with or without the help of professionals and/or self-help groups.

Regardless of your own viewpoint about Alcoholics Anonymous, the Rational Recovery movement poses another alternative that may help a specific population. However, the approach may also cause others to continue to deny their alcoholism and drug addiction and continue to suffer the negative consequences of their alcohol/drug use.

Drug Addiction Treatment, 1960–80

⚔ History of Alcohol/Drug Treatment

The four basic kinds of treatment that had federal, state, and local government support in the 1960s were

1. Therapeutic communities
2. Outpatient methadone clinics
3. Outpatient drug-free programs
4. University-affiliated clinical research centers

Therapeutic Communities

In 1958, Synanon was established as a model for most therapeutic communities, and the approach was expanded to other programs, including Day Top Village, Phoenix

House, and Odyssey House in New York, and Delancey Street and The Family in California.

By 1978, a national organization, Therapeutic Communities of America, was organizing and unifying the goals of more than 300 therapeutic communities.

These communities were essentially residential programs, where alcoholics/ addicts lived together in a family atmosphere, which promoted

- Addicts helping addicts to recovery in a structured lifestyle
- Confrontational and group therapies
- Adherence to the principles of AA and the 12 steps
- Honesty, drug abstinence, self-reliance, and personal responsibility through example

Methadone Treatment

The monumental methadone treatment work of Dole and Nyswander (1965) became a treatment model that spread throughout the United States. In 1980, 48 out of 50 states had methadone treatment programs.

Dole and Nyswander believed that heroin addiction is a metabolic disease and that a single administration of a narcotic can change a person's metabolism. There-fore, multiple administrations of the narcotic has even more potency in changing the person's nervous system. Dole and Nyswander searched for a medication to replace the metabolic need and craving for opiates (heroin). They found methadone, a long-acting, orally administered drug that eliminates the craving for heroin and other opi-oids. By successfully reducing the need for heroin, methadone reduces the antiso-cial, crime-related behavior of many addicts.

Methadone treatment involves detoxification and maintenance. *Detoxification* helps patients gradually reduce their dependence on opiates by giving them decreas-ing doses of methadone over 21 days. After detoxification, the individual is then drug free.

Maintenance essentially helps addicts develop a productive nondrug-using lifestyle. In effect, methadone replaces the devastating addiction to heroin and other opiates. Methadone does not affect the pleasure centers as do opiates, and addicts do not experience highs. The craving for heroin is stopped with the rather benign de-pendence on methadone. There is still some controversy with methadone mainte-nance because addicts are still dependent on another drug—methadone.

The treatment methods in both methadone detoxification and methadone maintenance include individual and group education, counseling sessions, self-help 12-step recovery, and rehabilitative services.

Outpatient Programs

A variety of outpatient treatment clinics existed in the 1970s and 1980s, including medically supervised programs and storefront centers. Medically supervised pro-grams provided crisis-oriented medical services for alcohol/drug detoxification and overdose. At storefront drop-in/crisis counseling centers, treatment was unstruc-tured, often focusing on crisis intervention, legal and criminal-justice counseling, medical care and/or health-related services, welfare and social services, employ-ment, and counseling for family and interpersonal problems. The outpatient clinics served as a community-based entry point into the health care system for drug users in low-income communities.

University Research Centers

The drug revolution of the 1960s saw some significant changes. Drug use was no longer confined to inner-city, lower socioeconomic groups. When drugs began affecting the campus population, government spending increased for alcohol/drug research and treatment. During the same period, the government foresaw that large numbers of soldiers returning from Vietnam would need treatment for heroin addiction.

As a result, university-based research treatment centers opened, and many affiliated with the Veterans Administration. These centers tested new pharmacological aids. They evaluated medications, such as naltrexone, propoxyphene, levo-alpha-acetylmethadol (LAAM), and clonidine, for treatment of opiate craving and addiction.

Alcohol Treatment, 1970–80

Private commercial, inpatient, and residential 28- to 30-day treatment programs rapidly expanded during the 1970s. Their tremendous financial success caused these programs to become a major standard of alcohol treatment. The 28- to 30-day length of stay was developed as a standard, not as a result of empirical study but, instead, as the negotiated arrangement between the hospital-based inpatient providers and the insurance companies. These inpatient programs were also successful because they were modeled after AA 12-step principles and integrated AA self-help meetings as part of the program.

When former first lady, Betty Ford, entered an alcohol treatment facility, public disclosure of her alcoholism did much to bring this kind of treatment into public view and acceptance (Ford 1987). "Her forthright discussion of her alcoholism and addiction and subsequent sponsorship of the Betty Ford Treatment Center provided a turning point in the alcoholism field" (Rawson 1991).

Disinterest in Alcohol/Drug Treatment, 1970s and 1980s

In the late 1970s, public interest in therapeutic communities, methadone treatment, outpatient programs, and university research centers seemed to wane. A variety of factors caused this loss of interest. First, the anticipated epidemic of heroin addicts returning from Vietnam was not realized. Many returning soldiers withdrew from heroin on the long boat and plane ride back home. For many of these young men, heroin use was inconsistent with their lifestyles back home. Others did not have the connections at home to maintain their addiction to heroin. Most discontinued opiate use without significant involvement in the treatment system.

Second, a dramatic reduction took place in the use of hallucinogens, sedative-hypnotics, and amphetamines. The primary nonopiate drugs used by the white population shifted primarily to marijuana and cocaine. At the time, the treatment community and general public thought marijuana and cocaine had a low risk for dependency. Most experts were still referring to marijuana and cocaine as psychologically dependency-producing rather than addicting. That mistake caused one of the major drug problems of the 1980s.

Third, the confrontive strategies of some therapeutic communities got out of control. Many therapeutic communities were exposed as dysfunctional systems much like the alcoholics/addicts' dysfunctional families of origin. Fourth, there was also opposition and public disenchantment with methadone maintenance on the principle that, rather than recovering, heroin addicts were addicted to a new drug—methadone.

Fifth, the efficacy and success of drop-in counseling centers was questioned. The criminal-justice system was often in conflict with these centers because clients were protected from criminal prosecution. Funding misappropriation and failure to adequately document client charts created tremendous conflict between centers and various government funding sources.

Due to these developments, public interest in drug addiction problems had decreased by the late 1970s. Although a treatment network had been established and some promising new treatments were in development, there appeared to be a societal loss of interest in drug addiction treatment. The one drug problem that obviously was going to persist was heroin. However, heroin was predominately a lower-income, inner-city, minority problem. Since middle-class Americans did not appear to be significantly at-risk from heroin problems, there was to be a loss of commitment to continued funding for new treatments. Funding levels in many of the programs dropped, resulting in a reduction in treatment slots and a reduction in ancillary services for the remaining slots. Research funding decreased, and many of the clinical strategies developed during the 1970s were put on the back burner. As the 1980s began, the drug treatment system appeared to have lost momentum (Rawson 1991).

Changes in the 1980s
Cocaine Epidemic

The explosive emergence of cocaine addiction in the 1980s challenged the alcohol/drug treatment system to develop new treatment strategies. In 1984, Mark Gold and Arnold Herman described cocaine as a major public health concern. What experts thought was a rather benign, psychologically dependency-producing drug became known as the most addicting drug to date.

Animal studies, human studies, and clinical human reports all validate cocaine as the most highly addicting drug. Thus, warnings not to try it even once are not scare tactics but frightening reality. Sidney Cohen, the most prolific writer in the drug field, predicted in the early 1980s that "if cocaine were readily available and inexpensive, this would create the biggest drug epidemic we had ever known." His prediction has come true with crack cocaine.

In the early 1980s, there were no treatment programs for cocaine addiction. This new addict population, however, soon found treatment at inpatient alcohol treatment facilities. Facility directors responded to the need by developing cocaine treatment programs. Financial reward motivated these inpatient facilities, which saw a tremendous treatment population developing. Their television commercials added taglines stating, "We treat cocaine addiction, too." The constant flow of sports figures, celebrities, and other public figures further created an attractive notoriety for these treatment programs.

The cocaine epidemic was even further catapulted into the public consciousness with the development of freebase cocaine. In the mid 1980s, crack cocaine use made cocaine available to all socioeconomic levels. Crack cocaine was marketed to new populations: those who could not afford cocaine in the inner city and young people. "Smokable cocaine, preprocessed in ready-to-smoke dosage units flooded major American cities from 1985 to today. Use of the drug in this form produced addiction very rapidly, and the availability of the drug in lower-cost dosage units made cocaine available to lower-income users. This combination produced a fire storm of addiction among lower income, minority, inner-city residents" (Rawson 1991).

Risk of AIDS

Exacerbating our crack cocaine epidemic is the AIDS crisis. The fact that the AIDS virus can be spread by high-risk sexual practices and the sharing of needles used to inject drugs has identified intravenous drug users as being at high risk for the spread of the HIV virus.

Treatment Trends

Some research has indicated that intensive outpatient alcohol/drug treatment is as effective as inpatient treatment. Ritson (1968) found no significant difference in effectiveness between inpatient and outpatient alcoholism treatment programs and questioned the routine hospitalization of alcoholics.

Due to the high cost of inpatient treatment, the trend in the 1990s was to refer more patients to outpatient treatment. Instead of the expensive, traditional, hospital-based 28-day inpatient chemical dependency treatment program, the alternative is intensive outpatient programs for 30 to 180 days. This is a more appropriate recovery period because it allows support during the time when the recovering alcoholic/addict is most vulnerable to relapse. It also minimizes the costly aspects of inpatient hospitalization.

Managed care is the trend today. Inpatient treatment programs are becoming part of a managed care network in order to survive. Approximately 40 percent of inpatient alcohol/drug treatment programs have gone out of business or have been consumed by managed care operations. Certainly, the preferred trend for managed care of alcohol/drug problems is outpatient counseling to minimize cost. As a result, the entire fields of alcohol/drug recovery, mental health, and treatment of co-occurring disorders have been affected by managed care. In his workshops "Brief Targeted Strategic Therapy for Relapse Prevention," Terence T. Gorski (1996) emphasizes treatment that is brief (up to 20 sessions), targeted (What is the problem?), strategic (What am I going to do about it? Step by step plan), and outcome-focused.

In the 1990s, there was a major focus on cognitive-behavioral therapies, solution-focused therapy, motivational interviewing, and other techniques that allow for brief, targeted therapies.

Arnold Washton, in his introduction to the book *Psychotherapy and Substance Abuse* (1995), comments on solution-focused, brief therapy: "along the way we have discovered that regardless of what the problems are, the solutions to them seem to be so similar and yet so mundane; to do what will be good for clients and their families, such as talking to each other, being open and honest with each other, doing kind deeds, working hard, developing healthy habits, and looking for ways to change tomorrow by creating a vision of what they want."

✖ Treatment in the New Millennium

Inpatient/residential programs are now extending care beyond the traditional inpatient 27- to 30-day (insurance reimbursable) stay. Many patients are requiring extended care (31 to 180 days). The model is usually 30 days of inpatient/residential care followed by 31 to 150 additional days in an extended-care facility (usually a less expensive residential setting).

Following are some of the elements most drug/alcohol treatment programs are now focusing on:

- Treatment for co-occurring disorders
- Specialized treatment for trauma
- Adjunct tracks for eating disorders.
- Specialized treatment for sexual addictions and sexual disorders
- Cognitive-behavioral therapies
- EMDR and other techniques for trauma
- Dialectical behavior therapy (DBT) for borderline personality disorder
- More emphasis on family members and family systems (e.g., family week at the residential program)
- Medications to reduce craving and for affective disorders
- Outpatient treatment as an alternative to inpatient/residential treatment when appropriate
- Specialized tracks for gambling addiction

✖ Stages of Alcohol/Drug Recovery

Richard Rawson and associates (1988) outlined five basic stages of cocaine recovery, which also apply to alcohol/drug recovery. (See Table 11.3.) The time periods for each stage vary from individual to individual and based on the kinds of drugs used. The stages are

0–15 days—withdrawal
16–45 days—honeymoon
46–120 days—the wall

TABLE 11.3

Stages of Recovery

Stage	Time Course*
Withdrawal	0–15 days
Honeymoon	15–45 days
The Wall	45–120 days
Adjustment	120–180 days
Resolution	180–360 days

From Richard Rawson et al., "Neurobehavioral treatment for cocaine dependency" in *Journal of Psychoactive Drugs* 22 (2): 159–71. Haight-Ashbury Publications, San Francisco, CA. Reprinted by permission.

*These generalized categories are rough estimates for periods of time when alcohol/drugs are not used. The actual time course for each stage of recovery may be quite different for each individual and alcohol or drug used.

T A B L E   1 1 . 4

Withdrawal Stage (0–15 Days)

Behavioral Symptoms	Cognitive Symptoms	Emotional Symptoms	Relationships
Increased need for sleep	Difficulty concentrating	Depression	Hostility
Behavioral inconsistency	Cravings for alcohol/drugs	Anxiety	Confusion
Impulsive, erratic behavior	Short-term memory	Self-doubt	Maladaptive coping
Anergia (lack of energy)	disruption	Shame	responses (inappropriate actions and behavior)
			Fear

From Richard Rawson et al., "Neurobiological treatment for cocaine dependency," in *Journal of Psychoactive Drugs* 22 (2), 159–71. Haight-Ashbury Publications, San Francisco, CA. Reprinted by permission.

T A B L E   1 1 . 5

Honeymoon Stage (16–45 Days)

Behavioral Symptoms	Cognitive Symptoms	Emotional Symptoms	Relationships
High energy (perhaps manic)	Inability to prioritize	Optimism	Denial of addiction disorder
Poorly directed behavior	Abbreviated tension span	Overconfidence	Desire for things to return to normal
Excessive work and/or play	Inability to recognize	Feelings of being cured	Conflict between spouse or partner, family, and treatment
Return to alcohol, marijuana, or other drug use	relapse potential		

From Richard Rawson, et al., "Neurobiological treatment for cocaine dependency," in *Journal of Psychoactive Drugs* 22 (2), 159–71. Haight-Ashbury Publications, San Francisco, Calif. Reprinted by permission.

121–180 days—adjustment
181+ 365 days—resolution
1 year—after resolution and beyond

Withdrawal Stage

Most of the physical aspects of withdrawal clear up after 3 to 7 days. Emotional feelings of anxiety, fatigue, pain, and depression persist throughout the first 15 days. Patients require education and direction during the withdrawal phase. Once patients go through the initial physical withdrawal, they want to leave treatment to avoid the emotional issues. (See Table 11.4.)

Honeymoon Stage

The honeymoon stage is the opposite of the withdrawal stage. (See Table 11.5.) The neophyte to recovery has gone through the difficult withdrawal stage and now feels energetic, confident, and optimistic. Cravings for alcohol/drugs are usually reduced and moods improve. This may lead clients to believe that recovery is easier than they thought it would be. Unwittingly, they begin to stray from the elements of their recovery program that helped them stay sober. Their behavior becomes more unstructured, inconsistent, and at times frenetic. They may go through a manic cycle, doing many things and overextending themselves. These behaviors then disrupt their recovery. This is the time when patients are most at risk to return to alcohol use, marijuana use, or other drug use. They may convince themselves that they had a problem with a particular drug, not that they are at risk with all alcohol/drugs.

The Wall Stage

After 45 days of sobriety, the largest percentage of relapses to alcohol/drugs occur, as shown in Table 11.6. Personal and interpersonal issues are emotionally experienced more fully during this stage. Relapse vulnerability increases as patients start feeling these emotional issues and begin to further sort out some of the problems in their lives and in their relationships. Patients often get discouraged and may verbalize that they "feel this will go on indefinitely." Patients may lose hope, strength, and motivation to continue in their process of recovery. This is a time when the supportive elements of their recovery program need to be strengthened, even though patients may attempt to alienate those who can help. Group counseling can be especially helpful at this stage. Others in the group who have gone through this difficult stage can share their struggle and ultimate success and lend support.

TABLE 11.6

The Wall Stage (46–120 Days)

Behavioral Symptoms	Cognitive Symptoms	Emotional Symptoms	Relationships
Sluggishness, anergia (lack of energy)	Cognitive rehearsal of relapse, thinking, planning, or playing over the idea of relapse	Depression	Mutual blaming
Sexual disinterest/dysfunction	Euphoric recall, remembering the feelings and good times of drug/alcohol use	Anxiety	Irritability
Insomnia		Fatigue	Devaluation of progress
Discontinuation of treatment, recreational, exercise, diet, and/or occupationally appropriate behaviors	Increased frequency of drug/alcohol thoughts, dreams, and cravings	Boredom	Threatened separation or expulsion from home
Resumption of alcohol, marijuana, and/or other drug use	Denial or rationalization of emotional feelings and reactions	Anhedonia (inability to feel pleasure with things that normally give pleasure)	
	Difficulty concentrating	Irritability	

From Richard Rawson, et al., "Neurobiological treatment for cocaine dependency," in *Journal of Psychoactive Drugs* 22 (2), 159–71. Haight-Ashbury Publications, San Francisco, Calif. Reprinted by permission.

Adjustment Stage

The achievement of working through the intense feelings of the wall stage gives patients new hope and energy for recovery. Patients begin to accept that this is a life-long struggle. The achievement of being sober for 120 or more days affirms the addicts' ability to be sober for a long time. This is the longest time that most patients have ever been sober. (See Table 11.7.)

Resolution Stage

Completion of an intensive six-month program signals a shift from learning new skills to monitoring for relapse signs, maintaining a balanced lifestyle, and developing new areas of interest. Some clients may need individual psychotherapy or relationship work. (See Table 11.8.)

Period After the Resolution Stage

After the resolution stage, the individual may need to do more in-depth counseling on family of origin and family systems issues. Issues of underlying affective disorders and other psychiatric disorders may also be more fully explored during this stage.

TABLE 11.7

Adjustment Stage (121–180 Days)

Behavioral Symptoms	Cognitive Symptoms	Emotional Symptoms	Relationships
Return to activities that may have been inappropriate and had relapse potential in early stages Return to normal behavior	Reduced frequency of drug/alcohol thoughts, dreams, and cravings	Reduced depression, anxiety, irritability Continued boredom Loneliness	Emergence of long-term relationship problems Resistance to assistance with relationship problems

From Richard Rawson, et al., "Neurobiological treatment for cocaine dependency," in *Journal of Psychoactive Drugs* 22 (2), 159–71. Haight-Ashbury Publications, San Francisco, Calif. Reprinted by permission.

TABLE 11.8

Resolution Stage (181+ Days)

Behavioral Symptoms	Cognitive Symptoms	Emotional Symptoms	Relationships
Emergence of other excessive behavior patterns: gambling, sex, work, eating, alcohol use	Questioning of the need for long-term monitoring and support	Emergence of psychodynamic material Boredom with abstinence	Conflict between recovery principles and relationship needs

From Richard Rawson, et al., "Neurobehavioral treatment for cocaine dependency," in *Journal of Psychoactive Drugs* 22 (2), 159–71. Haight-Ashbury Publications, San Francisco, Calif. Reprinted by permission.

The factor most predictive of alcohol/drug treatment success is the counselor's attitude about treatment. When counselors truly believe that they can help patients, and have the necessary insight and training, treatment tends to be more successful. The same holds true for treatment programs.

"Since the addictive alcoholic patient is fundamentally hostile, his behavior is unconsciously designed to arouse negative feelings and to invite retaliation. Hostility and retaliation must be constantly guarded against by all treatment personnel" (Chafetz, Blane, and Hill 1970). Many mental health counselors are uncomfortable working with alcoholics/addicts because of the hostility and resistance of these patients in complying with treatment. The alcoholic/addict's grandiosity and denial of reality causes him or her to always be just one step away from terminating treatment and to rationalize away the need for change. "The pervasive hopelessness that some clients feel regarding themselves and their lives is apt to be projected into the treatment process and the counseling relationship, so that the client feels, 'This is useless; it isn't going to get me anywhere'" (Marks, Daroff, and Granick 1987).

Breaking through denial and the evasive tactics of alcoholics/addicts and their families requires a special kind of counselor. M. Duncan Stanton described that counselor as needing to be energetic to engage clients/patients and their families into treatment.

Addicts and alcoholics are constantly testing counselors' competency by pushing boundaries and testing to see if counselors know what they are talking about. Denial is the defense mechanism of addiction; alcoholics/addicts wonder if counselors are strong enough to break through their denial system. Counselors also need to conduct an accurate assessment of alcohol/drug problems, affective & personality problems (see Figure 11.1).

Due to shameful feelings about self, alcoholics/addicts naturally seek or provoke rejection, hostility, anger, frustration, and even rage. Alcoholics/addicts test the

"Basically, what I hear you saying, Mr. Smith, is 'Help!'"

FIGURE 11.1   *The Need for a Good Assessment*

counselor, as they do everyone in their own family systems. If counselors become provoked, alcoholics/addicts can play familiar "bad child at odds with authority" roles.

To effectively engage alcoholics/addicts and their families in treatment, counselors must exhibit a combination of both patience and boundary setting. Counselors need to be powerful yet sensitive, while recognizing both the need for limit setting and the inner vulnerability and sensitivities of the patients. Counselors must establish control of the therapeutic process, while being flexible to the patients' weak ego-strength and sensitivity to shame.

Group counseling is an effective treatment modality because alcoholics/addicts can be confronted in a caring way by other alcoholics/addicts. Each person in the group observes other group members struggling with similar issues and modeling growth and success in that struggle to maintain abstinence and sobriety.

Early Phases: Safety and Stabilization

⚹ Counseling and Chemical Dependency

In the early phases of counseling with substance abusers, the therapist must be concerned with *safety* and *stabilization*.

Safety and stabilization focus on a variety of factors that help the recovering alcoholic/addict maintain sobriety and a basic sense of balance in his or her life. Mistakenly, in their zealousness to uncover traumatic content, therapists may open up wounds without first determining if the individual has the emotional strength, resources, and support network to help him or her heal these wounds. Opening up these wounds may exacerbate already fragile relationships with family members and the spouse or partner. The result inevitably is a relapse to alcohol/drug use.

Not long ago, psychoanalytically trained therapists maintained that they could cure alcoholics/addicts. Psychoanalysts tended to approach alcohol/drug users with the fixed, often rigid perception that all addicts have personality and/or affective disorders, such as narcissism, depression, bipolar disorder, and borderline personality disorder. The psychoanalysts then tried to treat alcoholics/addicts by personality reorganization and lumped all of the disorders together. The psychoanalysts attempted to show the addicts that the etiology of their drinking/drugging was due to personality disorders. "Analysts had unreal expectations of their patients, such as that they could give up their drug use immediately while in therapy, come in at fixed times, fit into the fifty-minute sessions, and adhere to the requirements of therapy" (Brill 1981).

Probing into feelings so early in recovery often caused alcoholics/addicts to re-experience traumatic emotional issues that they were not emotionally ready or able to deal with. As a result, alcoholics/addicts did what they had done before when feeling emotionally vulnerable—go back to using alcohol/drugs.

Unfortunately, this treatment still continues today, as professionals try to validate their theoretical models, without insight into when and how it is appropriate to deal with underlying issues and feelings. These psychoanalytical issues are best dealt with when alcoholics/addicts have maintained a significant period of sobriety (usually 1 to 5 years), have a strong support system, have the ego strength to tolerate the feelings, and have the insight and motivation to work on these issues. This

TABLE 11.9

Stages of Drug Alcohol Treatment

Stage of Treatment	Patient Status	Treatment
1	"I can't drink." (need for external control)	Alcohol detoxification, directive psychotherapy, AA, Al-Anon, family therapy, Antabuse
2	"I won't drink." (internalized control)	Directive psychotherapy, supportive psychotherapy, AA, consider discontinuing Antabuse
3	"I don't have to drink." (conflict resolution)	Psychoanalytically oriented psychotherapy

From S. Zimburg, "Principles of Alcoholism Psychotherapy" in *Practical Approaches to Alcoholism Psychotherapy,* 2d ed, edited by S. Zimberg, J. Wallace, and S. B. Blume, Human Science Press, 1985.

happens during Stage 3 of alcohol/drug treatment, as Table 11.9 shows. The first phase of counseling, therefore, focuses on strengthening both the alcoholic/addict's alcohol/drug recovery support system and the therapeutic alliance.

In the early stages of counseling with alcoholics/addicts the therapist needs to be extremely active, focusing on relapse prevention, helping the client overcome fears of and resistance to AA or other self-help programs, facilitating the development of a sponsor relationship, focusing on stress and anger management, and using other factors that will meet safety and stabilization needs. The need for interventions to stop the drinking and drugging and a solid period of sobriety are prerequisites for successful counseling/psychotherapy (Fox 1958; Tiebout 1962).

Affect (Feeling), Recognition, and Modulation

Once stabilization and safety needs are addressed, the next stage of counseling may focus on affect, recognition, and modulation. The therapist slowly works with the client in labeling and tolerating feelings. The counseling can then take many forms, exploring a variety of issues relevant to the chemical dependency. Throughout this process, regular review of relapse dynamics and support for a stable and secure recovery from alcohol/drugs are maintained.

Counseling approaches explore both the conscious and the unconscious levels of feelings. The Johari window (Table 11.10) is a training model that describes the domain of counseling. Counseling focuses on all four of these areas of self. These areas cover the following:

1. *Public self:* The public self includes all the aspects about the individual that are known by the individual and others close to the individual (e.g., age, marital status, hobbies, job, interests, basic personality type).
2. *Private self:* The private self involves information that the individual is aware of but others don't know (e.g., sexual practices, mistakes in the past or present, private feelings or thoughts, family of origin issues).
3. *Blind self:* The blind self includes things the individual is not consciously aware of that others are aware of about the individual (e.g., personality

TABLE 11.10

Johari Window

Others	Self	
	Things You Know About Self	**Things You Don't Know About Self**
Things They Know About You	1. Public	3. Blind
Things They Do Not Know About You	2. Private	4. Discovery

Adapted from *Group Processes: An Introduction to Group Dynamics* by Joseph Luft. Mayfield Publishing Company, Copyright © 1984, 1970, and 1963 by Joseph Luft. Reprinted by permission.

characteristics; denial about others' behavior or own behavior; lack of awareness of interpersonal, occupational, social, and marital issues).

4. *Discovery self:* Discovery self is the category of the future. These things are not in the conscious awareness of the individual or of others and will be discovered in the future (e.g., the natural changes that occur in life's unexpected journey).

By placing a major emphasis in counseling on Category 2, the private self, and Category 3, the blind self, individuals can see changes in Category 1, the public self, and Category 4, the discovery self. When individuals are defensive or unwilling to deal with their feelings about their private selves and blind selves, there are limitations to progress and personal change. Clients would do well to follow Louise Hay's (1984) advice: "If you think of the hardest thing for you to do and how much you resist it, then you're looking at your greatest lesson at the moment. Surrendering, giving up the resistance, and allowing yourself to learn what you need to learn, will make the next step easier."

Other techniques that are often included as part of the counseling approach to chemical dependency recovery include relaxation training (e.g., biofeedback), stress reduction, anger management, problem-solving/coping skills, communication skills, exercise, nutrition, life management (i.e., balance in activities), relationships, and work.

The common goals of all counseling approaches are education; the provision of information and resources; catharsis (patients' release of emotion and feelings); connectedness and trust, which facilitates disclosure of feelings and concerns; support for positive growth; awareness and insight; and personality change (reorganization).

Family Treatment

Peter Steinglass (1979) outlined five major family modalities for alcohol/drug treatment:

1. Pure family therapy is based on a family systems mode, in which all family members are present at the same time in therapy sessions.
2. Individual or group treatment approaches fulfill specific criteria suggested by a family therapy theory of alcoholism, such as the concept of homeostasis.

3. Therapies involving concurrent therapeutic work with both the alcoholic and family members rely on a more traditional, individual, psychodynamic theoretical base.
4. Specific therapies designed for the spouses or partners of alcoholics
5. Supportive treatments assist nonalcoholic family members in dealing with common problems related to having an alcoholic family member.

Following are some of the goals of the family treatment modality:

1. Develop family commitment for recovery.
2. Identify enabling behaviors and counter them.
3. Encourage leveling or open communication.
4. Validate members' reality and feelings regarding the chemical abusing member and the negative consequences of chemical abuse.
5. Educate the family to the family disease concept.
6. Elaborate on concrete rules and consequences.
7. Plan and define family leisure activities.
8. Solidify the parental coalition.
9. Specify attitudinal and behavioral changes for each member.
10. Prepare relapse prevention guidelines and family response.

According to Steinglass (1979), the advantages of a family systems approach are the following:

1. It bridges the disparity between psychodynamic and stress-reduction explanations of drinking.
2. It explains diversity in alcoholic families by redirecting the focus from common etiological characteristics in alcoholic families to the common function of alcohol to maintain imbalanced family systems.
3. It gives therapists an understanding of alcoholism as a total system's behavior.

Group Therapy

Therapy groups have the same guidelines as individual counseling. Members adhere to strict confidentiality and do not socialize outside of the group. The group's purpose is to provide a safe environment to explore individual and interpersonal issues.

Most therapy groups are led by professional counselors trained in group therapy and experienced in the dynamics of chemical dependency recovery, family systems, and related areas of expertise. Some therapy groups have co-therapists, usually male-female counseling teams that co-lead and clarify issues in the group.

Therapy groups can take many forms. I have found more success leading all-male recovery groups, and female therapists have seen a benefit to all-female therapy groups. This avoids some of the sexual and gender-specific issues that may distract from the focus on alcohol/drug recovery. Most groups have from four to eight members to allow adequate opportunity for interaction by all group members.

As discussed in Chapter 7, Yalom outlined 11 curative factors of group psychotherapy:

1. Instilling hope
2. Sharing universality
3. Imparting information
4. Fostering altruism
5. Recapitulating the primary family group
6. Developing socializing techniques
7. Imitating behavior
8. Sharing interpersonal learning
9. Developing group cohesiveness
10. Sharing catharsis
11. Exploring existential factors

Intensive Treatment

Intensive treatment modalities include intensive outpatient treatment, inpatient detoxification, and residential and inpatient treatment. These programs use a variety of treatment methods too lengthy to describe here.

An integral component of counseling alcoholics/addicts is relapse prevention. The traditional inpatient, residential alcohol/drug treatment program has people leave the program after 28 days. They leave because this is the usual time period that insurance companies have established as reimbursable. Unfortunately, from 30 to 120 days is the time when alcoholics/addicts are most at risk for relapse. The initial glow of the alcoholic's first 30 days of recovery is soon replaced with awareness of the reality of struggling to stay sober in the real world. After the first 30 days, the alcoholic/addict faces the first pivotal relapse point, or the wall. In the next 90 days, there are repeated situations that threaten the addicts' sobriety. "About two-thirds of relapses occur within the first 90 days following treatment" (i.e., between 30 and 120 days of sobriety) (Marlatt and Gordon 1985).

Case Study 11.1 presents an example of an individual who needs extended residential and out patient care.

Recognizing the Signs of Relapse

One must be trained to recognize the signs and problems that may cause relapse. (See Table 11.11.) The defense mechanisms of denial (rationalization and minimization) may be invoked to avoid looking at the potential for relapse. Many alcoholics/addicts tend to discount the stressful situations and distressful lifestyles and behaviors that contribute to relapse. The alcoholic/addict trained in relapse prevention can recognize these problem areas and avoid being blindsided by high-risk relapse situations. (See Table 11.12 and Figure 11.2.)

⚔ Relapse Prevention

Habit

Alan Marlatt and Judith Gordon (1985) described the following stages in changing a habit:

Case Study 11.1

A Need for Extended Care

Jerry

Jerry recognized he had an alcohol and drug problem. Two years earlier, he had been through treatment at a local program (27 days) and he had stayed sober for several months before going back to drinking. Recently he rationalized that the recession had caused much stress at his work and in his finances, and he quieted that anxiety with some marijuana each day. It was actually quite some time before he began using cocaine again. Although he knew he couldn't handle cocaine, he tried several times to stop without much success. His wife was the one who first suggested he get back into AA, but he refused. When his boss told him he would let him go if he didn't get into a program, Jerry voluntarily committed himself to a residential program for professionals. The employer had referred employees to this program before, with good results.

Jerry knew all the lingo and the routine, having been in treatment before. The first 2 weeks he was an ideal patient, and it was Jerry's intention to be the "best" patient and get back to work. His bubble was burst in the third week, when counselors began to confront his "ideal patient" scam. It got Jerry's attention, as he soon realized that although he might know a lot about recovery on a cognitive level, he knew very little about it on a gut or emotional level. During family week Jerry became even more aware of the depths of his feelings, when confronted by the impact of his drinking and drug-taking on the children. In his first inpatient program, he had seemed oblivious to the impact on his family, and the program had treaded lightly on those issues.

His new awareness that he needed to focus more on his "inner" recovery was a big "first step" for Jerry. He remained in the residential program and did significant work. Upon his graduation from the program, he spoke of his gratitude for the staff and the program, and said he was proud that he had spent the additional time working on his recovery. He eagerly followed through with his aftercare plan, including an outpatient group with other addicts/alcoholics who had attended the same residential and extended care program.

Discussion Questions

How long do you think addicts/alcoholics need for recovery?
Do you think extended care or an intensive outpatient follow-up is necessary in Jerry's case?
What benefits does extended treatment provide?
What problems need to be overcome for extended care to be effective?
What are the drawbacks of extended care?

1. Preparation for change, involving commitment, desire, and motivation to change
2. Implementation of the specific behavioral change (such as to eat healthy, balanced meals or to stop using alcohol/drugs)
3. Maintenance of change in long-term goals

TABLE 11.11

Relapse-Prone vs. Recovery-Prone

Denial and Evasion	Recognition and Problem Solving
Relapse-Prone	*Recovery-Prone*
Evade or deny the sticking point	Recognize a problem exists
Stress	Accept that it is O.K. to have problems
Compulsive behavior	Detach to gain perspective
Avoid others	Ask for help
Problems	Respond with action when prepared
Evade/deny new problems	

© Terence T. Gorski, The Cenaps Corporation, Homewood, IL., 708-799-5000. Published by Herald House Press, Independence, MO., 1-800-767-8181.

TABLE 11.12

Analysis of Situations for Relapse

Situations	Example	Sample Number	Percentage
Frustration/anger	Patient tried to call his wife (they were separated); she hung up on him; he became angry and took a drink.	14	29%
Social pressure	Patient went with friends to a bar after work. They put pressure on him to join the crowd, and he was unable to resist.	11	23
Intrapersonal temptation	Patient walked by a bar and just unconsciously walked in for no real reason; could not resist the temptation to take a drink.	10	21
Negative emotional state	Patient living alone, no job, complained of feeling bored and useless; could see no reason he should not take a drink.	5	10
Miscellaneous other situations	Patient reported that everything was going so well for him that he wanted to celebrate by having a drink.	5	10
No situation given or unable to remember		3	7

Source: Data from Alan Marlatt and Judith Gordon, *Relapse Prevention*, Guilford Press, New York, 1985.

FIGURE 11.2 *Caution: Relapse Ahead*

Drawing by Ed Arno; © 1980 The New Yorker Magazine, Inc. Reprinted with permission.

Marlatt and Gordon quote Mark Twain: "Quitting smoking is easy; I've done it hundreds of times." Deciding to change a habit is easy. However, implementing the change is a bit more difficult, and maintaining change is the most difficult stage because it's an ongoing, long-term goal.

For alcoholics/addicts, the beginning step is admitting that they are powerless over alcohol/drugs and have the desire to stop using. Quitting is just the beginning of the journey; implementing the change by working a program of recovery is the next difficult step. Maintaining that program despite stressful situations and life events is the most difficult, day-at-a-time struggle for recovering alcoholics/addicts.

The first 120 days of chemical dependency recovery are the most difficult because it is a significant period of time to establish a period of maintenance. Even after this primary period of maintenance, there is still no guarantee. Stressful situations, places, times, and interpersonal interactions may still cause a relapse. Even after a year of maintenance, there are pressures, as evidenced by the many alcoholics/addicts who have problems at their 1-year anniversary of sobriety. After 2 to 5 years of sobriety, alcohol/drug use is not a choice for most, even during stressful periods.

Case Study 11.2 describes the difficulties of addiction and recovery when both partners in a couple have substance addictions.

Causes of Relapse

Marlatt and Gordon (1985) identified three major categories that cause recovering alcoholics to be vulnerable to relapse:

1. *Negative emotional states* cause 35 percent of all relapses. In these situations, individuals experience negative emotional states, moods, or feelings, such as frustration, anger, anxiety, depression, or boredom. (See Table 11.13.)

Case Study 11.2

The Ideal Coupling

Alcohol and Cocaine

Alice was 35 and Gary was 29 when they first met. He was struggling to be a movie producer and she was working as the office manager in an off-Broadway theater. They were opposites in many ways.

Gary grew up in the shadow of his father's accomplishments as a major Hollywood movie producer. His family was Jewish, wealthy, and had no history of problems with drugs/alcohol. Alice grew up on the east side of New York. Her father was an alcoholic, and her mother was dependent on Valium and pain medication. She grew up in a rigid, abusive family system, with strong Catholic indoctrination.

Gary began smoking marijuana at age thirteen and used hallucinogens throughout the early 1970s. Despite his drug use, he was bright enough to graduate high school and was accepted to a college film program that he failed to complete. Gary was talented and bright. His underlying shyness stemmed from a fear of rejection and a fear of failure. He would vacillate between grandiosity and hopelessness.

Alice began drinking alcohol at the age of ten and had adverse reactions when she tried marijuana. Her drug of choice was alcohol. An extremely rebellious child, Alice had a tough time in Catholic school and barely graduated. Alice was bright, aggressive, and resourceful. Despite their different backgrounds both Gary and Alice had fathers who were emotionally unavailable, and smothering mothers who were enmeshed and needy of their affection.

The differences between Alice and Gary initially made them a good team. Gary was working on a film project in New York City when they first met. She was the perfect partner, someone who could encourage him when he was feeling insecure or down. He was the sensitive partner who represented everything that Alice didn't have when she was growing up. Alice was also able to bridge the relationship with Gary's father, which enabled Gary to get support and contacts for film projects and allowed Alice to access the powerful father figure that she never had growing up. Things were going well as Alice and Gary struggled in New York City. They enjoyed their friends, the lifestyle, and the exposure to the inner workings of the city.

Unfortunately, New York City also represented Alice's shame-based childhood; contact with her mother triggered sad memories. As a result, Alice pressured Gary to move back to Los Angeles where the major studios were and where his father's contacts could move his career faster.

Once in Los Angeles, other things moved faster, but not Gary's career. Alice quickly moved into the fast-lane lifestyle. Her flirtations and attention to others made Gary extremely jealous and angry. Before too long, Alice was again drinking heavily, and Gary's attempts to have her cut back only escalated further conflicts. At the same time, Gary was again smoking marijuana heavily. A short time later, he was snorting cocaine and eventually smoking freebase cocaine. Periodically, they swore off alcohol and cocaine. However, in a few days they would have an argument and return to using. The conflicts between Gary and his family created feelings of shame and rage. Initially, Alice was close with his family but when she began drinking and hanging out, she was snubbed by them. This brought back her feelings of rejection, shame, and feeling lesser than everyone else. Next, they taught each other about their drugs of choice, and soon they both were using alcohol and cocaine on an addictive level. With her entrepreneurial aggressiveness, Alice began dealing cocaine to support their habit, and Gary scammed

(continued on next page)

Case Study 11.2 (*continued*)

The Ideal Coupling

Alcohol and Cocaine

his parents for additional money to keep them in cocaine, alcohol, and the fast-lane lifestyle. They continued to abuse cocaine and alcohol; after a 24- to 36-hour cocaine binge, they drank alcohol to counteract the depressive crash of the cocaine. Many times they drank alcohol excessively, which lead to cocaine use. Most of these binges were followed by 2 to 5 days of sleep, excessive food binges, and a generally reclusive existence. Once a partnership of different backgrounds, now their partnership was based on alcohol and cocaine addiction.

My contact with them began when Alice was trying to get sober and struggling to get Gary into treatment. Alice finally got out of this dysfunctional codependent relationship based on alcohol and cocaine. She entered an inpatient drug/alcohol treatment program. Two years later, Alice told me that she was the director of marketing for a drug/alcohol treatment program. She had not been in contact with Gary but suspected that he was doing drugs/alcohol with a new girlfriend and going through the same addictive cycle.

Discussion Questions

What problems occur when couples try to get sober at the same time?

Do you think couples should enter the same treatment? Explain.

Explain the codependency issues in this case.

TABLE 11.13

Negative Emotional States

Difficulty Managing Negative Emotional States	Difficulty Managing Stress Effectively	Difficulty Dealing with Feelings from Family of Origin	Difficulty with Blocked Goal-Directed Activities	Physical States That Contribute to Negative Emotional States
Feelings of depression, anxiety, rage, and distress exacerbated by feelings of shame and a poor sense of self	Feelings of confusion and overreaction to problems and conflicts	Feelings of emotional pain, loss, grief, separation, abandonment, violation, rejection, and isolation	Feelings of aggressiveness and rage Feelings of being hassled by normal daily living Feelings of boredom, loneliness, isolation, uselessness, helplessness, or hopelessness; lack of purpose in life	Physical health problems, pain, illness, injury, fatigue, specific physical disorders (e.g., chronic or recurrent pain caused by headaches, menstrual cramps, back pain) Physical states associated with prior substance abuse

2. *Interpersonal conflict* causes 16 percent of all relapses. These situations involve an ongoing or a relatively recent conflict associated with any interpersonal relationship, such as marriage, friendship, relationships with family members, employer-employee relations. Arguments and interpersonal confrontation occur frequently in this category. (See Table 11.14.)

3. *Social pressure* causes 20 percent of all relapses. In these situations, individuals respond to the influence of another person or group of people exerting pressure on them to engage in the taboo behavior. (See Table 11.15.)

Sometimes recovering alcoholics/addicts do not develop or maintain all aspects of their recovery program. Table 11.16 lists some of the reasons certain persons are more prone to relapse. These factors may lead people to make impulsive decisions to test their recovery by using alcohol/drugs. In effect, this testing of their willpower to go back to controlled alcohol/drug use frequently leads to relapse.

Cravings and Urges

Thoughts, desires, even dreams about using alcohol/drugs are very common in chemical dependency recovery. A variety of things can trigger this craving for alcohol/drugs, and cravings acted on can lead to relapse. The most effective way of coping with cravings and urges is to detach from the craving. "Instead of identifying with the urge (e.g., I really want a cigarette right now) the client can be trained to monitor the urge or desire from the point of view of a detached observer (I am now experiencing the craving/urge to smoke). By externalizing and labeling the craving/urge and

---

TABLE 11.14

Interpersonal Conflicts

Conflicts with Partner/Spouse	**Conflicts with Family**	**Other Stressful Interpersonal Conflicts**
Once sober, the recovering person begins to see dysfunctional aspects of the relationship.	Recognition of family dysfunction may lead to unresolved feelings of loss, abandonment, violation, and rejection; then these issues are stuffed and not worked out.	Separation; divorce; or continued physical, sexual, or emotional violations
Different stages of recovery: one person is working on her recovery program and the other is not actively working on his issues	Family system does not change or adapt to alcoholic/addict's recovery but maintains some dysfunctional patterns of communication and interaction.	Conflicts with employer, employees, friends, and other social situations
New adjustment in relationship due to recovery		Pattern of excessive fighting, arguments, and conflicts that go unresolved and are a repetitive cycle
Fear that the relationship will not be maintained or improve		Pleasing people, avoiding conflicts, not telling others how one feels, acquiescing, and avoiding anger and other feelings associated with conflict

TABLE 11.15

Social Pressure

Peer Group	Isolating
Return to old alcohol/drug–using peer group	Withdrawing from friends who support recovery; nonattendance or passive involvement with support group, such as AA or NA
Hang out with alcohol/drug users	Not maintaining contact with sponsor, counselor, or aftercare program
	Emotionally shutting down, not sharing feelings with others who are trusted and supportive of recovery; AA's motto is "Silence is the enemy of recovery"

TABLE 11.16

Other Risk Factors for Relapse

Miscellaneous Factors

High-stress personality type

Mood swings, temper, rage

Shutting down, withdrawing emotionally

Overseparation and overattachment

Difficulty establishing intimacy and maintaining appropriate boundaries in relationships

Personality disorders: narcissism, bipolar disorder, borderline personality, codependent personality, depression (affective disorder), anxiety disorders, obsessive-compulsive disorders, and others

High-risk lifestyle: constant changes, high-stress job (i.e., always wheeling and dealing), financial and employment roller coaster, partner/spouse relationship changes and/or conflicts, always around others who use alcohol/drugs (entertainment industry, business-related drinking, bars, nightclubs, etc.)

Financial: problems in managing finances, inability to control spending, making inappropriate financial commitments and taking on inappropriate financial obligations

Problems in employment, career change with poor planning

Trouble with back taxes and the Internal Revenue Service or other previous debt

Thinking and Perceptual Factors

Self-defeating or self-sabotaging thoughts

Painful memories and/or euphoric recall of alcohol/drug use

Return of denial and inability to consciously recognize loss of control over alcohol/drugs

Poor judgment and negative or grandiose thinking, which leads to impulsive self-destructive decisions

Overreacting, crisis building, and creating problems when things are beginning to go better

Spiritual Factors

Feeling at a loss, not feeling that life has meaning

Difficulty maintaining sobriety or having a reason for staying sober

Existential despair: not seeing a function of or reason for living watching it come and go through the eyes of the observer, there will be a decreased tendency to identify with the urge and feel overwhelmed by its power" (Marlatt and Gordon 1985).

Recovering alcoholics/addicts can identify triggers leading to cravings for alcohol/drugs and develop an awareness as to why cravings occur. Then the alcoholics/addicts can structure their lives either to avoid these triggers or to desensitize themselves to the trigger.

A trigger is "a stimulus which has been repeatedly associated with the preparation for, anticipation of, or the actual use of alcohol/drugs. These stimuli include people, places, things, times of day, emotional states, and alcohol/drugs" (Rawson 1989). The following lists of time, place, thing, and people triggers show how diverse triggers are:

Time

- Periods of idle or leisure time
- Periods of extended stress
- Payday, holidays, Fridays, and Saturdays
- Birthdays and anniversaries
- Specific times of the day or evening
- Vacation
- Periods of unemployment

Place

- Drug dealers' home, bars, and parties
- Neighborhoods where drugs are dealt
- Clubs, concerts, and social events
- Places where alcohol/drugs have been used before

Things

- Drug dealers' car, telephone number, or name
- Large amounts of cash, $100 bills, and bank machines
- Paraphernalia: pipes, syringe, and rolling papers
- Movies, films, and television shows about alcohol/drugs and alcohol/drug lifestyle
- Particular music
- Alcohol and tobacco advertisements
- Conferences or seminars on alcohol/drugs
- Sexually explicit movies or magazines

People

- Alcohol/drug using friends
- Drug dealers and bartenders
- Partner/spouse, relatives, and family members who use alcohol/drugs
- Sexual encounters
- Groups of people talking about or using alcohol/drugs

Case Study 11.3

Let's Bury the Cocaine

Cocaine Addicts

Cocaine is so addicting that negative consequences often do not deter continued use. In one situation, three men who were using and dealing cocaine decided that the situation was getting out of control. They lived in a large mansion with high walls and a sophisticated security system. Late one evening, because things were getting out of hand, they dug a 6-foot-deep hole in their backyard and stored all their cocaine in this hole. They covered it up and put an extremely heavy cement statue on top. By only 3 A.M., the allure of the cocaine had gotten to them. Flashlights and shovels in hand, they were busy digging up their stash.

Discussion Questions

How strong do you think the allure of "cocaine" is?
Have you ever found yourself hiding drugs, food, etc. so you can't get to it?
What happened?
Can an "addict" have a small quantity of a drug?

Case Study 11.3 illustrates the power of cravings over individuals with substance addictions.

Drug Relapse Induced by Alcohol Use

Some individuals in recovery test their recovery by using alcohol instead of drugs. They rationalize that they were addicted to drugs but never had a problem with alcohol. This rationalization is unfounded. Once addicted to drugs, people have an addiction potential to all drugs, including alcohol. It is only a matter of time before individuals build tolerance and become addicted to alcohol or alcohol use impairs judgment and they return to drugs.

Richard Rawson (1988) has established that a return to alcohol use by cocaine addicts increases their cocaine relapse vulnerability by an astounding 800 percent. (See Table 11.17.) Case Study 11.4 illustrates the revolving-door relapse cycle.

TABLE 11.17

Percentage Return to Regular Cocaine Use, Matrix Study, 1988

Did return to alcohol use	50%
Did not return to alcohol use	6%
Sierra Tucson, 1988	
Did return to alcohol use	61%
Did not return to alcohol use	8%

> ## Case Study 11.4
>
> ### *Alcohol-Induced Relapse—A Need for a Stronger Team Approach*
>
> #### Mary
>
> Mary, 42 years old, married with three children, was hospitalized for severe depression, panic reactions, and post-traumatic stress. She was also assessed as having an addiction to pain medication and tranquilizers. As part of her treatment plan, Mary worked with the team for co-occurring disorders (alcohol/drug and psychiatric problems) on her addiction to pills. Gradually, she was physically withdrawn from the tranquilizers and pain medication, while she received individual and group counseling on alcoholism and drug addiction. Mary also attended AA meetings and educational classes on various aspects of the disease model of alcoholism and drug addiction.
>
> Approximately 6 weeks after her discharge from the hospital, Mary's aftercare nurse asked if it was appropriate for Mary to be drinking wine with dinner each evening. Despite in-service training on alcoholism and drug addiction with the hospital staff, Mary's psychiatrist had approved her use of wine with dinner. When asked about his counsel, the psychiatrist felt that Mary had no history of alcoholism and her problem was with drugs (medication).
>
> Despite interventions by the treatment team, the psychiatrist insisted that Mary's use of alcohol with dinner was appropriate. Mary was only able to maintain this use of wine with dinner for a short time. Two weeks later, under the influence of alcohol, Mary tripped and broke her leg. She then lapsed back to using pain medication and alcohol. Six weeks later, she was readmitted to the hospital.
>
> Unfortunately, there are many Marys who continue on this revolving-door cycle with treatment facilities.
>
> #### Discussion Questions
>
> Explain: "A drug is a drug, is a drug."
> Do you think a person with a drug problem can drink?
> What problems may occur?

Once recovering alcoholics/addicts understand which factors contribute to relapse, they can try to prevent relapses. Also, all chemical dependency treatment programs have the responsibility to conduct relapse prevention to help maintain the client/patient's chemical dependency recovery. Alan Marlatt and Judith Gordon (1985) developed a very organized model of global self-control strategies in relapse prevention (see Figure 11.3).

✖ Relapse-Prevention Strategies

Lifestyle Imbalance

You may recall that homeostasis is an organism's natural tendency to seek a balanced state. If a life is imbalanced, the individual experiences too much or too little

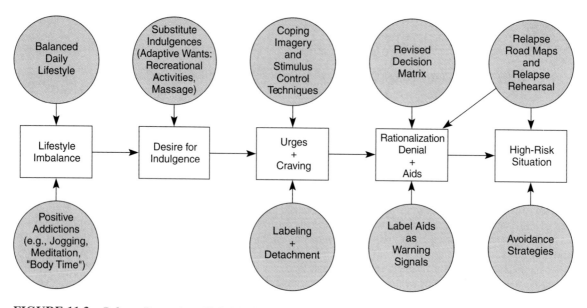

FIGURE 11.3   *Relapse Prevention: Global Self-Control Strategies*

stress; eventually, that results in a compensation in some area of life, or a breakdown. The imbalance can be evidenced by

- Too much work (workaholism) or overresponsibility, resulting in a neglect of self
- Difficulty relaxing; lack of spontaneity; and an inability to have fun, enjoy others, and feel emotions (shut down or emotionally unavailable to self or others, especially spouse and family)—"too many shoulds, too many wants"
- Too much play or irresponsibility, resulting in procrastination, laziness, avoidance of conflicts and pain, and avoidance of life-maintaining activities (passively forgetting or avoiding responsibilities)—"too many wants, not paying attention to needs"

Both workaholic and playaholic behavior have common root issues: the avoidance of taking up painful issues of self-concept interpersonal and life situation displeasure and the avoidance of recognizing and integrating true feelings. Usually, some deeper family of origin issues that have not been worked through are recapitulated (duplicated) in present-day life situations.

The alcoholic/addict has lived a life structured around alcohol/drugs. Removing the alcohol/drugs is a challenge to the individual and family's systemic organization. Triggers for alcohol/drug cravings, and potential relapse, are frequently related to the lack of organization and structure in the lives of the newly sober alcoholic/addict and the family. Structure promotes a variety of important recovery functions. First, structure redirects idle time through time scheduling, goal setting, and planning of activities. This includes work, play, vacation, recreation, and leisure time. Structured time maintains a focus on activities and is based on an integration of feelings.

Case Study 11.5

Physically Strong Addict

Kim

Kim, 31, was able to outdrink and outdrug the best of her friends, male and female. She was thin, tall, blond, and attractive with beautiful delicate features. Not only was she physically able to tolerate drugs/alcohol with no significant hangover but despite thin arms, she was also one of the best arm wrestlers in the state.

Her normal weekend behavior was to drink and drug at a local bar. Due to her good looks, she was frequently approached by men at the bar. Often these men had drunk beyond their capabilities and could be quite obnoxious. To stop their advances and obnoxious behavior, Kim would challenge them to arm-wrestling matches. The stakes of the arm-wrestling match were simple: if she lost, she would buy him a drink; if he lost, he would buy drinks for the house. Suffice it to say, she was extremely popular at the bar.

Discussion questions

Explain the role of tolerance as relates to this case.
What role did "set & setting" play in this case?
Do you know someone like Kim? What are their behaviors?

Second, structure teaches balance in daily activities, balance between work and play, balance in responsibility, and balance in establishing effective boundaries in relationships. Third, structure promotes self-concept by placing emphasis on moving from passive dependence to proactive involvement in life. Structure reduces fears and anxieties, and it promotes self-reliance and preparedness. *Freedom* is a word often misused to represent lack of responsibility. Freedom is choosing your own version of responsibility to self and others and the structure necessary to achieve such freedom. Case Study 11.5 illustrates a common sort of bravado alcoholism. Case Study 11.6 illustrates periodic relapses in an individual who keeps very busy.

The following pitfalls of structure are adapted from Richard Rawson (1989):

- A rigid dysfunctional approach, overdoing, scheduling unrealistically
- Burnout from workaholism and overextending of self
- Neglecting recreation and leisure activity
- Being perfectionistic and/or overly zealous about recovery
- Talking a program, rather than working a program of recovery
- Alienating others by preaching your program of recovery
- External control—structure that is not self-imposed; pleasing the counselor, sponsor, spouse, parent, instead of working a program for self; blind adherence without self-involvement in program
- Failure to maintain spontaneously to others, and life in general

Areas of structure for the recovering alcoholic/addict include the following social, health, and cognitive facets of life.

Case Study 11.6

High-Functioning Cocaine Addict/Alcoholic— "For a While"

Ralph

Ralph, 37, is a high-functioning addict/alcoholic for a while. When his cocaine use became a problem, he signed himself into outpatient treatment through an employee assistance program at work. He did extremely well in the intensive outpatient treatment program, which involved both individual and group counseling. Ralph stopped using cocaine completely. When told that he must also stop using alcohol and attend regular Alcoholics Anonymous or Narcotic Anonymous meetings, Ralph resisted. He candidly admitted that he felt the issue was his cocaine use, not his alcohol use. He admitted that he was a cocaine addict but believed that he was not an alcoholic because he never drank alcoholically.

As the normal pressures and stress of work, family, and marital life intensified, Ralph periodically got drunk to fall asleep. After this pattern persisted for a while, he cut back his alcohol consumption and exercised on a regular basis. Ralph enjoyed the diversion of long-distance running and was in remarkable shape considering his use of alcohol. Running also allowed him to get out of the house and release the pressure from work. Ralph maintained this cycle of control and then release for over a year. Meanwhile, he still attended counseling sessions although not heeding the warning by the counselor about the potential for relapse to cocaine.

During the following 6-month cycle, Ralph returned to cocaine use. A pattern of cocaine binges then occurred for 6 months before Ralph concluded that alcohol often led to these binges.

Discussion Questions

> How long do you think before Ralph is sober?
> How long before his next relapse?
> Explain the "narcissistic" traits that Ralph possesses.

Interpersonal and Social Recovery Support System

- Drug-free friends who understand and support recovery from alcohol/drugs
- Self-help groups, such as Alcoholics Anonymous, Narcotics Anonymous, Adult Children of Alcoholics, and Co-Dependents Anonymous
- Spouse/partner and family members who understand recovery and are involved in their own recovery and counseling
- Support of an AA or NA sponsor; someone who has strong personal recovery is available and active in pointing out relapse vulnerability
- Support from an aftercare program, group, or individual and family counseling on a regular basis

Health and Physical Well-Being

- A regular program of exercise: athletic activities, slow long-distance walking, or jogging/running, minimum three to five times per week

- Balanced, nutritionally sound, and structured diet
- Adequate sleep, functional stress level, appropriate balance between work and play and activity and rest

Cognitive, Emotional, and Spiritual Self

- Good sense of self, as a person (1) who is unique and worthwhile with emerging talents and skills; (2) who can accomplish things, has good decision-making and problem-solving skills—no self-sabotaging; (3) who can trust and be trusted while setting appropriate boundaries in relationships; and (4) who has the ability to resolve conflict and communicate feelings
- Ability to be aware of feelings and thoughts and to integrate feelings and thoughts in taking appropriate action
- Ability to adapt to life changes and stresses and to choose to grow emotionally, intellectually, occupationally, and interpersonally
- Ability to achieve at work, at school, at home, and in the community
- Spiritual orientation and growth with others and to spiritual life in general

Desire for Self-Indulgence

Frustration and anger are feelings that result from not attaining personal long-range goals. After losing hope and motivation, the recovering alcoholic/addict decides to take the short-range, immediate relief by using alcohol/drugs.

The immediate gratification of drugs needs to be countered with the understanding that things change, feelings can be felt, and time changes the way one views things. The entire chemical dependency recovery program is designed to get the person back on track by using new recovery skills to instill feelings of hope. Those in recovery should follow the AA saying "Take it one day at a time."

> Waiting is not mere empty hoping. It has the inner certainty of reaching a goal. Such certainty alone gives that light which leads to success. This leads to the perseverance that leads to good fortune and bestows power to cross the great water.
>
> One is faced with a danger that must be overcome. Weakness and impatience can do nothing. Only a strong man can stand up to his fate, for his inner security enables him to endure to the end. This strength shows itself in uncompromising truthfulness (with himself). It is only when we have the courage to face things exactly as they are, without any sort of self-deception or illusion, that a light will develop out of events, by which the path to success may be recognized. This recognition must be followed by resolute and persevering action. For only the man who goes to meet his fate resolutely is equipped to deal with it adequately. Then he will be able to cross the great water—that is to say, he will be capable of making the necessary decision and of surmounting the danger. (*I Ching,* Hexagram 5)

AA Serenity Prayer as a Relapse-Prevention Technique

The serenity prayer of AA is an extremely valuable relapse-prevention technique that is easily invoked:

God grant me the serenity
To accept the things I cannot change,
Courage to change the things I can,
And wisdom to know the difference.

Accepting the things I cannot change means accepting what can't be controlled. Those in recovery need the skills to let go, to not control others or project their wishes on others. As a result, recovering alcoholics/addicts avoid the negative emotional feelings of anger, rage, anxiety, depression, and intolerable frustration.

Courage to change the things I can means controlling what can be controlled. Those in recovery need the skills to focus on today, to take action, and to work on themselves. As a result, recovering alcoholics/addicts develop positive affirmations, progress toward long-term goals, and develop a stronger sense of self.

Wisdom to know the difference means learning to discriminate between the impossible and the possible. Those in recovery need the skills to talk about feelings, accept limits, and ask "Can I change this?" As a result, recovering alcoholics/addicts can achieve a balanced lifestyle, can develop the ability to deal with urges and cravings, and can learn to avoid impulsive, destructive decisions and interactions.

> Recovery is facilitated by the individual's ability to adapt to change and integrate feelings related to change. Striving for progress rather than perfection is a healthy goal.

✖ Controlled Drinking Controversy

Widespread controversy has arisen over the issue of the controlled drinking of alcohol. Controlled drinking has been defined as monitoring one's own drinking in order to prevent a return to problem drinking. "With the trend has come a maelstrom of controversy. Many traditional figures in the alcoholism field have bitterly attacked the concept of controlled drinking, maintaining that a disease model and total abstinence represents the only true hope for alcoholics" (Miller 1980).

Ruth Fox (1963) has asserted that, "among my own approximately 3,000 patients, not one has been able to achieve moderate drinking, although almost every one of them has tried to."

Once someone has been diagnosed as being addicted to alcohol/drugs, experts predominantly agree that a return to controlled alcohol or drug use is extremely difficult and could lead to a tragic outcome if pursued.

Proponents of controlled drinking agree with this position that controlled drinking is not a viable option for alcoholics, especially alcoholics already in successful abstinence recovery. They stress that controlled drinking is a viable treatment approach only for some problem drinkers. Controlled drinking is considered only when individuals have a stable marital and occupational background and do not have a family history of alcoholism.

William Miller and G. R. Caddy (1977) identified controlled drinking as an appropriate treatment approach in situations involving resistant clients who view abstinence as unachievable or undesirable. The major criteria are (1) their refusal to consider abstinence as a goal; (2) their strong external demands to drink or lack of social support for abstinence; (3) an early-stage drinking problem without a history of physiological addiction; and (4) prior failure of competent abstinence-oriented treatment.

The problem with these criteria is that denial may be ignored. Almost every alcoholic/addict would like to continue using alcohol/drugs in a controlled fashion.

Refusal to consider abstinence, failure in abstinence-oriented treatment, and preference for controlled drinking may all be part of the alcoholic/addict's denial system.

Miller (1980) identified additional criteria that would favor choosing the abstinence model instead of moderation:

1. Evidence of progressive liver disease or other medical problems
2. Psychological problems of sufficient magnitude to render even moderate drinking harmful
3. Personal commitment to abstinence or strong external demands for abstinence
4. Pathological intoxication
5. History of physiological addiction and severe withdrawal symptoms
6. Use of medication considered dangerous when combined with alcohol
7. Current successful abstinence following severe problem drinking
8. Prior failure of competent moderation-oriented treatment

Additional risk factors for controlled drinking include a current addiction, a family history of addiction, a high-stress individual, a high-stress lifestyle, an inability to cope effectively with stress, and other relapse dynamics present, such as poor health, negative emotional states, or psychiatric problems.

Vernon Fox (1976) and others agree that abstinence remains the viable and conservative recommendation for alcohol/drug recovery while research and guidelines establish accurate means for identifying clients appropriate for controlled drinking as an optimal treatment modality. The primary goal of recovery is complete abstinence from alcohol/drugs.

✄ Harm-Reduction Approach

Controlled drinking is just one example of a harm-reduction approach. The harm-reduction approach has its roots in The Netherlands public health, or sociomedical, perspective. In 1984, the Dutch were concerned with "reducing the harm" of drug use, abuse, and dependence and implemented the first needle exchange program to reduce the harm of hepatitis due to injecting drugs. They saw the greater risk of hepatitis and had public support. This is very different from the moral and political perspective, in the United States, that needle exchange programs are not addressing the substance dependence problem.

The harm-reduction approach takes a more realistic perspective—that people are going to use drugs, so why not reduce the risk that they will also contract and spread other diseases? The success of the needle exchange program in The Netherlands is due to the support of the government and the Dutch people. In the United States, the limited needle exchange programs lacked that support. It is believed that the epidemic levels of HIV/AIDS in Europe never reached those levels in The Netherlands due to the needle exchange program. Other countries have successfully implemented needle exchange programs to prevent hepatitis and HIV/AIDS—England, Switzerland, and Australia.

The United States has maintained "supply reduction" as the dominant approach to the drug problem. Recent efforts to expand the methadone treatment programs is another effort at harm reduction. Methadone treatment is being expanded to primary care physicians, rather than being limited to the methadone treatment center. LAAM, a longer acting methadone, is being used as well.

FIGURE 11.4 *Spectrum of Drug Control Policies*

Source: In *Harm reduction,* edited by A. Marlatt. New York. Guilford Press.

Harm reduction includes a wide range of programs and policies, including the following (Inciardi and Harrison 2000) (see Figure 11.4):

1. *Advocacy for changes in drug policies*—legalization, decriminalization, ending the drug prohibition, changes in drug paraphernalia laws, reduction of penalties for drug-related crimes, and treatment alternatives to incarceration
2. *HIV/AIDS-related interventions*—needle/syringe exchange programs, HIV prevention/intervention programs, bleach distribution, referrals for HIV testing and HIV medical care, and referrals for HIV/AIDS-related psychosocial care and case management
3. *Broader drug treatment options*—methadone maintenance by primary care physicians, changes in methadone regulations, heroin substitution programs, and new experimental treatments
4. *Drug-abuse management for those who wish to continue using drugs*—counseling and clinical case-management programs that promote safer and more responsible drug use
5. *Ancillary interventions*—housing and other entitlements, healing centers, and support and advocacy groups

The harm-reduction perspective is totally different from the perspective of traditional alcohol/drug counseling and this has made it controversial. Following are some elements of the harm-reduction approach in counseling (Denning 2000):

- The harm done, not the drug use itself, is the focus.
- Any reduction in drug-related harm is a success (a change in the right direction).
- Confrontation is to be avoided.

Legalization, controlled availability, medicalization, and decriminalization are drug-control policies that are seen as having a harm-reduction nature (see Figure 11.4).

✖ An Effective Alcohol/Drug Recovery Strategy

The following steps can help those in recovery achieve their goal:

1. *Break the bonds of denial.* Recovery is an ongoing process often facilitated by the support of others—friends, others in recovery from alcohol/drugs, family, or a counselor. All of these people can help alcoholics/addicts work through their denial and maintain sobriety.
2. *Actively work and apply the 12 steps and other AA principles in recovery.*

This provides guidelines, structure, and support for recovery efforts. Developing a relationship with an AA or NA sponsor is a key element in effectively helping the newly recovering person understand and implement the principles of AA.

3. *Seek nonchemical altered states of consciousness.* The innate human drive to alter one's sense of consciousness can be attained through healthy and balanced activities, not the use of alcohol/drugs. These activities enhance the individual's sense of self and well-being.

4. *Work through negative emotional states and control destructive impulses.* Negative life experiences commonly result in emotions that get out of control and cause additional problems. The individual in recovery can learn new coping skills and gain support in working through impulses that may lead to destructive decisions and interactions.

5. *Move from passive to active decision making in all aspects of life.* Most addictive behaviors are passive, automatic, ritualistic, and habitual. This includes workaholism, gambling, eating disorders, and many other behaviors that fit our behavioral definition of addiction. Recovering individuals need to be involved and active in their recovery. Most learning comes from doing.

6. *Resist social or peer pressure.* When it endangers welfare or inhibits growth, peer pressure can cause those in recovery to make the wrong choices. Recovery is maintained by being and talking with others in recovery, rather than isolating. Associating with people who don't understand or, more important, don't respect the individual's recovery could require changing relationships. Recovering alcoholics/addicts should develop and maintain relationships that support a healthy alcohol/drug-free lifestyle.

7. *Improve and continue to work on the sense of self.* Those in recovery need to be involved in activities and relationships that promote a positive sense of self. To develop a sense of self, they must believe they are unique, worthwhile individuals with emerging talents and skills; individuals who can accomplish things; individuals who can trust and be trusted while setting appropriate boundaries in relationships and avoiding codependency and dysfunctionality.

8. *Deal more effectively with stress.* Recovering addicts/alcoholics must develop awareness in recognizing stressful situations and the need for support (attachments), coping skills, and resources to deal with or adapt to the stress.

9. *Maintain the structure of the recovery program.* Recovering alcoholics and addicts should consistently attend self-help meetings, aftercare, counseling sessions, and other elements of the recovery program.

10. *Have patience and direction.* Those in recovery must have a road map, while maintaining a day-at-a-time perspective in recovery.

11. *Learn how to enjoy life and others.* By developing the capacity to relax, enjoy, and have fun with others, recovering persons can establish leisure activities, hobbies, and personal interests.

12. *Maintain a sense of humor.* Those in recovery very much need to keep things in perspective, and remember, "I'm not O.K. You're not O.K. But that's O.K."

13. *Take responsibility for self.* No matter what the event is, those in recovery have the freedom to choose their response to it. Taking responsibility for self leads to awareness, which in turn helps the individual make effective choices.

14. *Maintain physical, emotional, and spiritual well-being.* Recovering alcoholics/addicts need regular exercise, balanced nutrition, and adequate sleep and rest. Recovery also involves effective communication in relationships, especially intimate relationships. One must work on spiritual values in life and strive to experience the joy and creativity of life, while exploring one's own sense of spirituality.

15. *Avoid shame.* Mistakes may occur, but alcoholics/addicts can return to recovery without a burden of shame. Shame generated by others or themselves inhibits personal recovery and growth from situations that may be painful.

16. *Work on relapse-prevention strategies.* Those in recovery need to deal with urges and cravings to use alcohol/drugs, imbalanced lifestyles, negative emotional states, social pressures, high-risk situations, and other factors that may make them vulnerable to relapse.

17. *Adapt to changes in life.* Alcoholics/addicts can remind themselves that they are human and subject to human feelings and emotions. Life is not perfect and always involves change. Recovery is facilitated by the individual's ability to adapt to change and integrate feelings related to change. Striving for progress rather than perfection is a healthy goal.

✖ Treatment of Co-occurring Disorders

As outlined in Chapter 10, a person who has *co-occurring disorders* is chemically dependent and has a psychiatric disorder. Affective (feeling) or mood disorders and personality disorders were the major focus in Chapter 10. However, any psychiatric disorder classified in the fourth edition of the *Diagnostic and Statistical Manual of Mental Disorders (DSM-IV)* combined with a chemical dependency is considered a co-occurring disorder.

Traditionally, patients with co-occurring disorders are viewed as difficult, distracting, and disorganized in treatment. Many patients with co-occurring disorders are multiple users of psychiatric, medical, and chemical dependency treatment facilities and are often described as "revolving door" treatment users, moving from agency to agency. Such patients are reported to be difficult, noncompliant, and resistant to treatment. They tend to become crisis users of the emergency room and of inpatient and medical detoxification services (Hellerstein and Meehan 1987).

Boundaries with Patients Who Have Co-occurring Disorders

Groves (1978) identified some of the troublesome behavior patterns in describing four categories of patients who arouse negative feelings in the counselor.

1. Dependent Clingers
    - Need a great deal of "attention"
    - Perceive the therapist as "inexhaustible"
    - Express gratitude to therapist, causing feelings of specialness and power in therapist (set up to continue giving to client)

Guidelines for counselor:
- Establish boundaries (limits of time, knowledge, skill, and stamina)
- Avoid promises that can't be kept
- Avoid supporting illusions that will be shattered

2. Demanders
   - Intimidate, devalue, and try to instill guilt in the counselor
   - Are unaware of their deep dependency needs and terror of abandonment

   Guidelines for counselor:
   - Resist the temptation to make a devastating response
   - Support entitlement but direct it to needed treatment ("You are entitled to the best help we can give you, but we can't give good treatment unless you help")
   - Avoid tireless debates
   - Repeat theme or acceptance that they deserve good treatment

3. Manipulative Help-Rejectors
   - Try your recommendations but nothing works
   - Seek an undivorcible marriage with an inexhaustible caregiver who will maintain the relationship as long as symptoms/problems exist
   - Intense dependency needs but fear closeness

   Guidelines for counselor:
   - You are putting out "fires"—band-aid treatment
   - Use gentle, simple reasoning rather than complicated explanations
   - Establish clear boundaries
   - Agree that progress is slow

4. Self-Destructive Deniers
   - Continue drinking/drugging, despite significant negative consequences
   - Have given up hope to have needs met
   - Seem to enjoy defeating recovery attempts

   Grove gave these guidelines for counselor:
   - Fight the impulse to abandon these clients
   - Recognize your own limitations, get help through consultation
   - Intervene to try to "raise their bottom"

Many clients with co-occurring disorders present these kinds of troublesome behaviors, which make treatment difficult. However, the counselor skilled in setting appropriate boundaries and having clear expectations for these clients can be more effective.

Counseling for Co-occurring Disorders
Breaking Denial—Educating and Empowering Patients

These patients tend to have strong denial that can be difficult to break through. The client may focus on one co-occurring disorder as the primary cause for his or her problems while ignoring the impact of the other disorder. The family may also focus on one cause of the problem (i.e., his or her drinking/drugging or manic-depressive behavior) to avoid recognizing the painful dimensions of the co-occurring disorder.

Education and intervention are needed to help the client and family members recognize that they are dealing with not one but two interrelated disorders. The counselor can establish rapport by educating clients with co-occurring disorders and helping them recognize the dimensions and impact of their disorder. The primary treater is the patient. Once educated, patients become experts on their diagnosis. They are then empowered to take personal responsibility for their recovery.

Developing Skills in Patients Who Have Co-occurring Disorders

Feelings and Emotional Buildup   Like most counseling approaches with individuals who have an alcohol/drug problem, counseling for co-occurring disorders involves helping the client identify feelings, especially feelings of anger, guilt, and shame. It is important to help these clients also identify how these feelings may build up and eventually result in psychiatric relapse.

Methods to reduce stress and deal with these feelings are an integral aspect of the counseling (e.g., redirection to recreational activities, exercise and relaxation, stress-reduction techniques).

Cognitive-Behavioral Approaches   Cognitive-behavioral techniques help in the recovery from co-occurring disorders. One major focus is to instill hope and to change depressive thinking.

The way a person thinks plays a major role in feelings of depression, mood disturbances, and personality problems. The individual's perception of events in life colors his or her emotional reaction dramatically. This can be described as depressive thinking. Although one should not ignore one's feelings, overreacting to situations may develop into a pattern or habit of depressive thinking, or thinking the worst. If the individual is already depressed, it may significantly deepen his or her depression.

Some of these negative and depressive ways of thinking may have their roots in childhood. Parents may have modeled depressive thinking and depressive patterns of behavior. Parents who shame their children with negative statements (e.g., "You are stupid") teach them to internalize these depressive messages, which are then carried into adulthood. Cognitive-behavioral approaches can teach the individual to change these unhealthy ways of thinking and of reacting to life situations by countering these negative thoughts.

Alcoholics Anonymous has a number of slogans that trigger cognitive-behavioral change from depressive thinking:

Shame statement: "No matter what I do, it's never good enough."
AA slogan: "Progress not perfection" reminds us that we don't have to see ourselves as either successes or failures, or be perfect all the time.
Shame statement: "I am aggressively argumentative, and always have to be right. I feel especially bad when I behave this way with those close to me."
AA slogan: "Would you rather be right or happy?" reminds us that always having to be right or prove another wrong is often alienating, and isolating, behavior.

The following are some examples of common depressive thinking patterns:

- Black-and-white or right-wrong thinking: "If you're recovering, you can't take any medication, because all medications are drugs."
- "Awfulizing," or making things seem worse than they really are: "I'm probably going to get fired because I missed that deadline."

- Overgeneralizing: "Boy, I'm really stupid because I made that mistake."
- Catastrophizing: "What if they tell me I've got cancer?"
- Disqualifying the positive: "Oh, anybody could've done it."
- Jumping to conclusions: "He looked upset when I walked past his office. He probably saw me come in late."
- Feeling that temporary situations are permanent: "I'm never going to find a job."
- Shaming ourselves with "should" and "why" statements: "Why didn't I study harder?" or "I should have known the answer to that."
- Negative labeling: "I'm stupid." "I'm hopeless." "I'm a failure."
- Personalizing, or taking responsibility for things we're not responsible for: "We probably lost the account because I wasn't aggressive enough."

Depression feeds on inactivity and depressive thinking. Clients can interrupt the depressive inactivity and depressive thinking by taking action. Physical activity is the remedy prescribed most often for mood disorders. I will joke with my patients by telling them to use "LSD"—*l*ong, *s*low, *d*istance, walking for clients recovering from alcohol/drugs and/or depression. The first step is to make *taking action* as easy as possible by eliminating the obstacles. For example, to be successful, an exercise program needs to be realistic and allow little room for procrastination.

Taking action can also mean eating in a healthy manner, taking a class, working on relationships at work and home, taking a vacation, playing with friends, and so forth. All of these things help clients recover from the co-occurring disorders of chemical dependency and mood disorder.

Both chemical dependency and affective disorders are diseases that grow with isolation and withdrawal. The metaphor of the dragon in the corner, eating its own tail, describes their crippling effects. The AA motto "Silence is the enemy of recovery" applies here. Clients must develop relationships with others in recovery. They can find friends and support by being active in Twelve-Step recovery programs, educational groups, counseling (both individual and group), and community and church groups.

Treatment Compliance—Medications

Frequently, antidepressant medication is an integral part of the recovery from co-occurring disorders. The selective serotonin reuptake inhibitors (SSRIs) category of antidepressants are most frequently used with patients who have co-occurring disorders. As their name implies, these drugs work in the brain by blocking the reuptake of serotonin into nonactive storage areas, thus increasing its availability, which has an antidepressant effect. (See Table 11.18.)

Interestingly, in double-blind studies, with nondepressed alcoholics who were given an SSRI antidepressant, approximately 20 percent reported a decrease in alcohol craving and were therefore aided in maintaining abstinence (Jancin 1994).

Unfortunately, many patients with co-occurring disorders do not comply with the directions given by their psychiatrist regarding medication. The counselor who may have more ongoing contact can help monitor medication compliance.

The common noncompliance behaviors include stopping medications abruptly, reducing dosage, and stopping and starting or forgetting to take medication on schedule. Some patients will discontinue medication before they have given the medication

---

TABLE 11.18

Generic and Proprietary Names of Psychiatric Medications

Antidepressants	**Antianxiety (continued)**
Imipramine (Tofranil, Presamine)	Oxazepam (Serax)
Doxepin (Sinequan, Apapin, Sinequan)	Alprazolam (Xanax)
Desipramine (Norpramin, Pertrofrone)	Clonazepam (Clonopin)
Amitriptyline (Elavil)	Buspirone (BuSpar)
Nortriptyline (Pamelor, Aventyl)	Hydroxyzine (Vistaril, Atarax)
Protriptyline (Vivactil)	**Antipsychotic**
Chlomipramine (Anafranil)	
Fluoxetine (Prozac)	Haloperidol (Haldol)
Trazodone (Desyrel)	Chlorpromazine (Thorazine)
Maprotiline (Ludiomil)	Fluphenazine hydrochloride (Prolixin)
Amoxapine (Asendin)	Trifluoperazine (Stelazine)
Bupropion (Wellbutrin)	Perphenazine (Trilafon)
Tranylcypromine (Parnate)	Thioridazine (Mellaril)
Phenelzine (Nardil)	Thiothixene (Navane)
Antianxiety	**Mood Cycling**
Diazepam (Valium)	Lithium
Chlordiazepoxide (Librium)	Carbamazepine (Tegretol)
Chorazepate dipotassium (Tranxene)	Valproic acid (Depakote)
Lorazepam (Ativan)	Clonazepam (Clonopin)

Not all medications in each group are listed.

---

time to begin working (usually 2 or more weeks). Working closely with the psychiatrist prescribing medication can assure the proper dosage, and the type of medication can be adjusted to best serve the patient with co-occurring disorders.

The Family of the Client Who Has Co-occurring Disorders

The behavior (e.g., suicide attempts, psychotic episodes, grossly disturbed behavior, feeling disorders) of the patient with co-occurring disorders may expose other family members to tremendous stress and trauma. The severity and length of the problem may emotionally, physically, financially, and spiritually exhaust family members. Some family members (e.g., brothers, sisters) may have felt that their needs were not being met. Family members can benefit from supportive counseling.

Often, family members have unique perceptions of the family member who has co-occurring disorders. This causes tremendous conflict and tension between parents and other family members.

Frequently, the mother sees her son as ill and needing acceptance and understanding (e.g., "If only we could get him the right help he will be O.K."). The father, on the other hand, sees the son as lazy and irresponsible and that the problem stems mainly from the son's drinking/drugging too much (e.g., "If he only would stop using alcohol/drugs, things would get better."). Unfortunately, they are both wrong—the problem involves both alcohol/drugs and psychological problems, and both need to be addressed.

Educating the family and engaging them in treatment early often positively effects treatment outcome. Families are more likely to cooperate if approached in a supportive manner by clinicians. Clinicians can be viewed as people who understand their experience and don't blame them. The counselors' ability to demonstrate their expertise regarding co-occurring disorders (both the psychiatric and alcohol/drug aspects of recovery) can help in establishing trust and rapport with the family.

The goals of family treatment are these:

1. Acquiring knowledge about co-occurring disorders
2. Increasing self-awareness, especially each family member's role in the family
3. Helping individual members make changes in the family system
4. Maintaining family members' involvement in ongoing recovery efforts (e.g., Alanon, individual and family counseling, groups)

It is estimated that 29,000 Americans commit suicide each year. Suicide is the eighth leading cause of death in the general population and the third among adolescents. Less than 1 percent of the general population commits suicide, yet studies reveal that between 7 and 27 percent of all deaths of alcoholics are by suicide. A percentage of these suicides by alcoholics are probably due to other underlying or comorbid psychiatric disorders (e.g., primary affective disorders, antisocial personality disorder, borderline personality disorder). The San Diego Suicide Study (SDSS) of 283 consecutive suicides in San Diego County (1981–83), found that 58 percent of the suicides had diagnoses of drug addiction, and psychiatric diagnoses frequently overlapped with the addiction diagnoses.

✖ Suicide and Alcohol/ Drugs

Frequently, alcohol or drugs impair judgment and influence suicidal ideation and behavior. The right combination of trauma, stress, loss, depression, isolation, health problems, interpersonal/spouse conflict, financial/occupational problems, and alcohol/drug use may lead to feelings of hopelessness, helplessness, and shame, making the individual vulnerable to suicide.

The following facts have been drawn from the research literature to help you understand and possibly help someone thinking of suicide.*

- Most people who commit suicide give some clue or warning of their intent; therefore, suicidal threats, gestures, or attempts should always be treated seriously.
- Suicide tends to "run in families," due, most likely, to genetic vulnerabilities to depression or other forms of mental or emotional illness.
- Having fallen out of love with life, most suicidal people remain ambivalent about dying. Thus, most can be talked back into living.

---

* This section was developed by, and permission was granted by, Paul Quinnett, Ph.D., Spokane, Wash. Dr. Quinnett is the author of *Suicide: The Forever Decision* and *Suicide: Intervention and Therapy.*

- Some depressed people appear to be "suddenly" happy after they decide to "resolve" all their problems at the same time.
- Alcohol/drug abuse greatly enhances the short- and long-term risk of suicide—even in people who are not alcoholic.
- If the person in a suicide crisis receives the proper assistance and support, he or she will probably never be suicidal again. Only about 10 percent of suicide attempters go on to complete a suicide.
- Asking someone directly about suicidal intent does not increase the risk of suicide. Rather, the question lowers anxiety, opens up communication about the problems worth dying for, and lowers the risk of an impulsive act.
- The majority of suicidal people will visit a physician within three months of an attempt to kill themselves. Too often, their thoughts of suicide are neither expressed to the doctor, nor asked for.
- Twenty to 40 percent of patients with affective disorder (depression) exhibit nonfatal suicidal behavior, including thoughts of suicide.
- Fifteen percent of patients with severe depression for at least one month eventually commit suicide.
- Sudden unemployment is associated with increased risk of suicide.
- Suicide occurs more often in midweek.
- Suicide rates decline during major holidays, such as Thanksgiving and Christmas.
- Drinking alcoholics have a lifetime suicide rate much higher than the general population and are 60 to 120 times more likely to die by suicide.
- In America, suicide rates are higher on the East and West coasts.
- Suicide increases with age, reaching a peak among older white males. Older people are at greater risk for suicide than teenagers.
- Most suicidal people plan their self-destruction in advance and leave clues indicating they have become suicidal.
- Of those who die by their own hand, men outnumber women 3 to 1.
- Women make gestures or attempts on their lives three times as often as men.
- As age increases, so does the risk that a first attempt at suicide will end in death.
- Contrary to popular myth, those who talk about suicide often do make an attempt on their own lives.
- The most common emotional states of the suicidal person are ambivalence and hopelessness.
- People are not acutely suicidal forever; rather, the actual crisis during which the person may act typically lasts only a few minutes or a few hours.

Clues to Suicidal Intentions

People thinking of suicide often give clues to their thoughts and feelings and plans to deal with their growing sense of hopelessness. One clue may or may not mean a great deal, but *any* clue is worth asking about. (See Table 11.19.)

There are many motivations for suicide and suicidal behavior. Some of them include the following:

T A B L E   1 1 . 1 9

Suicidal Clues

Direct Verbal Clues*

- "I've decided to kill myself."
- "I wish I were dead."
- "I'm going to commit suicide."
- "I'm going to end it all."
- "If [such and such] doesn't happen, I'll kill myself."

Indirect or Coded Verbal Clues*

- "I'm tired of life."
- "What's the point of going on?"
- "My family would be better off without me."
- "Who cares if I'm dead, anyway?"
- "I can't go on anymore."
- "I just want out."
- "I'm so tired of it all."
- "You would be better off without me."
- "I'm not the person I used to be."
- "I'm calling it quits—living is useless."
- "Soon I won't be around."
- "You shouldn't have to take care of me any longer."
- "Soon you won't have to worry about me anymore."
- "Goodbye. I won't be here when you return."
- "It was good at times, but we must all say goodbye."
- "You're going to regret how you've treated me."
- "You know, son, I'm going home soon."
- "Here, take this [cherished possession]; I won't be needing it."
- "Nobody needs me anymore."
- "How do they preserve your kidneys for transplantation if you die suddenly?"

Behavioral Clues

- Donating body to a medical school
- Purchasing a gun

Behavioral Clues (continued)

- Stockpiling pills
- Putting personal and business affairs in order
- Making or changing a will
- Taking out insurance or changing beneficiaries
- Making funeral plans
- Giving away money and/or possessions
- Making changes in behavior, especially episodes of screaming, hitting, or throwing things or failure to get along with family, friends, or peers
- Acting suspiciously, such as going out at odd times of the day or night and waving or kissing goodbye (if not characteristic)
- Showing sudden interest or disinterest in church or religion
- Scheduling appointments with a doctor for no apparent physical causes or very shortly after the last routine visit
- Losing of physical skills; general confusion; or losing of understanding, judgment, or memory
- Relapsing into drug or alcohol use after a period of recovery

Situational Clues

- Sudden rejection by a loved one, (e.g., girlfriend or boyfriend) or an unwanted separation or divorce
- Recent move—especially if unwanted
- Death of a spouse, child, friend (especially if by suicide or accident)
- Diagnosis of terminal illness
- Flare up with friend or relative for no apparent reason
- Sudden, unexpected loss of freedom (e.g., about to be arrested)
- Anticipated loss of financial security
- Loss of cherished counselor or therapist

Sources: Marv Miller, *Suicide After Sixty,* Springer, New York, 1979; Edwin Schneidman and Norman Farberow, *Clues to Suicide,* McGraw-Hill, New York, 1957; David Spain, *Post-Mortem,* Doubleday, New York, 1974; Louis Wekstein, *Handbook of Suicidology,* Brunner/Mazel, New York, 1979.

*Many of the following statements were made by people who subsequently went on to kill themselves.

- Wanting to end psychological pain
- Wanting to escape an unacceptable situation
- Wanting to join a deceased loved one
- Wanting to gain attention
- Wanting to control others
- Wanting to avoid punishment for a crime
- Wanting to control when death occurs
- Wanting to become a martyr
- Wanting to punish the survivors
- Wanting to avoid loss of face
- Wanting to avoid becoming a burden to others
- Wanting to take revenge
- Wanting to avoid social ridicule
- Wanting to please a cult leader

It is good to remember that the risk of acting on a suicidal thought or feeling shifts over time and that, although persons who have been considering death believe they are no longer at-risk, something terrible or unexpected can hit them from "out of the blue." Whatever this new source of stress is, it is essential that suicidal per-

TABLE 11.20

Do's and Don'ts with Suicidal People

Do's

- Get involved. If in doubt, ask questions. Don't wait for a call from someone in trouble; make the call yourself. Examples of how to ask the question: Are your problems so big you are thinking of harming yourself? Do you wish you could end it all? Have you been thinking of suicide?
- Be accepting and nonjudgmental. Don't offer simple solutions (they sound like brush-offs). Be realistic about the problems, but offer reassurance (hope).
- Be confident and bold. As a solution, suicide can wait. What needs fixing may take a little time, but, at least for today, suicide can wait. Buy time—any way you can.
- Remove the means of suicide. Get rid of guns, pills, razors, whatever. Suicidal people are running red lights without a seat belt; buckle them up.
- Always take a positive, hopeful approach. Suicidal people feel hopeless. Fortunately, hope is infectious, so assure them things will get better because, in fact, they usually do.

Don'ts

- Don't act shocked, dismayed, or frightened. Suicide is drastic, but it's only a solution to a problem. What's the problem worth dying for? Try to understand this and you can save a life.
- Don't ignore the person's threats. Even if he or she doesn't really intend to die, can either of you afford to ignore this cry for help?
- Don't point out the shock, embarrassment, or suffering the family or loved one will endure if the person dies, unless you are sure that isn't exactly what the person wants.
- Don't get into a debate on the merits of living or dying. You might lose the argument.
- Never put yourself at risk of injury (taking a gun or knife away) unless you are highly trained in this area.

sons know there is someone whom they can call, someone who will listen, someone who will care enough to help. If you happen to be that person, Table 11.20 lists some things you can do.

Remember, if you feel that any persons you know may be thinking about suicide, go ahead and ask. If they weren't thinking of suicide, the worst they can do is be a little offended that you would think them capable of such an act; however, if they were thinking of suicide, they may be forever grateful.

Resources

Every community has many resources to help prevent death by suicide. The mental health center, the crisis hot line, the hospital emergency room, the police or sheriff's department, firefighters, clergy, school counselors and teachers, doctors, nurses, social workers, psychologists, and psychiatrists all should and will respond to a request for help.

⚔ Conclusion

At the start of this textbook, we saw that there are no simple solutions to the problems of alcohol/drug dependence and addiction. Remember the wisdom of philosopher H. L. Mencken, who said, "The solution to big problems that are simple, are usually wrong."

There will always be some level of alcohol/drug problem in the United States. Despite our best efforts, many people will still choose not to get help. This is not a war on drugs but, instead, a crusade—a crusade to help people who need and want alcohol and drug treatment; a crusade to prevent the next generation from developing alcohol/drug problems; and a crusade to help those who care to intervene, when appropriate, on those who may benefit from alcohol/drug treatment.

Clinicians' efforts can help many people with alcohol/drug problems and prevent others from suffering the same devastating life of addiction. Most important, they can work on the current problems that make the next generation at risk for chemical dependency.

References

Armor, D. J., J. M. Polich, and H. B. Stambul. 1978. *Alcohol and treatment.* New York: Wiley.

Bateman, N. I., and D. M. Peterson. 1971. Variables related to outcome of treatment for hospitalized alcoholics. *International Journal of Addictions* 215–24.

Bishop, F. Michler. 1995. Rational-emotive behavior therapy and two self-help alternatives to the 12-step model. In *Psychotherapy and substance abuse,* edited by Arnold Washton. New York: Guilford Press.

Brill, Leon. 1981. *The clinical treatment of substance abusers.* New York: Free Press.

Browne-Mayers, A. N., E. E. Seeley, and D. E. Brown. 1973. Reorganized alcoholism services: Two years after. *Journal of the American Medical Association* 23–35.

Chafetz, Morris E., Howard T. Blane, and Marjorie Hill. 1970. *Frontiers of alcoholism.* New York: Science House.

Denning, Pat. 2000. *Practicing harm reduction therapy: An alternative approach to addiction.* New York: Guilford Press.

Dole, V. P., and M. E. Nyswander. 1965. A medical treatment of diacetylmorphine (heroin) addiction. *Journal of the American Medical Association* 193:646–50.

Ford, B., with Chris Chase. 1987. *A glad awakening.* Garden City, N.Y.: Doubleday.

Fox, R. 1958. Antabuse as an adjunct to psychotherapy in alcoholism. *New York State Journal of Medicine* 58:1540–44.

Fox, R. 1963. Normal drinking in recovered alcohol addicts: Comment on the article by D. L. Davies. *Quarterly Journal of Studies on Alcohol* 23:117.

Fox, V. 1976. The controlled drinking controversy. *Journal of the American Medical Association* 236:893.

Gorski, Terence T. 1996. *Brief targeted strategic therapy for relapse prevention.* Paper presented at the Third Annual Florida Dual Disorder Conference, March 16.

Groves. 1978. Troublesome behavior patterns. *New England Journal of Medicine* 4.

Hay, Louise L. 1984. *You can heal your life.* Santa Monica, Calif.: Hay House.

Hellerstein, D., and B. Meehan. 1987. Outpatient group therapy for schizophrenic substance abusers. *American Journal of Psychiatry* 144:1337–39.

Inciardi, James A., and Lana D. Harrison, eds. 2000. *Harm reduction: National and international perspective.* Thousand Oaks, Calif.: Sage.

Jancin, Bruce. 1994. SSRIs help drinkers reduce, but not eliminate, alcohol consumption. *Clinical Psychiatry News* (April).

Kish, G. B., and H. T. Herman. 1971. The Fort Meade Alcoholism Treatment Program: A follow up study. *Quarterly Journal of Studies on Alcohol* 32:628–35.

Lawson, Gary, James S. Peterson, and Ann Lawson. 1983. *Alcoholism and the family: A guide to treatment and prevention.* Rockville, Md.: Aspen.

Marks, S. J., L. Daroff, and S. Granick. 1987. Basic counseling for drug abusers. In *Treatment services for adolescent substance abusers.* Washington, D.C.: U.S. Dept. of Health and Human Services.

Marlatt, Alan, and Judith Gordon. 1985. *Relapse prevention.* New York: Guilford Press.

Miller, W. R. 1980. *Addictive behaviors: Treatment of alcoholism, drug abuse, smoking, and obesity.* New York: Pergamon Press.

Miller, W. R., and G. R. Caddy. 1977. Abstinence and controlled drinking in the treatment of problem drinkers. *Journal of Studies of Alcohol* 38:986–1003.

National Institute of Drug Abuse [NIDA]. 2002. Over 1 million people receiving addiction treatment: Annual survey of substance abuse treatment facilities released [SAMHSA press release]. Rockville, Md.: NIDA, Substance Abuse and Mental Health Services Administration.

Rawson, Richard. 1989. *Cocaine recovery issues: The neurobehavioral model.* Beverly Hills, Calif.: Matrix Institute on Addictions.

Rawson, Richard. 1991. Chemical dependency treatment: The integration of the alcoholism and drug addiction systems. *International Journal of Addictions.*

Rawson, Richard, J. Obert, M. McCann, and David Smith. 1988. *Treatment of cocaine dependence: A neurobehavioral approach.* Beverly Hills, Calif.: Matrix Institute on Addictions.

Ritson, E. B. 1968. The prognosis of alcohol addicts treated by a specialized unit. *British Journal of Psychiatry* 114:1019–29.

Robson, R. A., H. I. Paulus, and G. G. Clark. 1965. An evaluation of the effect of a clinic treatment program on the rehabilitation of alcoholic patients. *Quarterly Journal of Studies on Alcohol* 26:264–78.

Steinglass, Peter. 1979. An experimental treatment program for alcoholic couples. *Journal of Studies on Alcohol* 40:159–82.

Tiebout, H. M. 1962. Intervention in psychotherapy. *American Journal of Psychoanalysis* 33:1–6.

Trimpey, Jack. 1985. *The small book: A revolutionary alternative for overcoming alcohol and drug dependence.* New York: Delacorte Press.

Trimpey, Jack. 1996. *Rational recovery: The new cure for substance addiction.* New York: Pocket Books.

Washton, Arnold M., ed. 1995. *Psychotherapy and substance abuse.* New York: Guilford Press.

APPENDIX

Risk Factors for Adolescent Substance Abuse with Corresponding Prevention Findings

	Risk		Intervention		
Risk Factor	Etiological Study	Evidence (Findings)	Implications	Study	Effects on Risk Factor or Use/Abuse (Findings)
1. Laws and norms (a) Taxation	Levy and Sheflin 1985	1% increase in tax on alcohol led to ½% decreases in consumption.	Raise taxes on alcohol.	Levy and Sheflin 1985; Cook and Tauchen 1982; Saffer and Grossman 1987	Higher alcohol taxes were related to decreases in consumption and accompanying effects.
	Cook and Tauchen 1982	Increase in alcohol tax led to sharp decrease in consumption and cirrhosis mortality.			
	Saffer and Grossman 1987	Higher taxes associated with lower teen drinking and fatalities. Higher tax more salient than drinking age.			
(b) Laws regulating to whom liquor is sold	Saffer and Grossman 1987; Krieg 1982; Cook and Tauchen 1982; Joksch 1988	Higher drinking age associated with fewer teenage traffic fatalities, driving while intoxicated citations.	Increase and enforce age restrictions on purchase of alcohol.	Decker et al. 1988; Krieg 1982; Saffer and Grossman 1987; Cook and Tauchen 1982; Joksch 1988	Increasing age restrictions on alcohol purchases can reduce alcohol-related traffic fatalities.
(c) Laws regulating how liquor is sold	Holder and Blose 1987; Blose and Holder 1987	Liquor-by-the-drink sales increased consumption of distilled spirits but not proportion of drinkers in the population.	Discourage liquor-by-the-drink sales.		
(d) Criminal laws making drugs illegal	Polich et al. 1984	Neither doubling of interdiction nor increased arrests of drug dealers would affect retail prices or availability of illegal drugs.	Deemphasize interdiction and criminal sanctions.		
(e) Cultural norms	Watts and Rabow 1983; Flasher and Maisto 1984; Robins 1984; Vaillant 1983	Alcohol consumption and other alcohol-related effects are associated with sociodemographic factors, ethnic and other group norms.	Foster social norms opposing drug use.	Johnson and Solis 1983; Perry et al. 1988	Community health promotion associated with cessation or reduction of smoking.

Risk factor	Reference	Findings	Prevention/intervention	Reference	Findings
	Atkin et al. 1984	More exposure to ads promoting alcohol among teens reporting higher drinking levels.		Black 1989	Saturation advertising accompanied increases in negative attitudes toward drugs, drug users; talking about drugs with parents, teachers, siblings among college students, children but less for 13- to 17-year-olds.
				Pentz, Brannon et al. 1989; Moskowitz and Jones 1988	Comprehensive school policies emphasizing prevention; restrictions on opportunities for use may reduce smoking.
				Hansen et al. 1988; Perry 1986; Pentz Dwyer et al. 1989; Botvin 1986; Klepp et al. 1986	Some social influence resistance programs include normative-change components (e.g., depicting drug use as socially unacceptable, use of peer leaders to teach curriculum).
				Robins 1984; Johnston 1991	Norms antithetical to use are associated with reductions in prevalence of frequent marijuana, other illicit drug use.
					(Risk factors 1b and 2 are related, all involving social influences to use.)
2. Availability	Gorsuch and Butler 1976	Increased alcohol availability led to increases in drinking prevalence, amount of alcohol consumed, heavy use of alcohol.	Enforce drug and alcohol laws; resistance skills training.		
	Maddahian et al. 1988; Dembo et al. 1979; Gottfredson 1988	Availability affected use of alcohol and illegal drugs.			
3. Extreme economic deprivation	Bursik and Webb 1982; Farrington et al. 1985; Bachman et al. 1981; Zucker and Harford, 1983; Murray et al. 1987	Poverty associated with childhood conduct problems, delinquency, chronic offenses.	Target intervention to economically disadvantaged children.	Lazar et al. 1982; Ramey et al. 1988; Seitz et al. 1985	Interventions with low-income families, including day care, preschool, parenting, home visitors, health care, show promising effects on antisocial behavior in adolescence, aggression, special education placements, criminal involvement.
		Parental education and occupation positively correlated with teen alcohol and marijuana use.			

APPENDIX (*continued*)

Risk Factors for Adolescent Substance Abuse with Corresponding Prevention Findings

Risk			Intervention		
Risk Factor	**Etiological Study**	**Evidence (Findings)**	**Implications**	**Study**	**Effects on Risk Factor or Use/Abuse (Findings)**
	Robins and Ratcliff 1979	Extreme poverty one of three factors increasing risk of adult alcohol and drug abuse in adults who were antisocial as children.		Swift 1988: Olds et al. 1986; Bronson et al. 1984; Pierson et al. 1983; Seitz et al. 1985	Early family support interventions have shown positive effects on child abuse, early school performance and attendance, family size, maternal employment.
				Berrueta-Clement et al. 1984	Follow-up of low-income 5- to 6-year-olds form Perry Preschool Program at age 19 reveals less mental retardation, school dropouts, crime, and welfare reliance and greater literacy, employment, college/vocational school for participants.
	Brook et al. 1990	Low socioeconomic status in childhood related to greater drug use in adolescence.			
4. Neighborhood disorganization	Murray 1983; Herting and Guest 1985; Wilson and Herrnstein 1985; Fagan 1988; Simcha-Fagan and Schwartz 1986; Sampson et al. 1981; Sampson 1986; Cloninger et al. 1988	Characteristics of neighborhoods such as population density, mobility, physical deterioration, low attachment, high crime are related to juvenile crime and drug trafficking.	Target families in high-risk neighborhoods.	(See studies under Risk Factor 3, economic deprivation.)	

	Reference	Finding	Implication
5. Physiological factors		Sensation seeking and low harm avoidance predict early-onset alcoholism.	Target youngsters with certain central nervous system disorders or biochemical levels and with low socioeconomic status and central nervous system disorders.
(a) Biochemical	Zuckerman 1987; von Knorring et al. 1987; Tabakoff and Hoffman 1988;	Sensation-seeking, early-onset alcoholism linked to platelet monoamine oxidase activity.	
	Suwaki and Ohara, 1985; Schuckit 1987	Aldehyde dehydrogenase differences found in Asians with lower rates of alcoholism than controls.	
(b) Genetic factors	Blum et al. 1990	Genetic susceptibility to at least one form of alcoholism suggested by polymorphic pattern of dopamine D2 receptor gene.	Target interventions to children of alcoholics, especially boys.
	Pollock et al. 1983	More slow-wave electroencephalogram activity in children of alcoholics than nonalcoholics.	
	Schuckit et al. 1983; Schuckit 1980; Schuckit and Rayes, 1979; Schuckit 1987	Differences between children of alcoholics and nonalcoholics in serum prolactin response, muscle response, and levels of acetaldehyde after administration of alcohol.	
	Kaij 1960; Hrubec and Omenn 1981	Monozygotic twins were more than twice as likely as dizygotic twins to be concordant for alcoholism (all males).	

APPENDIX (continued)

Risk Factors for Adolescent Substance Abuse with Corresponding Prevention Findings

Risk			Intervention		
Risk Factor	Etiological Study	Evidence (Findings)	Study	Implications	Effects on Risk Factor or Use/Abuse (Findings)
6. Family drug behavior	Cotton, 1979; Goodwin, 1985; Cloninger et al., 1985; Johnson et al., 1984; Kandel et al., 1978; McDermott, 1984	Parental and sibling alcoholism, use of illicit drugs increase risk of alcoholism, drug use initiation, drug abuse in children.	DeMarsh & Kumpfer, 1986	Target interventions to children whose parents or siblings are users/abusers	Narcotic- and polydrug-abusing parents given parenting skills training developed more effective discipline methods; their children had fewer behavior problems after treatment and reported decreased intention to smoke, use alcohol.
	Ahmed et al., 1984	Drug salience in the household best predictor of children's expectations to use and actual use of alcohol, tobacco, and marijuana.			(Social influence resistance interventions can also target family drug use. See studies and results under Risk Factor 14, association with drug-using peers.)
	Hansen et al., 1987	Parental modeling directly related to friends' use of drugs, which in turn was related to adolescent subjects' drug use.			
	Brook et al., 1988	Oldest brothers and parents each had independent effect on younger brother's use. Both drug modeling and drug advocacy by older brothers had independent effects and interacted with parental drug use to provide a risk/protective effect.			
	Brook et al., 1990	Fathers' nondrug use, emotional stability enhanced effects of peer nonuse of drugs.			

	Reference	Approach	Findings/Outcomes
7. Family management practices		Teach family management skills to parents	
	Lazar et al., 1982; Ramey et al., 1988; Seitz et al., 1985; Berrueta-Clement et al., 1984; Swift, 1988		Early childhood interventions including a parenting skills component produced positive outcomes for high-risk, low-income children.
	Patterson et al., 1982; Baum & Forehand, 1981		Parent skills training improved family interaction, reduced child problem behaviors.
	Alexander & Parsons, 1973; Klein et al., 1977		Functional family therapy reduced delinquency for juvenile offenders; prevented delinquency for their siblings.
	Patterson & Fleischman, 1979; Fleischman, 1981; Patterson & Reid, 1973; Peed et al., 1977		Parenting skills training taught parents to monitor children's behavior, to use contingent discipline for undesired behavior, and to reward prosocial behavior.
	Tremblay et al., 1990		Parenting skills, social skills for kindergarten boys reduced school adjustment problems, delayed delinquent behaviors.
	Pentz, Dwyer, et al., 1989		Parents participated in Midwestern Prevention Project; 80% of experimental families involved in homework assignments. Parenting component not assessed separately, but program package associated with lowered rates of tobacco, alcohol, and marijuana use.
	McDermott, 1984; Hansen et al., 1987; Barnes & Welte, 1986; Brook et al., 1986; Jessor et al., 1980		Perceived parent permissiveness toward drug, alcohol use more important than actual parent drug use in determining adolescent drug, alcohol use.
	Kandel & Andrews, 1987; Baumrind, 1983; Penning & Barnes, 1982		Lack of or inconsistent parental discipline, low parental educational aspirations for children predict initiation into drug use.
	Ziegler-Driscoll, 1979; Kaufman & Kaufman, 1979		Overinvolvement by one parent accompanied by distance or permissiveness by the other associated with risk.
	Baumrind, 1983		Parent authoritativeness related to children's prosocial, assertive behaviors; parent nondirectiveness, permissiveness associated with higher drug use.
	Reilly, 1979		Common characteristics of families of adolescent drug abusers: negative communication patterns, inconsistent, unclear behavior limits, unrealistic parental expectations.
	Norem-Hebeisen et al., 1984		Drug users saw fathers as more hostile, adversarial; parents as less caring, more rejecting.
	Tec, 1974		Parental drug use in unrewarding family structure more linked to marijuana use than in a rewarding family context.

APPENDIX (*continued*)

Risk Factors for Adolescent Substance Abuse with Corresponding Prevention Findings

Risk				Intervention	
Risk Factor	Etiological Study	Evidence (Findings)	Implications	Study	Effects on Risk Factor or Use/Abuse (Findings)
	Brook et al., 1990	Parent-adolescent attachment related to less marijuana use.		Biglan, Glasgow, et al., 1987	No effect on child smoking of four parent messages mailed home for students involved in social influence resistance program. Parent compliance level not measured.
	Shedler & Block, 1990	Quality of mothers' interactions with 5-year-olds related to marijuana use at 18.			
	Brook et al., 1990	Psychological stability of mothers offset effects of peer drug use.		Karoly & Rosenthal, 1977; Martin, 1977; Patterson et al., 1982; Walters & Gilmore, 1973	Parenting skills training reduced preadolescents' problem behaviors, suggesting that parenting skills training can buffer risk factor of childhood behavior problems.
				Dishion et al., 1989	Parent training groups improved parent-child interaction, level of tobacco use, reduced depression.
8. Family conflict	Baumrind, 1983; Penning & Barnes, 1982; Robins, 1980	Children from homes broken by marital discord are at higher risk of delinquency, drug use.	Reduce family conflict; services to children whose families are in conflict		(See studies on parent training, family interventions above, Risk Factor 7).
	Wilson & Herrnstein, 1985	No independent contribution of parents' marital dissolution to delinquent behavior.			

Risk factor	References	Findings	Intervention strategy	Intervention references
9. Low bonding to family	McCord, 1979; Rutter & Giller, 1983; W. McCord & McCord, 1959; Porter & O'Leary, 1980; Hetherington et al., 1979; Wallerstein & Kelly, 1980; Simcha-Fagan et al., 1986	Family conflict stronger predictor of delinquency than family structure (intact parental marriage).	Strengthen family bonding	(Effective early childhood and family support programs and parent training programs have been found to increase parent-child bonding. See studies and findings under Risk Factors 3 (economic deprivation) and 7 (family management).
	Kandel et al., 1978; Brook et al., 1980; Braucht et al., 1978; Penning & Barnes, 1982	Lack of parent-child closeness, lack of maternal involvement related to drug initiation.		
	Hirschi, 1969; Elliott et al., 1985; Brook et al., 1990	Bonding inhibits delinquency. Family bonding interacts with peer variables to influence delinquency and drug use.		
	Jessor & Jessor, 1977; Kim, 1979; Norem-Hebeisen et al., 1984; Gorsuch & Butler, 1976; Selnow, 1987; Brook, Brook, et al., 1990; Brook, Gordon, et al., 1986; Hundleby & Mercer, 1987	Family involvement and attachment discourage youth drug initiation and level of use.		
10. Early and persistent problem behaviors	Robins, 1978	More variety, frequency of child antisocial behavior portends adult antisocial behavior.	Intervene early with children with problem behaviors. Strategies include parent training, social competence training for children	Patterson et al., 1982; Baum & Forehand, 1981; Fleischman, 1981; Patterson & Reid, 1973; Peed et al., 1977

Risk Factors for Adolescent Substance Abuse with Corresponding Prevention Findings

Risk			Intervention	
Risk Factor	Etiological Study	Evidence (Findings)	Study	Effects on Risk Factor or Use/Abuse (Findings)
	Lerner & Vicary, 1984	"Difficult" temperament in 5-year-olds contributes to drug problems in adulthood.		
	Shedler & Block, 1990	18-year-old frequent marijuana users had emotional distress in childhood.		
	Kellam & Brown, 1982; Lewis, Robins, & Rice, 1985; Nylander, 1979; Loeber, 1988; Spivack, 1983	Aggressiveness in boys age 5–7 predicts frequent drug use, delinquency in adolescence; drug problems in adulthood.	Battistich et al., n.d.; Bierman & Furman, 1984; Gesten et al., 1982; Ladd, 1981; Ladd & Asher, 1985; Rotheram 1982b; Shure & Spivack, 1982; Bierman et al., 1987; Weissberg & Caplan, 1989; Weissberg et al., 1981; Weissberg & Allen, 1985	
	Loeber & Dishion, 1983	Only 30–40% of boys with problem aggressive behavior maintained it 4 to 9 years later.		
	Loeber, 1988; McCord, 1981; Barnes & Welte, 1986; Kandel, 1982	Early aggressive or antisocial behavior persisting into early adolescence predicts later adolescence aggressiveness, drug abuse and/or alcohol problems.		
	Loney et al., 1979	Hyperactivity, attention-deficit disorder raises delinquency risk if combined with conduct problems.	Allen et al., 1976	No effects on adjustment of social competence skills intervention.

Risk factor	Reference	Finding	Intervention reference	Intervention
	Gittelman et al., 1985	Hyperactivity in children, especially accompanied by conduct problems, increases substance abuse risk in late adolescence.	Lochman, 1988	Aggressive boys given anger management program had lower alcohol, marijuana use, fewer negative consequences of alcohol at age 14 (3 years postintervention, compared with matched group of untreated boys). No positive 3-year follow-up effects on aggression or general deviance.
	Brook et al., 1990	Children who are irritable, distractible, have temper tantrums, fight with siblings, engage in predelinquent acts more likely to use drugs in adolescence.	Ketchel & Bieger, 1989; Kim et al., 1989.	Social competence, skills training in 4th grade produced lower use of alcohol, cigarettes, marijuana, especially in Grades 5–7.
11. Academic failure (a) Intelligence	G. D. Gottfredson, 1981	Intellectual ability and delinquency have inverse relationship, after controlling for socioeconomic status.		Target interventions toward some higher ability youths
	Fleming et al., 1982	High reading and IQ scores in Grade 1 predicted earlier, more frequent adolescent alcohol use in African-American inner-city sample.		
	Kandel & Davies, 1991	Higher test performance associated with higher lifetime levels of cocaine use in young adults.		
	Block et al., 1988	Drug use in boys related to IQ decline from age 11 to age 18.		

APPENDIX (*continued*)

Risk Factors for Adolescent Substance Abuse with Corresponding Prevention Findings

	Risk			Intervention	
Risk Factor	**Etiological Study**	**Evidence (Findings)**	**Implications**	**Study**	**Effects on Risk Factor or Use/Abuse (Findings)**
(b) School failure	Jessor, 1976; Smith & Fogg, 1978; Robins, 1980	Failure in school predicted adolescent drug abuse, frequency and levels of use of illicit drugs.	Promote academic achievement in a variety of ways.	Berrueta-Clement et al., 1984; Seitz et al., 1985; Horacek et al., 1987; Gotts, 1989; Lazar et al., 1982; Ramey et al., 1988	Early childhood education and family support interventions resulted in higher school achievement. (See Risk Factors 3 and 7 above.)
	Feldhusen et al., 1973	Early antisocial behavior may predict later academic failure.		Blechman et al., 1981, Bien & Bry, 1980	Parent involvement led to improved academic effort, grades, attendance in students with low school commitment.
	Hundleby & Mercer, 1987	Good school performance reduced likelihood of frequent drug use in ninth graders.		Brophy & Good, 1986	Student achievement gains linked to teacher's active instruction, direct supervision of learning.
				Hawkins & Lam, 1987; Hawkins, Doueck, & Lishmer, 1988	Interactive teaching, proactive classroom management, and cooperative learning led to greater math achievement gains in seventh-grade students.
				DeVries & Slavin, 1978; Madden & Slavin, 1983; Ziegler, 1981; Dolan et al. 1989	Controlled studies showed positive effect of cooperative learning on achievement and attitudes toward school and peers.
				Schaps et al., 1986	"Jigsaw" cooperative learning method did not prevent drug use.
				Coie & Krehbiel, 1984	Tutoring of socially rejected, low-achieving fourth graders produced improvements in reading, math achievement and reduced peer rejection, disruptive behavior.

		Reference	Finding
		Comer, 1988	Gains in student academic achievement demonstrated over 12-year period after creation of school governance and management teams in urban school district.
		Freiberg et al., 1989	Cooperative learning, classroom management, student–teacher motivation, parent contacts, interactive teaching, discipline prevention resulted in improved academic achievement.
		Felner & Adan, 1988; Felner, Adan, & Evans, 1987; Felner, Weissberg, & Adan, 1987	Intervention to ease transitions to middle, junior high, and high schools, with advocacy and schools-within-schools to decrease fragmentation. Participating students had better academic performance than nonparticipating student in the same schools.
	Promote commitment to school	Blechman et al., 1981; Bien & Bry, 1980	Parent involvement improved effort and attendance of students with low school commitment.
		Hawkins & Lam, 1987	Teacher interactive teaching, proactive classroom management, cooperative learning resulted in higher commitment to school and fewer suspensions, expulsions in seventh-grade experimental compared with control classrooms.
12. Low commitment to school		Johnston et al., 1985	Use of a variety of drugs is significantly lower among students expecting to attend college.
		D. C. Gottfredson, 1988	4–6% of variance in truancy was associated with drug involvement, controlling for ethnicity, parent education, delinquency.
		Kelly & Balch, 1971	How much students like school related to levels of drug use.
		Friedman, 1983	Time spent on homework, perception of relevance of course-work related to levels of drug use.

APPENDIX (continued)

Risk Factors for Adolescent Substance Abuse with Corresponding Prevention Findings

Risk Factor	Risk		Implications	Intervention	
	Etiological Study	Evidence (Findings)		Study	Effects on Risk Factor or Use/Abuse (Findings)
				DeVries & Slavin, 1978; Madden & Slavin, 1983; Ziegler, 1981	Cooperative learning produced positive effects on attitudes toward school and peers.
				Hawkins, Doueck, & Lishner, 1988	Cooperative learning produced reductions in suspensions, expulsion among low achievers.
				D. C. Gottfredson, 1986	Multicomponent school program promoting shared decision making, student services, academic innovations produced lower rates of drug abuse, delinquency, alienation; higher rates of attachment to school, educational expectations, belief in school rules in experimental than comparison schools.
				D. C. Gottfredson & Cook, 1986a, 1986b	Curriculum restructuring increased positive self-concept, attachment to school, belief in rules, math scores; decreased school rate of delinquency, drug use, suspensions.
				Felner & Adan, 1988	School transition study (see Risk Factor 11b, above) results show lower absenteeism, drop out for participating students compared with nonparticipating students in the same schools.

Risk factor	References	Findings	Protective factor/intervention	References	Findings
13. Peer rejection in elementary grades	Parker & Asher, 1987; Coie, 1990 Kellam et al., 1980	Low acceptance by peers seems to elevate risk for school problems and criminality. Children who had been aggressive as first graders or aggressive and shy had higher levels of drug use than those who were just shy.	Provide opportunities for socialization, social competence skills	Battistich et al., n.d.; Bierman & Furman, 1984; Gesten et al., 1982; Ladd, 1981; Ladd & Asher, 1985; Rotheram, 1982a, 1982b; Shure & Spivack, 1982; Weissberg & Caplan, 1989	Social competency studies have produced positive effects on children's interpersonal behavior. (See Risk Factor 10.)
	Brook et al., 1986	Childhood traits of social inhibition, isolation, and aggression not associated with adolescent drug use stage, but aggression, lower inhibition, and lower isolation in adolescence associated with higher drug use stage.		Lochman, 1988	In spite of positive alcohol and marijuana effects (see Risk Factor 10), there were no positive effects for aggressive behavior or general behavioral deviance at 3-year follow-up.
	Cairns et al., 1988; Hartup, 1983; Tremblay, 1988	Aggressiveness may be associated with acceptance by other aggressive peers who could foster drug use; similarly, socially rejected children may form friendships with other rejected children in adolescence, leading to later delinquent behavior.			

APPENDIX (continued)

Risk Factors for Adolescent Substance Abuse with Corresponding Prevention Findings

Risk			Implications	Intervention	
Risk Factor	**Etiological Study**	**Evidence (Findings)**		**Study**	**Effects on Risk Factor or Use/Abuse (Findings)**
				Ellickson & Bell, 1990	Social influence resistance curriculum for seventh graders with eighth-grade booster program. Results showed modest reductions in drinking for students at three levels of baseline use immediately after initial program (favoring teen leader over adult leader format) compared with controls. At follow-up in eighth grade, differences had disappeared. For smoking, significant reductions were observed across all subsequent smoking levels for baseline experimenters but not baseline nonusers or smokers. For the latter, smoking increased more for treatment than control students. For marijuana, both initiation and current use were 50% to 60% lower for the treatment group.
				Schinke, Botvin et al., 1988	Bicultural competence drug abuse prevention program for Native American adolescents found greater substance use knowledge, attitudes, interactive skills, lower self-report rates of drugs, tobacco, alcohol for participants than controls.

Risk Factor	References	Findings	Protective Factor/Skills	References	Findings
14. Association with drug-using peers	Barnes & Welte, 1986; Kandel, 1978, 1986; Kandel & Andrews, 1987; Elliott et al., 1985; Jessor et al., 1980; Brook et al., 1990	Peer use of substances is among the strongest predictors of substance use among youth.	Social influence resistance skills; social competence skills (see also Risk Factors 1, 2, and 6)	Botvin, 1986; Bukoski, 1986; Flay, 1985; Moskowitz, 1989, Tobler, 1986	Reviews of social influence resistance strategies have found modest but significant reductions in the onset and prevalence of cigarette smoking for groups receiving training in comparison with untrained controls.
	Newcomb & Bentler, 1986; Byram & Fly, 1984	Influence of peers on drug use stronger than that of parents for Whites, African-Americans, Asians, Hispanics.		McAlister et al., 1980; Botvin, 1986; Hansen et al., 1988; Pentz, Dwyer, et al., 1989; Perry, 1986; Johnson et al., 1984	Social influence strategies showed beneficial effects in preventing or delaying the onset of alcohol and marijuana use.
	Harford, 1985	Nondrinking African-American youths reported fewer drinking friends than African-American youths who drank.			
	Dembo et al., 1979	Friends' use of alcohol and marijuana was related to use by African-American and Puerto Rican youths.		Botvin et al., 1990; Klepp et al., 1986; McAlister, 1983; D. M. Murray et al., 1984	Social influence resistance training groups led by peers achieved greater reductions in drug use than non-peer-led groups.
	Brook et al., 1990	The most powerful linkage in causal pathway to marijuana nonuse was association with non-drug-using peers.		Botvin et al., 1989	Life skills training to prevent smoking for African-American urban junior high students resulted in fewer posttest smokers in treatment than control group on the basis of adjusted means for smoking status in past month.
				Flay et al., 1989	Six-year follow-up of social influence resistance smoking prevention program found no overall differences between program and control groups. Early program effects (Grade 8) had disappeared by Grade 12.

APPENDIX (*continued*)

Risk Factors for Adolescent Substance Abuse with Corresponding Prevention Findings

Risk			Intervention	
Risk Factor	**Etiological Study**	**Evidence (Findings)**	**Implications**	**Study**	**Effects on Risk Factor or Use/Abuse (Findings)**

				D. M. Murray et al., 1987, 1988; D. M. Murray, Pirie, et al., 1989	Follow-up of study comparing four smoking prevention strategies (three variations of social influences model and a health consequences model) and no intervention. Two to 5 years postintervention, mixed results favored peer-led social influences program (without videos) in restraining smoking for baseline nonsmokers and experimenters. At 5 and 6-year follow-up, differences had disappeared, with no program effects.
				Schinke, Bebel, Orlandi & Botvin, 1988	Smoking prevention program for children of blue-collar families compared skills-based with discussion-based and control groups. Skills-based program had lower use rates for participatants at 6, 12, 18, and 24 months follow-up.
				Vartiainen et al., 1983, 1986, 1990	Social influences smoking prevention program; two levels of intervention, one comparison condition. Two- and 4-year follow-up reported lower monthly smoking rates for intervention over comparison schools. By 8-year follow-up, only effects for baseline nonsmokers were evident.

Risk factor	Citations	Findings	Implication for prevention	Studies	Results
15. Alienation and rebelliousness	Jessor & Jessor, 1977; Kandel, 1982; Penning & Barnes, 1982; Jessor et al., 1980; Robins, 1980	Alienation from dominant societal values, low religiosity positively related to drug use, delinquent behavior.	Promote prosocial involvement	Schaps et al., 1986 Tobler, 1986	Operating a school store (combined with cross-age tutoring) did not prevent drug use in predominantly White middle-class eighth, ninth graders.
	Bachman et al., 1981; Kandel, 1982; Smith & Fogg, 1978	Rebelliousness, resistance to traditional authority positively related to drug use, delinquent behavior.			There is some evidence that intensive programs that empower high-risk youths to master new skills are associated with improved behavior and achievement.
	Jessor & Jessor, 1977; Jessor, 1976; Paton & Kandel, 1978	High tolerance of deviance, resistance to authority, strong need for independence, normlessness linked with drug use.			
	Shedler & Block, 1990	Interpersonal alienation at age 7 predicted frequent marijuana use at 18.			
16. Attitudes favorable to drug use	Kandel et al., 1978; Krosnick & Judd, 1982; Smith & Fogg, 1978	Initiation into substance use is preceded by values favorable to its use.	Foster antidrug-use attitudes and norms.		(See studies and results under Risk Factors 1e and 14 for social resistance and cultural norms interventions.)
17. Early onset of drug use	Rachal et al., 1982; Kandel, 1982; Fleming et al., 1982; Robins & Pryzbeck, 1985	Misusers of alcohol begin drinking earlier than users; earlier onset of drug use predicts greater and more persistent use of more dangerous drugs.	Direct intervention to younger children and their parents; target risk factors developmentally before initiation of drug use		(See Risk Factors 3 and 7 for early childhood, parent support, parent training interventions.)
	Brunswick & Boyle, 1979; O'Donnell & Clayton, 1979	Earlier initiation of drug use increases probability of deviant activities.			
	Kandel et al., 1976	Later onset of drug use predicts lower drug involvement and higher probability of discontinuation of use.			

From J. David Hawkins, R. Catalono, and J. Miller. "Risk and Protective Factors for Alcohol and Other Drug Problems in Adolescence and Early Adulthood: Implications for Substance Abuse Prevention." *Psychological Bulletin* 112 (1): (1992) 64–105.

Index